International Perspectives on Migration

South-South Migration

This book series serves the growing academic interests in South-South migration, offering a scholarly publication platform to scholars and practitioners globally. It advances a Southern perspective to migration studies. It encompasses distinct fields such as international migration, internal migration, remittances, migrant entrepreneurship, diaspora philanthropy, social cost of migration, political and environmental refugees, gender and migration, labor migration, migration policy, the political economy of migration, migrants' rights, and other migration-related issues in the global South. The series aims to address migration questions, employ critical analyses, and advance evidence-based migration scholarship. This book series takes an interdisciplinary approach to the causes, patterns, and implications of migration for countries and regions in the global South. This series invites original monographs and edited books. The series explicitly gives scholars from the global South more voice and visibility in academic publications.

Amrita Datta · S. Irudaya Rajan
Editors

Migration, Livelihoods and Gender

Insights from Odisha

Springer

Editors
Amrita Datta
Department of Liberal Arts
Indian Institute of Technology Hyderabad
Sangareddy, Telangana, India

S. Irudaya Rajan
International Institute of Migration and Development
Thiruvananthapuram, Kerala, India

ISSN 2214-9805 ISSN 2214-9813 (electronic)
International Perspectives on Migration
ISSN 2731-5045 ISSN 2731-5053 (electronic)
South-South Migration
ISBN 978-981-95-5464-5 ISBN 978-981-95-5465-2 (eBook)
https://doi.org/10.1007/978-981-95-5465-2

This Springer imprint is published by the registered company Springer Nature Singapore Pte Ltd.
The registered company address is: 152 Beach Road, #21-01/04 Gateway East, Singapore 189721, Singapore

Preface and Acknowledgements

Migration from Odisha is widespread and is understood to be rapidly increasing. This migration affects the economy, society, and everyday life of Odisha's population of nearly 50 million people. Despite its significance, Odisha migration remains an understudied area of research, and little is known about its magnitude, patterns, and processes. This book aims to address this gap.

The book is based on the Odisha Migration Study, undertaken in two phases in 2023–2024. In its first phase, based on a representative sample survey of 15,000 households spread across the 30 districts of Odisha, it estimates migration and remittances from the state and studies the characteristics of individual- and household-level migration, disaggregated by social group, land size, district, and region. It focuses on current migration as well as return migration to better understand various streams of migration from Odisha. It emphasizes the role of education and the spatialities of work migration and shows that the economic geography of work is gendered. It also explores several dimensions of human development. In its second phase, based on four sub-studies, the book examines the role of agriculture, non-agriculture, and remittances in rural household livelihood portfolios, studies the impacts of migration focusing on women's empowerment and well-being, and explores youth aspirations and the role of return migrants in agriculture and the rural economy.

Thus, this book presents new evidence and perspectives on migration and development in Odisha through the lens of rural livelihoods and gender. Its findings will be useful for both research and policy. We have been fortunate to have a multidisciplinary team of researchers—Gaurav Dhamija, Shubha Ranganathan, Haripriya Narasimhan, Sunitha S., Nandini Ramamurthy, Subhadarshee Nayak, Umi Daniel, Jayaprakash Mishra, Rohit Irudayarajan, Kunal Munjal, Pranita Kulkarni, Muhammed Thwoyyib K. P., Iswarya Priya Jagannathan, and Fahin Faras—on the project, who contributed to the various chapters in the book.

At the Government of Odisha, we are very thankful to Labor Secretary R Santhanagopalan's support for our study. At Aide et Action, our local research partner in Odisha, Umi Daniel and Jyoti Prakash Bramha provided critical research inputs and overall support to the study. Mr. Subhra Ranjan Swain provided administrative support. We are grateful for Aide et Action's collaboration with the project. Mr.

Ashok Panda, the state fieldwork coordinator, organized the fieldwork of the study and led the team of cluster coordinators and research investigators, who, despite several difficulties in the field, diligently collected the data. Lacqueen Jessica Paul painstakingly formatted the project report of this research.

Ethical approval for the Odisha Migration Study was obtained from the Institutional Ethics Committee at the Indian Institute of Technology Hyderabad (IITH). We would like to thank the Sponsored Research and Consultancy Office at IITH, in particular, Dean Chandrashekhar Sharma, and from the administrative team, Ashok Gajula, N. Srisailam, M. Eswar Reddy, Pradeep Jada, Ramanjaneyulu Narayana, E. Guruswamy, and Manasa Reddy. At the Department of Liberal Arts, Mr. Abani Das, Ms. Anjali Chintha, and Ms. Rojalin Panda provided able administrative support. Support from IITH's book-writing grant is also duly acknowledged.

We are indebted to Satvinder Kaur and her team at Springer, who patiently worked with us as we missed several deadlines, and to Pranita Kulkarni, who deftly and painstakingly copyedited the entire manuscript. Pritam Kumar Mandal's assistance in creating the maps in the book is duly acknowledged.

Last, and most importantly, we are grateful to the CGIAR Gender Platform for funding the study. In particular, we would like to thank Ranjitha Puksur and her team for their keen interest and involvement in the study. Mukund Variar's support at the IRRI Odisha office is also much appreciated.

Hyderabad, India
Thiruvananthapuram, India
August 2025

Amrita Datta
S. Irudaya Rajan

Contents

Editors and Contributors

About the Editors

Amrita Datta is an Associate Professor of Development Studies at the Department of Liberal Arts, Indian Institute of Technology Hyderabad. Amrita's research interests are in the areas of migration and mobilities, labour and employment, agrarian change and rural development, and gender and development. Amrita's book, *Migration and Development in India: The Bihar Experience* (Routledge), based on empirical research, studies out-migration from rural Bihar in the context of neoliberal economic development in India. Amrita has co-edited several edited volumes and published in journals such as the Journal of Development Studies, Journal of Gender Studies, Asian Journal of Women's Studies, Children's Geographies, Indian Journal of Human Development, Indian Journal of Labour Economics and the Economic and Political Weekly. Amrita has a PhD in Development Studies from the International Institute of Social Studies, Erasmus University Rotterdam, and an MPhil in the same subject from the University of Cambridge.

S. Irudaya Rajan is the chair, International Institute of Migration and Development. He is a former professor at the Centre for Development Studies (CDS), Kerala (close 40 years of post-graduate experience), and currently, the chair of the KNOMAD (The Global Knowledge Partnership on Migration and Development), World Bank working group on internal migration and urbanization. He is one of the expert committee members to advise the Government of Kerala on Covid-19. He has published in international journals on social, economic, demographic, psychological, and political implications of migration on individuals, community, economy, and society. He is the editor of the annual series India Migration Report since 2010 and South Asia Migration Report since 2017 published by Routledge. He is also the founder editor in chief, of the journal, Migration and Development (Sage).

Contributors

Umi Daniel hails from Odisha and has more than three decades of experience in the development sector across India and international locations. He specialises in migration studies, tribal development, disaster and climate vulnerability, and social protection. He has worked with several local and international NGOs and last served with Aide et Action as the Director of Migration and Education for South Asia. During his professional journey, he has led several social research, advocacy efforts, and policy initiatives on migration, labour rights, disaster response, and vulnerable communities. A regular contributor to newspapers, magazines, and blogs on social issues, Umi Daniel weaves together field experience, policy insight, practical solutions, and human stories in his writings, reflecting his long-standing engagement with vulnerable communities, survivors, and people affected by exploitation and human rights violations.

Gaurav Dhamija is an Assistant Professor in the Department of Liberal Arts at the Indian Institute of Technology Hyderabad, India. He is a member of the Center for Research on the Economics of Climate, Food, Energy, and Environment (CECFEE) and a Fellow of the Policy Edge. His research focuses on applied microeconometrics and development economics, with particular attention to the causal links between marital conditions and women's outcomes, the long-term impacts of early life conditions, and the socioeconomic determinants of health. His broader academic mission is to employ rigorous econometric methods to address pressing policy challenges.

Fahin Faras is a doctoral student in Development Studies at the Indian Institute of Technology Hyderabad. Trained in economics, his research interests include development economics, employment, and livelihoods. His current work focuses on platform-based gig workers.

Rohit Irudayarajan is a researcher at the International Institute of Migration and Development (IIMAD), working across migration, climate change, ageing, skills and social policy. He has contributed to major research projects, including the Kerala Migration Survey, Odisha Migration Survey, and the Horizon Europe Link4Skills project, with experience in survey design, field coordination, stakeholder interviews, data management, report writing, and policy-oriented research. He is also the Kobo Toolbox Ambassador based in India, reflecting his work in digital data collection and research capacity building.

Iswarya Priya Jagannathan has a PhD in Development Studies from the Indian Institute of Technology (IIT), Hyderabad. Her research interests lie in understanding and contributing to scholarship on women's informal labour through a heterodox economics lens, particularly in feminist economics and feminist political economy. Her doctoral research focuses on homeworkers in the leather footwear industry in Ambur, Tamil Nadu, examining homeworking through multiple lenses: informality and precarity in Global Value Chains (GVCs), women's work, the household, and social reproduction and care. Her work is qualitative, empirical, and rooted in a feminist methodological framework that foregrounds women's voices, narratives, and lived experiences. She has published her work in journals such as Gender and Development and the Economic and Political Weekly. Her broad research interests include the informal economy, gendered paid and unpaid labour, women's aspirations, and intra-household dynamics.

Pranita Kulkarni is an independent researcher with a background in Development Studies. Her work focuses on themes of labour, migration, trade unions, intersectionality, globalization, and political economy, with a particular interest in qualitative analysis. She aims to combine empirically grounded inquiry with critical perspectives, producing scholarship that speaks to questions of practice. She has also worked as a journalist and as an editor of academic manuscripts.

Jayaprakash Mishra is an Assistant Professor of Cultural Studies and Anthropology at the School of Liberal Arts in Thapar University, Patiala, Punjab, India. His research interests lie at the intersection of Critical Kinship Studies, Gender and Sexuality, Ageing and Reproduction, and Popular Culture. As the Principal investigator of both Ageing in Punjab (supported by Thapar Seed Grant) and Ageing, Care and Migration (supported by ICSSR major grant) projects, he leads a team of researchers doing literature review, ethnographic fieldwork and archival research. Some of his works have been published in the Journal of Family Issues, Asian Journal of Social Sciences, Sociological Review, South Asian Popular Culture etc.

Kunal Munjal is a Senior Research Fellow at the Economic Analysis Unit, ISI-Bengaluru, and a PhD scholar in Development Studies at the Department of Liberal Arts, IIT-Hyderabad. His broad research domain is agrarian studies, political economy, development economics and state-society relations. He employs an interdisciplinary frame for research using a mixed-methods approach. His work has been published in the Journal of Agrarian Change, Economic and Political Weekly, Review of Agrarian Studies, and Asian Studies Review. He has a degree in Rural Development from the Tata Institute of Social Sciences (TISS) and in Public Policy from the National Law School of India University (NLSIU).

Haripriya Narasimhan is an anthropologist. Her research interests are in gender, health, media and digital technologies. In her previous work, she has looked at education, employment choices, family and marriage, globalization and decision-making about health care. Her most recent research project is in medical anthropology of aging.

Subhadarshee Nayak is a researcher and development practitioner currently working with an NGO to improve Foundational Literacy and Numeracy (FLN) outcomes in selected districts of Odisha. He holds a PhD from the Tata Institute of Social Sciences (TISS), Mumbai, and has previously served as a Senior Research Fellow at the Economic Analysis Unit, Indian Statistical Institute (ISI), Bengaluru. His research interests focus on caste, education, social inequalities, school textbooks, and Dalit Studies.

Shubha Ranganathan is an Associate Professor in the Department of Liberal Arts, Indian Institute of Technology Hyderabad. Her research projects engage with health, gender, and disability from interdisciplinary perspectives. She has studied local healing practices among marginalized groups as well as mental health and disability-related issues in India. Currently, she is exploring questions about parenting and care in the context of autism as part of her engagement with the neurodiversity discourse. She is also a co-investigator in a project on aging, care, and migration in Punjab.

Nandini Ramamurthy is an independent researcher, based in Hyderabad, India, with an interest in the garment industry of southern India, particularly Tiruppur and Bengaluru. Her PhD, Local Clusters in Global Production Systems: Governance, Work and Value Share of Textile Industry in South India, was completed in 2022 at the Tata Institute of Social Sciences, Guwahati Campus. She has interest in wage disparity, migration and livelihood studies, precarity and has published in the Geoforum, The Indian Economic Journal, Indian Journal of Human Development, The Indian Journal of Labour Economics and contributed to the India Migration Report 2023.

Sunitha S. is a demographer and migration researcher with over two decades of experience in ageing, migration, health, and population studies. She currently serves as a Project Consultant at the International Institute of Migration and Development (IIMAD) in Thiruvananthapuram. She has worked extensively with leading institutions including the Centre for Development Studies (CDS), IIT Hyderabad, International Organization for Migration, and IIMAD, contributing to major migration and ageing surveys across India. Her research expertise includes demographic transition, elderly care, migration studies, social inclusion, and health among older adults. She has authored several book chapters and journal articles published by Springer, Routledge, Sage, and other reputed publishers.

Muhammed Thwoyyib K. P. has interdisciplinary training in Economics and Development Studies. He has contributed to research projects across Odisha, Gujarat, Kerala, and Haryana, with a focus on labour, migration, global value chains, education, and social transformation. His research experience spans mixed-methods approaches, qualitative fieldwork, and archival research. His interests lie in political economy, industrialization, and the historical dynamics shaping labour, industry, and development in India. He is currently working on a project examining the social history of engineering education in Kerala.

Chapter 1
Introduction

Kunal Munjal, Amrita Datta, S. Irudaya Rajan, Pranita Kulkarni, and Sunitha S.

Abstract This chapter provides the development context of migration from Odisha and briefly outlines the analytical framework and methodology of the Odisha Migration Study. Based on secondary data and literature sources, it finds that despite high economic growth, structural transformation in the state is lopsided, leaving labor largely dependent on agriculture. The neoliberal trajectory in agrarian and industrial transformation has not improved employment structures, exacerbating human development challenges for marginalized communities (from caste, tribe, gender, and regional lenses). This has led to the persistence of poverty, food insecurity, and vulnerability, driving a significant portion of the population to migrate in search of work and livelihood opportunities. The magnitude of migration is pronounced in Odisha, particularly for communities from certain regions (southern and western) and social profiles (Dalits and Adivasis). The patterns and streams are extremely heterogeneous, but vulnerability as a common factor leads to migrants working in precarious working conditions at destinations. The chapter examines gendered, demographic, and climate-induced aspects of migration, while also discussing the repercussions of unsafe migration, such as trafficking and bondage. It assesses state and non-state responses to migration issues, including COVID-19-induced reverse migration. The chapter underscores the necessity of policies integrating migration concerns into development strategies, with a specific focus on marginalized communities facing intersecting challenges of gender, caste, tribe, and region. In sum, the chapter sets the context for the empirical analysis, based on the Odisha Migration Study, in the subsequent chapters.

K. Munjal
Indian Statistical Institute, Bengaluru & Indian Institute of Technology, Hyderabad, India

A. Datta (✉)
Indian Institute of Technology, Hyderabad, India
e-mail: amritadatta@la.iith.ac.in

S. I. Rajan · Sunitha S.
The International Institute of Migration and Development, Thiruvananthapuram, India

P. Kulkarni
Independent Researcher, New Delhi, India

A. Datta and S. I. Rajan (eds.), *Migration, Livelihoods and Gender*, International Perspectives on Migration, https://doi.org/10.1007/978-981-95-5465-2_1

Keywords Migration and development · Remittances · Livelihoods · Gender · Odisha Migration Study

Odisha, situated on the eastern coast of India, is a state of paradoxes. Blessed with abundant natural resources and a rich cultural heritage, it has also been plagued by pervasive poverty and a history of recurrent natural disasters. One pressing issue that has defined the socio-economic landscape of Odisha in recent years is the complex interplay between development and migration. This introductory chapter provides a context for the empirical findings of the Odisha Migration Study, a multidisciplinary empirical research project.

The Odisha Migration Study was undertaken in two phases in 2023–2024. In the first phase, the Odisha Migration Survey (OMS), a quantitative survey covering 15,000 representative households across all 30 districts of Odisha, was conducted. Its primary goal was to determine the overall extent of migration from Odisha, including detailed breakdowns of intra-state (within the state), inter-state, and international migration flows. Additionally, the survey delved into several aspects of social and economic development, including education, work and employment, access to government programs, housing and amenities, land and asset ownership, household food consumption and security, and women's autonomy and mobility.

In the second phase, four standalone studies were undertaken to examine the role of agriculture, non-agriculture, and remittances in rural household livelihood portfolios, study the impacts of migration on women's empowerment and well-being, and explore youth aspirations and attitudes toward agriculture and the rural economy. Against this backdrop, this chapter first delves into the multifaceted relationship between migration and development in Odisha by exploring its development trajectory and migration-development nexus. It then presents the analytical framework of livelihoods and gender that anchors this empirical work and outlines the methodology of the study. The next section presents a population profile of the state based on the OMS, and the final section outlines the chapterization of the book.

1 Migration and Development in Odisha: An Overview

The complex relationship between development and migration in the Indian context becomes evident when one considers the role of development initiatives in influencing migration patterns. Conversely, migration plays a pivotal role in shaping a state/region's development trajectory. However, both these trajectories differ across regions because of the huge diversity in the country. For example, Kerala's development trajectory led to increasing international migration decades ago, which now has contributed back in the form of remittances, leading to enhanced incomes and well-being (Zachariah & Rajan, 2016). Bihar, on the other hand, remains one of the most backward states because of its development trajectory, even as it has high—mainly internal—migration (Rodgers et al., 2013). In this case, though migration led to support in incomes through remittances, it could not transform the Bihari migrants' economic conditions; rather, it led to the diversification of livelihood-generating activities through pluri-activity (Datta, 2022). In addition to development from an economic perspective, the interplay of migration trajectories with social structures, historical patterns, and processes of globalization is key. Tamil Nadu, for example, has had a very different trajectory than many other states in India, and as a result, has the persistence of both international and internal migration, which again differs from its neighboring states (Kerala or Karnataka) (Rajan et al., 2021).

Development in Odisha has been marked by significant strides in various sectors. The state, which had a predominantly agricultural economy during the 1970s, has witnessed a structural transformation over the past five decades, with the expansion of services as well as industry. However, this structural change in economic output did not correspond directly to a structural change in employment, as almost half of the population is still dependent on agriculture for employment. The state has witnessed high growth in the past two decades, but with inadequate distributional effects. As a result, the persistence of poverty, food insecurity, and vulnerability of various kinds impacts the poor, who still comprise a significant proportion of the population. The enhanced vulnerability in the wake of agrarian distress, employment crisis, and industrial expansion through land acquisition has adversely affected sections of the population. The survival strategy in such scenarios has been migration to other states (and intra-state as well) in search of employment opportunities to support livelihoods. Odisha is one of the primary source states for migration in India, and Odia migrants are found working in (mostly informal) establishments across the country.

The development trajectory of the state has remained skewed, leading to certain regions and communities lagging behind. These regions and communities overlap, with most deprived communities [Scheduled Tribes (STs), Scheduled Castes (SCs), and lower Other Backward Classes (OBCs)] predominantly belonging to the backward regions. The regional variations in caste-community demographics are such that SCs comprise one-fifth of the population in eight districts, whereas STs comprise more than half in six districts. Gender disparities are also stark, with females being disadvantaged in key social and economic indicators. It is thus necessary to incorporate women's perspectives in the state's development project in the context of neoliberal economic development—growth characterized by expanding inequalities and environmental degradation (Hans et al., 2021).

The political-economic perspective suggests a decline in agriculture and a lack of adequate non-agricultural livelihoods in the rural areas, despite increasing government welfare measures in some areas. An analysis by Sarkar and Mukherji (2025) points to a cycle of low capital investment in agriculture, degradation and diversion of cultivable land, stagnant crop and resource productivity, and underutilization of agricultural labor as some of the key challenges in reducing the state's development deficit. Many of these have stemmed from the colonial-era land revenue administration; abysmal land management practices of the time led to poor agricultural growth and rural poverty (Sarkar & Mukherji, 2025). However, the phenomena persisted even in the post-Independence era, notwithstanding the changes in the political and economic profile of the state. After Independence, all the forest land that was under the collective ownership of the tribal communities came under state ownership with restricted use of land as well as forest products (Ambagudia, 2010), which had significantly disruptive implications for the traditional tribal economy. Further, the neoliberal policies, in the later decades, of industrial extraction and corporate penetration were and continue to be legitimized through electoral processes, welfare measures, and media (Mohanty, 2014).

Over the years, tribal lands have been transferred to mining corporations. A draft report of the Comptroller and Auditor General (CAG) of India said that the land held by tribals in Odisha had decreased by 12% in the 10 years from 2005–06 to 2015–16 (Barik, 2023). Thus, the majority of Dalit, Adivasi, and rural poor (especially the laboring population) continue to remain at the periphery of development, reproducing labor fragmentation (Adduci, 2011).

Similarly, regional disparities have remained high—as is discussed in the course of the book—despite top-down investments by state and non-state actors. Tracing this back to British rule, the colonial governance focused primarily on the eastern (coastal) part of the state—owing to its fertility and fearing tribal resistance in the interior districts (Samal, 2000). This historical divide has been reinforced in the post-Independence period due to the continued political dominance by leaders from the coastal belt, contributing to uneven development and resource allocation (Mishra, 2011). In this context, with development policies not yet focusing on migration as the central concern, a deeper blind spot remains the conjugated oppression faced by migrant workers from marginalized communities (Dalits and Adivasis) from all sides—gender, caste, tribe, ethnicity, and region (Lerche & Shah, 2018).

2 Economic Profile

The first three decades after Independence (1950–80) witnessed a very slow rate of growth of Odisha's gross state domestic product (GSDP), at 2.8%—using the notional constant rate of growth at 1999–00 prices (Nayak et al., 2016b). This picture was not any better for the national statistics for the same indicators and period as well, with India's GDP growth at 3.6% at 1993–94 prices. The per capita net state domestic product (NSDP) for Odisha also saw a slow rate of notional constant annual growth at 1.1% between 1951 and 1981, largely aligning with the country-level estimates, which were not very different, at 1.3% (ibid.).

We analyzed simple year-on-year growth rates at constant prices (2011–12 back series) for Odisha's GSDP and NSDP from 1980 to 2025, and they reveal three distinct phases. The Phase I (1980–2000) saw 3.78% average growth but also high volatility, ranging from -15.01% (1990–91) to 20.03% (1988–89). In Phase II (2001–2011), growth rates were substantially stable at 7.98% average growth and no negative growth years. Phase III (2012–2025) witnessed a 7.22% growth showing steadiness, despite a -2.13% dip in 2020–21 (possibly COVID-19-induced), followed by a strong

16.42% rebound in 2021–22. Recent figures of 5.97% (2022–23) and 7.23% (2024–25) suggest that the economy has settled into a stable growth trajectory.

Investment in the industrial and mining sectors was one of the primary drivers of this growth in the post-2000s. Moreover, fiscal discipline led to Odisha becoming a revenue-surplus state, as it also overcame the problems of low revenue potential and large public expenditure responsibilities (Sen & Rout, 2016). Economic slowdown due to natural disasters has been a major deterrent to growth, but several disaster management measures (especially on cyclones and floods) have enhanced growth by minimizing the scope of economic slowdown, particularly after 2003 (S. Das, 2016).

Odisha's NSDP trajectory closely mirrors its GSDP path—marked by early volatility, moderate post-liberalization gains, and a high-growth phase from 2003 onward. Like GSDP, NSDP saw sharp swings in the 1970s–90 s, a stabilizing trend post-1991, and a major boom after 2003 (113.6% growth). The recent period (2016–2025) shows strong cumulative growth (97.4%), a pandemic dip (−3.3%), and a 17.4% rebound, reflecting a shared pattern of volatility to resilience. The per capita NSDP surged from Rs 27,895 (1999–2000) to Rs 106,918 (2024–25), growing at 5.8% annually. Notably, NSDP per capita doubled between 2003 and 2016 (+109.6%) and saw a strong post-pandemic recovery (16.6% in 2021–22). Recent growth (2022–25) averaged 6.9%, crossing Rs 1 lakh in 2024–25—now five times the 1990 level.

The proportionate change in the per capita NSDP of Odisha compared to per capita net national product (NNP) also shows a similar change: around 63.8% of the national NNP in 2001–02 and 70.8% of the national NNP in 2011–12 (Planning Commission, 2012). Based on the per capita NSDP ranking methodology for 16 major states, Samantaraya et al. (2014) show that Odisha's position has improved from the second poorest in 1994–95 to the fifth poorest in 2004–05 and the sixth poorest in 2009–10. Since 2011–12, the per capita NSDP of Odisha has been enhanced by more than three times (compared to 2.7 times nationally), and the gap between Odisha and India's per capita income has been reducing. In 2015–16, the per capita incomes (at current prices) of Odisha and India were Rs 64,835 and Rs 94,797, respectively (31.6% gap). The corresponding numbers for 2022–23 are Rs 150,676 and Rs 170,620, respectively, with the gap reduced to 11.7% (Government of Odisha [GoO], 2023).

The structure of the economy in 1982–83 was such that the primary sector (agriculture and allied) predominantly contributed to the GSDP (55.7%), followed by the tertiary sector (29.0%) and the secondary sector (15.3%) (Nayak et al., 2016b). Table 1 details the structural change in both GSVA and employment share, with a rural-urban divide. By 1993–94, the service sector gained steadily and contributed the highest in GSVA (50%), followed by agriculture (33%) and industry (17%). Since then, the industry's share has been expanding to reach 38% in 2019–20, whereas both agriculture and services declined to 22% and 40%, respectively.

In terms of employment, despite contributing only 22%, agriculture still employed 55% of the rural people in 2019–20, but its share has declined from 72% in 1993–94. The rural (and urban) agricultural laborers have moved to rural industry for employment as its share has increased from 9 to 26% in the corresponding period,

Table 1 Structural change in Odisha (employment and GSVA composition)

		Employment share (in%)				GSVA share (in current prices, in%)				
		1993–1994	2004–2005	2011–2012	2019–2020	1993–1994	2004–2005	2011–2012	2019–2020	2024–2025*
Agriculture	Rural	72	69	62	55	33	23	18	22	18.9
	Urban	10	14	14	5					
Industry	Rural	9	17	23	26	17	24	44	38	43.9
	Urban	26	27	23	33					
Services	Rural	18	14	15	19	50	53	38	40	37.1
	Urban	65	60	63	62					

Source Odisha Economic Survey, 2021–22 and 2024–25
*Advance estimates, MOSPI

whereas the share of services in rural (or even urban) employment has remained more or less the same.

Despite improvement, Odisha still has a long way to go, as its per capita income is almost half that of the richer states. A high growth rate does not ensure redistribution and can lead to high inequality if it is growth without inclusion—a phenomenon that Odisha has witnessed in the 1990s (Panda, 2008). Sen and Rout (2016) show that fiscal deficit has been eliminated often at the cost of curbing expenditure on education, health, and rural infrastructure. The former two have also become increasingly privatized.

Poverty and distress are high in the rural areas and for certain categories of the population. To study the differential impact of growth and development, let us look at different sectors and population groups to carefully analyze the differences in detail.

3 Development Trajectory of Odisha

3.1 Agrarian Scenario

Agriculture and allied activities were the dominant sectors of the economy during the 1980s, as noted in the previous section. Despite the declining share of agriculture and allied activities in GSVA, it still employs almost 60% of the state's working population (Table 1). However, its share in GSVA is a mere 22% in 2019–20 (declined from 33% in 1992–93). Nevertheless, agriculture still determines the state's per capita income changes and is therefore significantly important.

3.1.1 Agrarian Structure and Land Relations

Land relations vary regionally, as the present-day Odisha was subdivided and was part of three different land governance systems during the colonial period. Some regions (Cuttack, Puri, and Balasore) were under the Zamindari system, while some others (Ganjam and Koraput) were under the Ryotwari system. A few others (Sambalpur and Phulbani) were under the *Malguzari* and *Gountia* systems. Land ownership is skewed. In 2003, the top 5% owned 12% of the land, and the bottom 86% owned 42% of the total land (Gaurav & Mishra, 2016). The average operational holding size has been declining, and more than 72% are marginal operational holdings (ibid.). On operational holding, in 2015–16, the top 7% of the population operated 25% of the land, and the remaining 93% operated 75%.

Land ownership is also becoming increasingly fragmented, where the small and marginal landholdings are increasing and other big categories (semi-medium, medium, and large) are decreasing (Gaurav & Mishra, 2016; Swain, 2017). This has led to a reduction in inequality in land ownership, but with a preponderance of smallholdings.

According to National Sample Survey (NSS) data, one-tenth of the population is landless, and this proportion has been persisting since the 1970s.[1] The majority (proportionally and absolute) of landless households form a class that is highly intertwined with caste and tribe categories. A majority of SCs and STs are landless, and, as a result, they are proportionally very high in the class of landless households. The SCs also have a high proportion of marginal landholdings, both owned and operational. The STs have a relatively lower proportion of marginal holdings and operate as well as own small and semi-medium holdings more (Gaurav & Mishra, 2016). However, they face a big threat of land acquisition in the name of development, especially against extractive capital. Women's land operational holding is very low at 3.3% in 2010–11, much below the national average (12.8%). Therefore, land ownership and operational holding are skewed along the lines of region, class, caste, tribe, and gender.

The incidence of tenancy—both in terms of the number of plots and area—is quite high. As per NSS data in 2012–13, almost one-fifth of the operational area and one-sixth of the operational holdings were under tenancy arrangements (Swain, 2017). Odisha, with sharecropping arrangements in the majority (more than 70%), has the highest incidence of sharecropping tenancy among the top 15 states in India. Property rights on land are conflicting for tenant-cultivators with the prevalence of oral-seasonal nature of contracts. The coastal districts have a relatively higher incidence of tenancy, with almost half of the land under tenancy, with Cuttack at the top of this list.

As per the agricultural census 2015–16, the incidence of marginal landholdings is relatively higher for coastal districts and relatively lower for districts in western areas and the Sambalpur region.

Among the tribal-dominated regions, customary land tenure systems predominate. The land reform policy move, of declaring any land with a slope more than 9 degrees to be government property, was a key reason for unrest among the tribals since most of the hill slopes, where shifting cultivation and terracing had been practiced, fell in that range. The government realized this very late.

3.1.2 Crop Production

The benefits of the green revolution reached quite late in eastern India, particularly in Odisha. As a result, crop yields/productivity has remained low for a very long period and for most commodities. Crop diversification has been sluggish and still has much scope to increase farm incomes (Nayak & Kumar, 2019; Sarap & Sahu, 2016). Since the 1980s, the area under the respective crops has remained more or less the same at the category level (food grains, pulses, and cash crops), barring minimal changes at the crop level. Paddy is still the dominant crop cultivated in the

[1] The NSS, however, severely underestimates landlessness and land inequality. In 2003-04, while the incidence of landlessness reported by the NSS was 9.6%, Rawal (2008) estimates that the percentage of households *not holding any land other than homestead land* was as high as 38.5%.

state, but its absolute area has declined from 44.71 lakh ha. in 1970–71 to 39.41 lakh ha. in 2019–20 (GoO, 2020). The area under commercial and cash crops has remained as low as 1% over the last four decades. However, in terms of production, the food grain share has reduced from 47.58% to 41.18% between 1980–83 and 2007–10. A rise in fruit, flower, and vegetable production has driven this change mainly, along with an increase in traditional pulses and oilseeds. Only two coastal districts (Jajpur and Jagatsinghpur) have undergone a decent level of crop diversification. For other coastal districts, it has been minimal. However, in the KBK[2] region, many districts have high diversification. Nayak and Kumar (2019) found that the usage of high yielding variety (HYV) seeds and irrigation led to crop concentration, but an expansion of infrastructure and incomes has led to an increase in crop diversification.

Crop productivity has fluctuated across regions, time periods, and commodities grown. The overall crop productivity increased in the 1980s and witnessed a negative growth rate in the 1990s and 2000s. In addition to a much higher growth of some seasonal varieties of paddy, only a partial increase in rice, maize, groundnuts, cotton, chilies, and items under oilseeds was significant. There exists high regional variation in paddy productivity between the irrigated and dry regions. More than 10 districts have productivity lower than the state average (Sarap & Sahu, 2016).

Cropping intensity has increased from 121% to 167% between 1970–71 and 2010–11. Net sown area initially increased from 5652 thousand ha in 1950–51 to 6304 thousand ha in 1990–91, but has now been reduced to 5362 thousand ha in 2019–20, lower than that at the time of Independence. Of this, the net irrigated area is just 2592 thousand ha in 2019–20. Gross cropped area (GCA) has decreased to 8.5 m ha in the triennium ending (TE) 2016–17 from 9.6 m ha in TE 1992–93 (Hoda et al., 2021).

There exist high inter-district variations in agricultural productivity, especially for food grains (Patra, 2014). Agro-climatic conditions have a defining role to play since the coastal and central tableland regions are agriculturally advanced (crop diversification, commercialization, and technology adoption) because of better soils, high extent of irrigation and fertilizer application, and favorable rainfall (ibid.). The other regions have textured land, unfavorable climate, and rainfed, drought-prone habitats, leading to the prevalence of a backward form of agricultural systems.

3.1.3 Technology, Mechanization, and Infrastructure

The usage of HYV seeds and fertilizers has also increased. HYV seed supply expanded to 7.98 lakh quintals in 2015–16 from 1.42 lakh quintals in 1995–96 (Sarap & Sahu, 2016). Usage is very low in the Eastern Ghats and southern districts. The intensity of fertilizer usage has increased to 73.81 kg/ha in 2018–19 from a mere 20 kg/ha in 1990–91, but it is still well below the national average (133.12 kg/ha)

---

[2] Kalahandi-Balangir-Koraput (KBK) is a region comprising eight districts in southern and western Odisha, which is also the most backward part of Odisha.

(GoO, 2020). There are regional variations in fertilizer application, with the lowest in the Eastern Ghats and northern plateau at almost half of the state's average.

Odisha has the lowest gross irrigated area, lowest power intensity, and lowest surfaced road lengths (only 23.9%) among major states in India (Hoda et al., 2021). The source-wise irrigation potential is 2138 thousand ha through major and medium-sized irrigation projects, 823 thousand ha via minor irrigation (flow), 1815 thousand ha via minor irrigation (lift), and 1285 thousand ha from other sources. The mega-lift project started in 2015–16 but covers only 124.71 thousand ha as of 2019–20. Irrigation in the state is unevenly distributed, and the created potential is inefficiently used, where half of it is unutilized for flow and 37% for groundwater (Sarap & Sahu, 2016). Hoda et al. (2021) find that there is still much scope to realize the ultimate irrigation potential (UIP). Considering the strong association between irrigation and agricultural development in several districts of the state found in a study by Ghosh et al. (2012), the implications for livelihoods and poverty are serious.

Banking for the rural poor in Odisha has the following issues. The lending amount from the banks is very low compared to other states, and banks cite reasons such as not having enough viable proposals, poor recovery and high default rates, low credit absorption capacity, and inadequate workforce in financial institutions (Sarap & Sahu, 2016). The transaction cost and risk associated (with crop production/failure) with delivering a large number of small loans to poor households are very high. As a result, the rural poor are significantly dependent upon informal moneylenders for production as well as consumption loans. Interlinkages of input, credit, and output markets are very strong, as a result of which farmers have to undergo distress sales at lower (unremunerative) prices. These interlinkages become even more exploitative when mixed with tenancy relations.

Odisha stood 12th out of 15 states in the composite infrastructural development index as per the Eleventh Finance Commission Report (Government of India [GoI], 2000). Mohanty et al. (2016) have built a similar index at the district level and found that certain districts fare well (Khordha, Sundargarh, Cuttack, Mayurbhanj, and Ganjam) compared to others, which are lagging much behind (Boudh, Malkangiri, Sonepur [also known as Subarnapur], Gajapati, and Deogarh). They also find a positive effect of infrastructural development on human development indices, especially telecommunication, postal services, provision of drinking water, and banking.

3.1.4 Labor and Employment

As discussed earlier, despite the decline in the share of workers in agriculture over time, the sector continues to employ a majority of workers. At the same time, peculiarly, the share of workers in the services sector too has marginally declined, while that of industrial workers increased (Table 1). Underemployment is quite high compared to chronic unemployment and marginal unemployment (R. K. Panda, 2016). The unemployment and underemployment growth figures are higher for Odisha compared to all-India, both in incidence and intensity. The real wages of agricultural laborers have witnessed slow positive growth, but in absolute terms, their wages are lower than those of other rural workers. The gender disparity in wage rates has increased over time.

As per the Periodic Labour Force Survey (PLFS) 2018–19, the unemployment rate in Odisha was 7%, compared to 5.8% for India (NSO, 2020, as cited in Khan et al., 2021). However, there were regional variations with the central region reporting the highest unemployment rate at 9.2% followed by the southern (6.4%) and northern regions (5.8%) (Khan et al., 2021). Overall, as well as regionally, the unemployment rates are significantly higher in the urban areas, between 11 and 14%, compared to 4–9% in rural areas. Districts with high unemployment rates (ranging between 10 and 12%) are Cuttack, Kendrapara, Khordha, Ganjam, and Gajapati. With lower unemployment rates (ranging between 1 and 5%), there are seven districts from the southern region, two from the north, and one in the coastal region (ibid.).

As per the PLFS estimates (2021–22), the unemployment rate in Odisha was 6%, much higher than the national average (4.1%). It is even higher for the younger generation, 15–29 years age group, at 19.8% for the state compared to 12.4% for India (GoO, 2023).

On the distribution of the workforce, census data shows that there is a shift of main workers away from agriculture and allied activities (National Law University Odisha [NLUO], 2020). The NSO 67th report and PLFS data 2018–19 show that the labor force participation rate in Odisha is at 38.4%, and it is 40.9% for persons between 15 and 29 years of age. The worker population ratio is about 35.7%, with substantial gender differentials. Self-employed persons among workers constitute almost 60% of the workforce in rural areas and around 35% in urban areas. Casual wage work is higher for the rural population (28.8% and 30.4% respectively for males and females), whereas salaried/regular wage employment is high for urban workers (almost half of the workforce) (ibid.).

As per PLFS data (2023–24), the worker population ratio (15 + age) is 63%, higher than the national estimates (58%) (GoO, 2025). For males, it is 79% (India: 76%) and for females, it is 48% (India: 40%). Similarly, the labor force participation rate is also high compared to national estimates (Odisha: 64.9%, India: 60.1%), for both males (Odisha: 81.7%, India: 78.8%) and females (Odisha: 49.4%, India: 41.7%) (ibid.).

Odisha witnessed a structural change in employment between 1993–94 and 2011–12, with a decline in employment in the primary sector from 80.9% to 62.25%, and a rise in employment in the secondary and tertiary sectors from 9.4% and 9.8% to 22.64% and 15.13%, respectively. There are rural-urban differences in this structural change, wherein all or most of it is largely driven by changes in rural areas. Over this period, the growth rate of employment in agriculture was decreasing (−1.28%) for rural areas, whereas it was increasing for secondary (7.83%) and tertiary (3.02%) sectors (NLUO, 2020). The majority of the secondary sector's subsectors witnessed high positive growth in employment. In urban areas, however, the two sectoral growth rates were low: 0.7% for primary and 0.2% for tertiary. Only the secondary sector witnessed high growth (5.3%) in employment rates. Between 2011–12 and 2017–18, the employment crisis magnified in Odisha. The negative contribution of agricultural employment intensified during this period, leading to overall negative effects of the growth of employment on GSDP (Padhi & Panda, 2021). Even manufacturing and some other subsectors witnessed negative employment growth, except construction and a few service sectors (ibid.).

Between 2011–12 and 2023–24, based on the Employment-Unemployment Survey (EUS) and PLFS, the workforce distribution has further shifted from agriculture (56% to 49%) to industry (23% to 26%) and services (21% to 25%) (GoO, 2025). Among working individuals aged 15 and above, a majority—62% or about 135.2 lakh people—earn their living through self-employment. The remaining 38% work as either salaried employees (33.0 lakh) or casual laborers (53.8 lakh). Between 2017–18 and 2023–24, the share of the workforce in self-employed activities increased consistently (from 57.4% to 62%), whereas a decline has been witnessed for those in salaried employment (15.4% to 13.6%) and casual work (27.2% to 24.4%) (ibid.).

The conditions of employment are very poor in Odisha. The India Employment Report (IER) 2024 constructed an employment condition index to assess progress in quality and conditions of employment and found Odisha to be the worst performer (along with Bihar) across 22 major states in India for the reference years 2005, 2012, 2019, and 2022 (IER, 2024). Similar outcomes are noted for youth employment, where Odisha ranks among India's worst states, with high unemployment among educated youth, low regular jobs, and informal work exceeding the national average. Many youths are not in employment, education, or training. Slow economic growth limits job creation, driving outmigration. With a rising youth workforce, Odisha faces mounting pressure to generate employment opportunities.

With regional variations in economic indicators, R. K. Panda (2016) finds an inverse relationship between unemployment and poverty: high-poverty regions report low unemployment (since workers mostly do low-paid manual work, as they can't afford unemployment). Where poverty is low, people can afford to wait to find work, and therefore, unemployment is high. The Odisha government has launched an employment generation scheme in 2020, titled Mukhyamantri Karma Tatpara Abhiyan Yojana (MUKTA), for the urban poor and migrant workers. The urban local bodies (ULBs) are meant to develop ward-wise action plans annually to build projects that create job opportunities. The government has been allotting huge funding[3]; however, the OMS results show a general lack of awareness about this scheme, and less than 1% of urban households reported participating in the MUKTA scheme.

3.1.5 Agrarian Distress and Poverty

With the large number of small-marginal farms in Odisha, agrarian distress affects small-marginal farmers disproportionately. The exploitative and unequal tenancy relations, backward technology, limited crop diversification (mainly food grains, minimal cash crops), low private investment, along with vagaries of weather

[3] See: Odisha CM Sanctions Rs 184 Crore Under MUKTA Scheme, *Deccan Herald* (https://www.deccanherald.com/india/odisha-cm-sanctions-rs-184-crore-under-mukta-scheme-1227075.html).

(monsoon, floods, and droughts), lead to conditions of agrarian distress. The neoliberal policies were introduced in breaks and segments (1996, 2008, and 2013) with an initial (1996) focus on enhancing commercialization (competition and exports), followed by an emphasis on enhancing the marketing channels and agro-industries in 2008. The System of Rice Intensification (SRI), push for seed replacement (HYV adoption), expansion of the national horticulture mission, etc., were sped up in 2013. All these measures increased yields, but also raised the cost of cultivation. The profitability crisis eventually hit Odisha as well, resulting in higher indebtedness along with exploitative tenancy relations, in turn leading to an increasing incidence of farmer suicides (Mohanty & Lenka, 2019).

Agrarian distress has disrupted the agenda of poverty reduction. The returns from cultivation were significantly low two decades back, at a mere four rupees per day per capita in 2002–03 (Mishra, 2009). As a result, the high incidence of poverty is closely tied to the large share of people in agriculture trapped in chronic poverty. The returns from cultivation are still the lowest in Odisha across all the states as per the Situation Assessment Survey 2019, which has also declined in real terms between 2013 and 2019. The major source of income for an agricultural household is wage earning, followed by cultivation, which has less than half the income from wages (Munjal, 2021). Essentially, the proletarianization of peasants is being witnessed.

To support the distress-ridden agriculture, the Odisha government introduced a direct benefit transfer (DBT) scheme, Krushak Assistance for Livelihood and Income Augmentation (KALIA), in 2018–19, which would provide Rs 5,000 each for farmers of all size-classes, spread over five seasons till 2021–22. This amount was complementary to the national DBT scheme (PM-KISAN) amount of Rs 6000 per farmer per year. In addition, the KALIA scheme also provides livelihood assistance of Rs 12,500 to each landless household; interest-free crop loans and Rs 2 lakh insurance cover for each farmer. These cash transfers surely amount to an augmentation of incomes for the rural poor households, but it is a temporary measure that does not address structural problems and complexities in Odisha agriculture (Gaurav, 2023). Sustainability of agricultural incomes requires investment in irrigation, enhancing productivity, technology adoption, providing remunerative prices, and reforming agricultural markets. Despite changing economic and political contexts, low investment in agriculture remains a primary challenge (Sarkar & Mukherji, 2025).

3.2 *Industrial and Mining Scenario*

Industrialization in Odisha has been relatively slow in the twenty-first century, even as the Industrial Policy document of 2001 envisaged intensive industrialization through concessional rates for land, subsidies on interest, electricity waivers, tax concessions, and the so-called 'rationalization of labor laws' (GoO, 2001). The declining share of industry in GSDP in the 1980s started expanding after the liberalization period. Between 1980 and 2002, the growth rate of the aggregate industry was 5.1% and expanded to 9.3% between 2003 and 2013 (Bal et al., 2015). The state's focus has been primarily on manufacturing (registered and unregistered), but also on micro, small, and medium enterprises (MSMEs) (since 2009), as the latter is more important for employment. Industry in Odisha largely constitutes mining and quarrying (M&Q), manufacturing (registered and unregistered), electricity, gas and water supply (EGWS), and the construction sector. The investment for industrialization largely goes to steel, cement, power, aluminum, and chemical-petrochemical sectors. Nevertheless, the share of the industrial output of the construction sector in the overall secondary sector is still significantly high, despite a reduction from 49% in the 1980s to 26.3% in 2010–13 (ibid.). Marking a significant expansion, the M&Q sector's contribution to Odisha's GSDP has increased from 0.76% in the 1950s to 4% in the 1990s. It peaked in the 2000s at 6.5% and was at almost 6% in 2011–12 (Das & Acharya, 2016). With a steady rise during the early 2000s, the iron-ore and coal industries have contributed to the growth of the sector, whereas Bauxite and Chromite have witnessed volatility in growth trends.

Labor productivity in industry was low during 1980–2000, but has improved significantly since then. Capital accumulation shows a negative trend in all major industries except the chemical industry (Bal et al., 2015). However, the absolute number of employment generated has reduced from 53,000 to 48,000 between 1999–00 and 2011–12. Das and Acharya (2016) calculated employment elasticity (i.e., additional workers employed for an additional unit of output), which has remained negative for seven out of 12 years during the mentioned period. While industry has been witnessing positive growth rates, the employment figures have remained negative in the first decade of the twenty-first century (ibid.). Apart from the negative distributional effects of mining-led industrialization, there are other damaging consequences, such as deforestation, air and water pollution, and land acquisition and displacement, which remain inadequately addressed, predominantly due to regulatory failures.

Beyond manufacturing and mining, transport and power are two major sectors in Odisha's industrial economy that have significant spillover effects on other sectors, as well as contributions to communications and infrastructural development. However, despite their significant contribution to economic development, their full potential remains unrealized. Odisha fares better than national estimates on the average road density, but surfaced roads are still lagging (S. P. Das, 2016). The rail network is still poor in the KBK districts, as well as in the tribal belt of Mayurbhanj and Sundargarh. Despite undergoing structural changes in the power sector by dividing the generation, transmission, and distribution activities (with partial privatization of distribution), the electrification status of the villages was at 73% and of households at a mere 36%, as per the Census 2011. Our survey results show further improvement, discussed in detail in Chapter 2.

The expansion of large industries (mining, manufacturing) and MSMEs has sidelined the traditional industrial ecosystem, which plays a much greater role in generating employment and promoting local businesses, while holding cultural relevance to the communities. Some key traditional industries are handloom and textiles, handicraft and cottage, sericulture, and salt and coir industries. Their growth rates have been negative and on a downswing, as these industries are slowly reducing in number (shutting down), implying contraction in the sector (Mohanty, 2016).

The recent industrialization across the state has been led by mining (and extraction) and mainly situated in the forest belts. The industrialization process is strongly intertwined with ecological concerns, which raises serious questions about the sustainability of development. Given the presence of mineral-rich resources in Odisha, the state has pursued a policy of mining-led growth and industrialization. The impact of large industrial investments on unemployment or poverty has remained minimal. Rather, it has led to the loss of livelihoods through state-facilitated displacement and environmental disruption (Kumar, 2014; Padhi & Sadangi, 2020). Patnaik (2016) discusses the neoliberal trajectory of the development strategy of Odisha, which attracts big private players to the mining and manufacturing industries at the expense of the local population. Already facing rural distress, the population now also bears the brunt of the primitive accumulation of capital. A stark indicator explaining this scenario is the high growth in GSDP, but also increasing nutritional deprivation, vulnerability, and distress. Rather, he advocates for reforms in the agricultural sector to revive and improve the conditions of the farming population. Similarly, noting the political constraints to the current strategy, Nayak et al. (2016c) also suggest that the focus of the state should be on increasing agricultural productivity to improve the conditions of the tribal and rural population.

3.3 Communities and Human Development

This section discusses the demographic and human development indicators such as health, and educational outcomes, as well as poverty and deprivation faced by different community groups through the lens of caste, tribe, and gender.

The population of Odisha has expanded by almost three (2.9) times since Independence (Table 2). The decadal growth analysis shows that the population increased particularly during 1971–91, after which fertility rates, along with population growth, declined. (Tables 2 and 4). The projected figures from 2021 to 2051 reflect a further slowdown in growth, with the decadal growth rate falling to just 0.4% by 2051. The sex ratio at birth (SRB) in Odisha was favorable at the time of Independence (1022 females per 1000 males in 1951), but it has since consistently declined for half a century (1950–2000). It is only after the 2000s that the sex ratio improved somewhat, but still far below the level at Independence. While there has been no census since 2011, data from the Ministry of Health and Family Welfare shows that the SRB in the state fell to 948 in 2014–15 and, alarmingly, further declined to 926 in 2023–24 (GoI, 2024). However, projections by Rajan and Retnakumar (2025) indicate an overall upward trend in the general sex ratio, suggesting gradual demographic recovery, with the sex ratio expected to reach 1013 females per 1000 males by 2051.

Table 2 Trends in population growth rate and sex ratio, Odisha, 1951–2051

Census year	Persons	Males	Females	Decadal growth rate	Sex ratio
1951	14,645,946	7,242,892	7,403,054	–	1022
1961	17,548,846	8,770,586	8,778,260	19.8	1001
1971	21,944,615	11,041,083	10,903,532	25.0	988
1981	26,370,271	13,309,786	13,060,485	20.2	981
1991	31,659,736	16,064,146	15,595,590	20.1	971
2001	36,804,660	18,660,570	18,144,090	16.3	972
2011	41,974,218	21,212,136	20,762,082	14.0	979
2021*	46,054,629	23,196,847	22,857,782	9.7	985
2031*	48,784,527	24,476,760	24,307,767	5.9	993
2041*	50,190,660	25,063,578	25,127,082	2.9	1003
2051*	50,382,479	25,030,760	25,351,719	0.4	1013

Source Census of India, 1951–2011; *Rajan and Retnakumar (2025)

3.3.1 Health

On the verge of the twenty-first century, Odisha had the highest infant mortality rate (IMR) in India at 105 compared to the national average of 64 (Kurian, 2000). More than 10% of infants in Odisha, especially females, did not survive their first birthday. The lowest IMR was that of Kerala at nine. The second half of the post-reform period (after 2005) has witnessed improvement in indicators of poverty and human development in Odisha, and one can say that Odisha has become less poor between 2005 and 2015 (Samantaraya et al., 2014). The health indicators have largely corresponded to economic growth figures, both of which have been improving since 2003. Between 2005 and 2011, IMR declined from 75 to 57, crude death rate (CDR) from 9.5 to 8.5, crude birth rate (CBR) from 22.3 to 20.1, female life expectancy at birth was 64.9, up from 59.6, and the same for males was 62.3, up from 59.5 (Rout & Hota, 2016).

These figures have improved even more in the latest decade. IMR has further improved from 57 to 36 between 2011 and 2020 (Table 3). The decline was from 63 to 37 in rural areas and 43 to 28 in urban areas between 2010 and 2020 (GoO, 2023).

In 2021, Odisha's CBR decreased slightly to 17.4 per 1000 population, continuing the long-term trend of declining fertility. However, the CDR rose marginally to 8.6, potentially reflecting the lingering impact of the COVID-19 pandemic, including excess mortality during the second wave. Despite this, the IMR improved further, dropping to 35 infant deaths per 1,000 live births.

In 2022, the state saw a further decline in CBR to 16.5, reinforcing the demographic transition toward lower fertility. The CDR showed a modest improvement, falling to 7.8, indicating a recovery from pandemic-related mortality impacts. Most notably, the IMR declined to 32, marking sustained progress in reducing infant deaths.

Table 3 Crude birth rate (CBR), crude death rate (CDR), and infant mortality rate (IMR), 2009–2020

	CBR	CDR	IMR
2009	21.0	8.8	65
2011	20.1	8.5	57
2014	19.4	7.9	49
2018	18.2	7.3	40
2020	17.7	7.3	36
2021	17.4	8.6	35
2022	16.5	7.8	32

Source Sample registration system (SRS) bulletins

Table 4 Trends in fertility rate in Odisha, 1992–93 to 2019–21

TFR	Total	Rural	Urban
NFHS-1 (1992–93)	2.9	3.0	2.5
NFHS-2 (1998–99)	2.5	2.5	2.2
NFHS-3 (2005–06)	2.4	2.5	1.9
NFHS 4 (2015–16)	2.1	2.1	1.7
NFHS 5 (2019–21)	1.8	1.9	1.5

Source IIPS, NFHS-5, Odisha, 2019–21

Life expectancy has also improved to 70.3 years for Odisha (2016–20 period), higher than India now (70), for both males (69.1) and females (71.4) (Table 3). The CBR per 1,000 inhabitants has also declined from 20.1 to 17.7 between 2011 and 2020. In the same period, the crude death rate also declined from 8.5 to 7.3.

Still, mortality rates in Odisha continue to be high, and the demographic transition is led by the steep decline in fertility (see Table 4 for details), in the context of poverty and low levels of economic development. This is seen as a 'demographic dilemma' (Centre for Youth and Social Development [CYSD], 2024).

Health and mortality statistics from the state are alarming, especially for women. More than 25% of adolescent girls (15–19 years) have one surviving child, and there is an increasing occurrence of high-risk pregnancies. More than half of SC and ST women are anemic. The rates of institutional delivery are still very low among SC women (<33%) and much worse for ST women (<10%) (Acharya et al., 2021).

Regional and caste-wise variations are high in terms of access to healthcare facilities. As stated before, SCs comprise one-fifth of the population in eight districts, and STs comprise more than half in six districts. The districts having higher than one-fifth SC population have 40–70% institutional deliveries (ibid.). Access to institutional deliveries is generally higher for upper-caste groups (92%), compared to SCs (86%) or STs (72%) (ibid.).

Neonatal mortality rate is 2.7% as per National Family Health Survey (NFHS)-5 (2019–21), higher than the national average (2.5%). Neonatal and post-neonatal mortality rates are much higher for STs compared to others (ibid.). The same applies to infant mortality, child mortality, and mortality under five years of age.

Official statistics indicate that the government's health institutional infrastructure is much better positioned in Odisha compared to other states, but the investment in human capital is still low. Shortfalls in the recruitment and placement of professionals are huge: radiographers (89%), laboratory technicians (79%), nurses/midwives (73%), and specialist doctors (71%) (Rout & Hota, 2016). Odisha fares better than other states in health infrastructural terms for some other specific indicators (number of PHCs and CHCs, female health workers, assistants, as well as surgeons, gynecologists, and pediatricians). Yet, there is a need to expand the base of the government health services, especially given the lower investment by private players in the sector, compared to other states. A mere 10% of the total hospital-bed strength can be provided by the private hospitals, which is also regionally skewed and mainly situated in urban areas (ibid.). Regionally, the health infrastructure is much better and widely spread in the districts of Cuttack, Mayurbhanj, Ganjam, Sundargarh, and Keonjhar, whereas Deogarh, Subarnapur, and Boudh are some of the worst off.

Biju Swasthya Kalyan Yojana (BSKY) is a flagship universal health coverage scheme in Odisha, providing free healthcare at all government hospitals and special healthcare facilities in empaneled private hospitals for the poor households. Since healthcare is largely in the public sector in Odisha, positive changes have been observed in utilization since the launch of BSKY, with increasing uptake of Outpatient Department (OPD), lab services, and Inpatient Department (IPD) in government hospitals (Chandrasekhar & Naidu, 2021). Overall, it appears to have bolstered access to healthcare[4]; about 88% of the OMS households had the Biju Swasthya Yojana cards, and in the rural areas, this figure was nearly 90%.

3.3.2 Education

According to the Census 2011, the literacy rate of Odisha is 73.45%, with male and female literacy rates of 82.45% and 64.30%, respectively. The gender gap in literacy rates is much lower in urban areas. The SCs have a literacy rate a little lower than the state average, but females among the group have less than 60% literacy. *All of the districts* in the southern and south-western region of Odisha fall below the state's average literacy rate (Nabarangpur, Malkangiri, Koraput, Rayagada, Gajapati, Nuapada, Kalahandi, Kandhamal, Balangir, and Ganjam). Only four districts beyond southern Odisha reported similarly low rates: Debagarh, Boudh, Kendujhar, and Mayurbhanj (Fig. 1). The male-female disparity is particularly high in these districts, which have lower general literacy rates.

School attendance for the 6–14 age group is high at 92% but then drops significantly to 66% for the 15–17 age group (Acharya et al., 2021). While school attendance

[4] However, strong empirical evidence on the impact of BSKY in the reduction of household-level out-of-pocket expenditure can only be substantiated with the next round of NSS data.

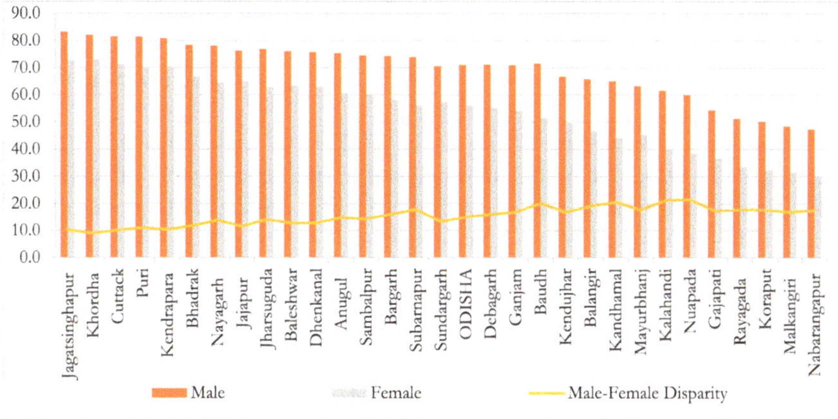

Fig. 1 Literacy rate and male-female gap by districts, 2011. *Source* Census of India (2011)

does not have high gender disparity, the duration of schooling is disparate, where 32% of women did not ever go to school compared to 16.3% of men. Drop-outs are huge after the upper primary level (before entering secondary school) in both rural and urban areas, but it is particularly remarkable to note that only 38% of rural females attend higher secondary schools (ibid.).

The transition rates at the elementary levels (primary to upper primary) are very low (84.5%) for both boys and girls in schools, implying poor access to transit from one level of education to another, or rather poor capacity for the next level to absorb the incoming batch of students (Nayak et al., 2016a). The transition from secondary to higher secondary is abysmally low at a mere 48%, much lower than other states such as West Bengal (74.6%), Tamil Nadu (78.7%), Maharashtra (63.6%), and Kerala (62.7%). Transition rates for Malkangiri and Koraput are significantly low. For girls, it is especially low in the districts of Mayurbhanj, Malkangiri, and Kalahandi (ibid.). Drop-outs among SC, ST, and girls are higher and a cause for concern.

Almost 37% of teachers in Odisha are employed on a contractual basis (Shiksha Sahayaks) and are possibly less trained and experienced. The student-classroom ratio (SCR) is more than 35 at the primary and upper primary levels. Female teacher availability is particularly low in the districts of Nuapada, Malkangiri, Kalahandi, Gajapati, and Rayagada.

3.3.3 Women

Despite the legal marriage age being 18 years for women, early marriages are a major concern in Odisha, where 20.5% of women aged 20–24 years get married before 18, as per the NFHS-5 (2019–21). For males aged 25–29 years, there are 13.3% who get married below the legal age of 21 years.

The female unemployment rate is higher (7.6%) compared to males (5.1%) or total (5.6%). Gender differential in unemployment rates holds for all caste categories, showing the disproportionate effect of unemployment on women (Acharya et al., 2021).

Fertility rates have declined from 2.9 in 1992–93 to 2.1 in 2015–16, further to 1.8 in 2019–21, as per the NFHS, now below the replacement level (Table 4). As of 2019–21, the rural fertility rate of 1.9 is what is still driving it higher because the urban fertility rate is well below 1.5 (Table 4).

More than half of the women are anemic in Odisha, of which almost 40% have severe anemia. In fact, the incidence of anemia among women and children has increased by roughly 10–20 percentage points in NFHS-5, compared to NFHS-4. The corresponding figures for men have remained the same. This is truly worrisome for the state of health among women and children in Odisha. SC and ST women have a higher incidence of all kinds of anemia (mild, moderate, severe).

3.3.4 Tribes

The indigenous communities in Odisha (STs) constitute almost one-fourth of the state's population and are heterogeneously spread across 62 tribes, the major ones being Kondhs (17.1%), Gonds (9.6%), and Santhals (9.54%). Other major tribes are Saora, Paraja, Munda, Oraon, Gadaba, Juanga, Bhuiyan, and Koya. The tribes can be differentiated by regions, ethnolinguistic features, and, broadly, levels of socio-economic development.

The STs are largely concentrated in southern Odisha. The OMS data illustrates how it's no coincidence that the southern region is the poorest and most deprived, with the worst social and economic outcomes, as is discussed in several chapters of this book. Their geographical location is mostly rural (95%), often the least accessible, and they face multidimensional deprivations (income poverty, food insecurity, poor health and sanitation facilities, and illiteracy and poor educational development). In addition, the loss of all types of land (agricultural, commons, and forests) to acquisitions has further deprived them of their means of livelihood, contributing to migration prevalence (especially seasonal). Health issues interlocking with indebtedness to local moneylenders for agricultural loans often lead them to lose out on assets and incomes (Skillshare International India [SII], 2014).

The sex ratio has always remained healthy among STs. On the other hand, chronic energy deficiency among them (38.6%) is higher than in Odisha overall (37.4%), and much higher for ST women (46%) compared to even women in Odisha (39.3%) (SII, 2014). Among the Particularly Vulnerable Tribal Groups (PVTGs), malnourishment among children is very high at 66%. All variants of mortality rates are high for STs, and institutional delivery rates are low. Districts with higher ST populations tend to also have lower than the average state Human Development Index (HDI).

The occupations and livelihood-generating activities of the STs largely come from agriculture, forests, and informal employment (in mining, manufacturing, and retail trade). Agricultural laboring also constitutes a major proportion of their work. Out-migration is common, for both males and females, and the nature of employment is highly precarious. Minor forest products (MFP) and non-timber forest products (NTFP) are two key livelihood-generating sources that the state has invested in to generate incomes. These have largely failed, except for maybe tendu leaves and the bidi-making industry (Padhi & Panigrahi, 2016).

Indigenous communities have struggled for self-determination over forest resources in a long fight against the extractive capital-state nexus (Xaxa, 2012). As a safeguard against the latter's push for investments via global finance-capital, the communities secured the Scheduled Tribes and Other Traditional Forest Dwellers (Recognition of Forest Rights) Act in 2006 to protect their interests and seek remedies for past injustices.

According to a report by SII (2014), roughly 546,794 individuals from ST communities have been displaced during 1951–95 in the name of developmental projects. Only around one-third have been rehabilitated. Displacement often reduces the sources of livelihood-generating activities and also makes accessing food entitlements (PDS) difficult. Displaced individuals face the disproportionate brunt of the seasonal vulnerabilities, such as crop failures and weather catastrophes.

The kind of welfare provisions put in place by the state has had a direct influence on policies of tribal development (Padhi & Panigrahi, 2016). The special packages for Kalahandi, Balangir, and Koraput (KBK) region, or the formation of the Western Odisha Development Council, are developmentally considered as politicized moves. Padhi and Panigrahi (2016) argue that such moves stray further from addressing structural issues—such as land-man-resource relations—and even end up being ignored later. Moreover, international funding in development channels has enabled the state to move away from providing welfare entitlements for tribals. This shift is also linked to fiscal adjustment, where public expenditure, particularly for health, was reduced during the mid-2000s (Sen & Rout, 2016).

3.3.5 Poverty and Food Insecurity

Odisha's poverty indicators have improved in the last two decades, but the persistence of vulnerability is significantly high. The head-count ratio (HCR) of poverty is higher in Odisha compared to India. In 2009–10, half of the rural population was still poor (Misra, 2016). As per the 2011–12 data, 32.6% of the state's population falls below the poverty line (Tendulkar measure) compared to the national average of 21.9% (Sahoo & Senapati, 2022). The proportion (HCR), depth (gap), and severity (squared gap) of poverty are higher in rural areas than in urban areas. The rural-urban differences are so high that the HCR is double for rural areas (35.64%) compared to urban areas (17.28%) (ibid.).

Poverty is particularly high for STs and SCs across all kinds of measures, and the incidence of poverty is almost twice for these groups compared to others. Regional variations in poverty are also high, with the southern region being the poorest, followed by the northern region. The coastal region has improved in poverty indicators and is now almost one-third less poor than the other two. The KBK region is still under abject poverty, which remains a cause for concern.

As per the multidimensional poverty index (MPI) prepared by the NITI Aayog, the proportion of multidimensional poor in Odisha reduced from 29.34% to 15.68% between 2015–16 and 2019–21 (GoI, 2023). It is among the five best-performing states that witnessed the steepest decline in poverty estimates. There are 16 districts with higher than the state-level estimate of poverty, and 14 below the state-level poverty estimates; most of the latter are tribal-dominated regions as well. More than 30% of the population in the Malkangiri, Nabarangpur, Rayagada, Koraput, and Mayurbhanj districts is multidimensional poor. The improvement along the specific indicators of health and education has not been impressive. However, the overall MPI has improved because of positive developments in sanitation, drinking water, housing, electricity, and banking.

Almost one-fifth of the population in both rural and urban Odisha is not able to meet their daily calorie needs as per the 2009–10 data. The OMS results show that one in four households in Odisha experiences food insecurity (see Chapter 5 for details). M. Panda (2016) highlights compositional problems in food intake. Notwithstanding the relatively higher per capita calorie consumption compared to the national average, the per capita fat and protein consumption is much lower. Moreover, Patnaik (2016) argues that the decline in per capita calorie consumption between 1993–94 and 2009–10 was due to a decline in Odisha's per capita food grain output. He hints at the changing pattern of land use and low agricultural productivity as the causes of low per capita output.

The impact of droughts on crop production leads to reduced household food consumption, and imbalances in diet (especially milk, fruits, and vegetables), which disproportionately affect the poor, women, and children. Sahu (2018) reported drought-led reduction in food intake among women: 71% in tribal areas and 59% in non-tribal areas.

Welfare schemes such as the PDS have been helpful in countering food insecurity and addressing poverty by increasing real income (Sahoo & Nayak, 2023). The Odisha government has partnered with the World Food Programme (WFP) to address food insecurity and launched six projects in 2021. The broad range of initiatives under this collaboration includes the transformation of the PDS and paddy procurement, grain ATM and smart mobile storage units, evidence-based interventions, partnering with the Odisha Millet Mission, and collaboration with the state's women's empowerment program, Mission Shakti.

4 Migration in Odisha

Development in Odisha is characterized by a key paradox: an improving economic profile with high growth rates, coexisting with the persistent and widespread poverty and unemployment. The expansion of industry has been accompanied by agrarian distress, dispossession, and vulnerability of the rural poor. With a lack of employment opportunities in the non-farm sector, the state has witnessed jobless growth. In this context, migration has become an essential channel for a substantial number of rural households.

Given the heterogeneity within migration, we use several parameters to distinguish between its types: (i) temporally, there is seasonal, circular, and permanent migration; (ii) regionally, there is intra-state, inter-state, rural-rural, rural-urban, and international migration; (iii) on the freedom front, there is voluntary and involuntary migration; and (iv) socio-economically, there is distress- and opportunity-driven migration. In eastern India, seasonal distress migration has been a known phenomenon for decades, wherein choosing to work in informal set-ups in destination regions is a practical decision rather than a strategic one for migrant workers (Rogaly et al., 2002). Deshingkar and Akter (2009) call for a shared understanding of distress migration among various agencies involved in research and action on migration.

The livelihood crisis, persisting because of agrarian distress and displacement, has led to substantial outmigration from Odisha. The forms of migration range from permanent to circular, with the most dominant one being seasonal migration. Seasonal migration is a strategy adopted by households to complement their incomes when agriculture and other non-farm employment do not suffice. Rural households are increasingly becoming 'migrarian', implying that the majority of work and incomes come from migration (remittances) and agriculture (Ali & Sharma, 2014). Remittances have become a significant component of household incomes, and Odisha's domestic remittance dependency has risen sharply, especially after the 1990s (Tumbe, 2011).

With large-scale migration, more and more intermediaries are being involved in its facilitation, making it an important feature of the local economy. The *Dadan* system of migration has prevailed in Odisha for a long time, wherein a labor contractor gives advances of money to the worker, against which the latter must migrate to other parts of the country for wage work (Acharya, 2021). Such contractors are commonly called 'Sardar' or 'Khatadar'. Initially, monthly payments are promised against piece-rated contracts, but once the worker is under the contractor's control in the destination state, the terms and conditions of the contract can change significantly. In the western districts of Nuapada, Kalahandi, and Balangir, these advances are usually paid in October-November during the *Nuakhai* festival to a family unit called *pathuria* (Mishra, 2016).

In the following subsections, we discuss the magnitude, patterns, and streams of migration, household vulnerabilities and sectional deprivation, women's migration, climate-induced migration, and unsafe migration.

4.1 Magnitude of Migration

The secondary data sources on migration—such as the Census—have limitations, as they cannot adequately capture temporary or seasonal migration, which is the most dominant pattern, especially among poor households. The definition of a short-term migrant worker in the EUS, as well as PLFS, limits the estimation of the actual magnitude of migrants (Deshingkar & Akter, 2009; Deshingkar & Farrington, 2009; Nayyar & Kim, 2018). These surveys rely solely on the place of birth or residence without incorporating any variable related to the multiple spatialities. Due to the lack of focus on worker mobility and employment, the scope of such surveys remains limited and fails to capture the actual processes of migration.

Setting aside these limitations, NSS data shows that in 2007–08, the rate of migration in Odisha was 302 per 1,000 persons, higher than the all-India average of 285 (GoI, 2010). NSS data also depicts the gendered nature of migration; while a majority of males from Odisha migrated for employment-related reasons and education (58.9%), a majority of females migrated for marriage (89.9%) (ibid). However, feminist scholars have highlighted that macro surveys such as the NSS record only one reason for migration, thus camouflaging—and invisibilizing—female migration for work among marriage migrants (Mazumdar et al., 2013). Based on the NSS data, it is estimated that there are 4.17 lakh short-term migrants from rural Odisha, of which 82% are men (Ali & Sharma, 2014).

Given the conceptual and methodological drawbacks of official statistics, surveys such as the India Human Development Survey (IHDS) provide more reliable estimates of migration. The IHDS in 2011, for Odisha, showed that 15.2% of households had one or more non-resident members (Srivastava, 2020a). According to the survey, the incidence of migration is also high, almost 10 times more than NSS estimates (Nayyar & Kim, 2018). In the OMS, the percentage of households with current migrants is 17.5 (see Chapter 3 for details), closer to the IHDS estimate.

On the other hand, the data from Odisha's labor department presents a gross underestimate of a mere 1.46 lakh people migrating for labor in 2015 (Srivastava, 2020a). The number refers to the workers migrating and registered under the Inter-State Migrant Workmen (ISMW) Act, which implies that they migrated with licensed contractors. However, the majority of migratory movements are autonomous or with unlicensed contractors.

As per a study conducted by Aajeevika Bureau in coastal (Nayagarh, Khordha, and Puri) and western (Kalahandi, Nuapada, and Balangir) districts of Odisha, covering almost one lakh migrant households, nearly 30% of the households had one or more migrant workers (Ali & Sharma, 2014). When extrapolated to population levels, this figure corresponds to 1.53 million migrant households from these two regions (ibid.). The OMS, conducted in all 30 districts of the state, estimates 2.9 million households with current migrants in 2023 (see Chapter 3 for details).

4.2 Patterns and Streams of Out-Migration

Historically, the Odisha region witnessed famine-led distress migration from the coastal areas to various plantation sites and tea gardens. Workers were also taken by the British colonial government as indentured laborers to tropical colonies (Bhowmik, 1981). Many Odia migrants have been living in the tea plantations of Assam to date. Large-scale migration to jute mills in Kolkata has also been noted; the closure of the mills in the 1970s shifted the trajectory of migration streams to Surat, where textile industries were expanding. Since the 1990s, a new migration corridor to Kerala has also emerged (Nag et al., 2023).

As discussed in Chapter 3 of this book, the main migration corridors from Odisha include Ganjam–Gujarat, Bhadrak–Karnataka, and Balangir–Andhra Pradesh. Nag et al. (2023) argue that caste dynamics in the source region are reproduced at the destination in the prominent Ganjam–Surat migration corridor. They find that just as in the village, dominant castes ill-treat lower-caste workers in Surat, which has led to the latter shunning Surat and instead moving to the southern states of Tamil Nadu and Kerala to escape caste-based harassment (ibid.).

The contemporary patterns and streams of migration follow distinct regional pathways. The southern region of Odisha appears to have the highest incidence of migration, followed by the western and coastal regions (Ali & Sharma, 2014). However, most studies have focused more on the coastal and western regions. More than half of the migrants from the western region comprise Dalits and Adivasis (ibid.). In the coastal region, OBCs comprise a majority of the migrating population.

Construction work in Chhattisgarh (Raipur and Durg), Gujarat (Rajkot), Goa, and peri-urban parts of metropolitan cities such as Mumbai, Delhi, Chennai, and Bengaluru draws the largest share of migrant workers from western Odisha. This is followed by brick kilns in Uttar Pradesh, Chhattisgarh, Andhra Pradesh, and Tamil Nadu (Ali & Sharma, 2014; Mishra, 2016). The migration to brick kilns exhibits a seasonal pattern—typically from November-December to June—pausing in the monsoon when the kilns are shut. Apart from this, informal work in the agriculture and transport sectors also employs migrants. Workers from the Mali caste have recently started migrating to horticultural farms in Chhattisgarh (Mishra, 2016). Beyond these, migrants are also working at several establishments informally, such as hotels, restaurants, security services, etc., in parts of south India. The prominent intra-state migration trajectory from the western region leads to brick kilns in cities (Cuttack, Bhubaneshwar, and Puri). This is followed by piece-rate agricultural work (paddy transplanting and harvesting) in Sambalpur and Bargarh, informal work in the mining and construction sectors in nearby regions (Bargarh, Sonepur, and Balangir), and stone crushing in Nuapada.

Nuapada from the western part of the state shows high migration estimates largely due to family migration to brick kilns. Field-based studies find that migration profiles from Kalahandi and Balangir comprise single males, largely working in the construction sector (Ali & Sharma, 2014).

In a survey of more than 31,000 people from Nuapada and Balangir, more than 19,000 reported being migrants (NLUO, 2020). Among the more than 7600 households interviewed, each had at least one member migrating for work. Of these, 24% were children. Major destinations were brick kilns and construction sites in states such as Andhra Pradesh, Chhattisgarh, Gujarat, and Maharashtra. Almost 90% of workers migrating from western Odisha choose inter-state migration compared to two-thirds in coastal Odisha (Ali & Sharma, 2014).

For coastal Odisha, major inter-state occupational trajectories lead to construction work in Kerala and Gujarat, followed by spinning mills and power looms in Surat, carpet weaving in eastern Uttar Pradesh, and head-loading work in warehouses of Jammu and Kashmir (Ali & Sharma, 2014; Vidyarthi, 2014). Tamil Nadu, Maharashtra, and Andhra Pradesh are other popular destinations for migrants. The intra-state destinations for the coastal region are Bhubaneshwar, Cuttack, and Puri—for work in the construction and transportation sector (NLUO, 2020). Minor streams of workers also work in the factories of the Sundargarh and Angul districts. Among coastal districts, Kendrapara and Khordha show a high incidence of migration largely due to their disaster-prone habitat (Ali & Sharma, 2014). The region sends a large number of skilled construction workers, especially plumbers and masons.

4.3 Vulnerabilities, Entitlements, and Livelihoods

Though migration may raise wages and incomes, it generally lacks job security and social protection. Losing out on government entitlements (especially PDS, education, and healthcare) and even basic amenities creates difficulties for most migrants in the destination sites. Socio-cultural challenges faced at the destination states—linguistic and cultural exclusion and alienation—further add to their stress. Injured workers have to return to their homes, often without any compensation.

While declining profitability in agriculture pushes rural households to seek other livelihoods (Gram Vikas & CMID, 2024), seasonal migration has been transforming the agrarian structure in the villages, allowing poorer households to move away from long-term work at the farms of the upper castes/classes and also reducing their dependency on exploitative moneylenders (Mishra, 2016). This is particularly due to the changing nature of the informal credit market, where contractors play a key role. Despite these silver linings, migrant workers often remain vulnerable, and there is little evidence of long-term social or economic mobility. Therefore, the argument that distress-based seasonal migration is a poverty-reducing strategy requires more deliberation and serious reconsideration, as it appears to be more of a coping and survival strategy (Meher, 2019). It may allow migrants to move away from one form of exploitation, but they often end up tied under another form of labor circulation arrangement without economic mobility, leading to what Breman (2019) calls 'neo-bondage'. Households engaged in low-productivity activities are specifically found to be sending out migrants (Mitra & Pradhan, 2016).

Credit and indebtedness are one of the primary drivers of distress-led migration, which often turns into a bondage-like situation. Advances are paid to workers by contractors, or loans are borrowed by workers, for reasons such as health concerns or marriage, which lead them into a debt trap with usurious interest rates. They have only the labor power to repay these debts and thus end up in neo-bondage-like conditions under the guise of seasonal migratory work (Vidyarthi, 2014).

Some of the other drivers of migration are destitution and social discrimination. Sengupta and Vijay (2015), in a detailed study on migration from Balangir to Telangana brick kilns, observed that high inequality of assets and incomes contributed to the 'systematic reproduction of social asymmetries' (p. 82).

One key reason for the high proportion of the migrant population in the informal sector and low-paying jobs is the persistence of illiteracy and lower levels of education. A survey of more than 45,000 migrant workers in coastal and western Odisha found 40% to be illiterate (Ali & Sharma, 2014). The survey also found that more than 50% of migrants from coastal regions had studied up to higher secondary level compared to only 26% from the western region (ibid.). As a result, incomes from migration tend to be higher among households in coastal Odisha compared to their western counterparts (Ali & Sharma, 2014), as the latter's limited skills often confine them to low-paying hard labor jobs.

Remittances constitute a significant share of the household consumption expenditure in the source region. Studies indicate that for poorer migrant households, remittances comprise almost half of the household incomes (Mitra & Pradhan, 2016). Migration and earning remittances, therefore, act as a risk-diversification strategy (Dandekar & Ghai, 2020). Given the highly seasonal nature of migration, earnings from remittances are also seasonal, particularly high in the *rabi* season. Mitra and Pradhan (2016) find that remittances of higher amounts are found more frequently in the transactions of educated and literate people. Households receiving remittances that amount to about half of their income primarily use them for consumption and health, while those receiving smaller remittances spend them mainly on health. Relatively better-off households benefit from remittances for overall well-being rather than daily survival (ibid.).

4.4 Gender, Age, and Family Concerns in Migration

Most discussions on migration in India center on male migration, with women seen as dependent followers. The singular focus on associational female migration underplays migrant women's work and employment. There has been limited research examining migration from a gender lens. Migration can play a key role in enhancing women's agency through new opportunities and by distancing them from patriarchal relations prevalent in the source region. However, the patriarchal elements might be embedded within the migration process, and therefore, this issue requires careful attention. The secondary data (with all its limitations) show that women's migration in Odisha is largely marriage-related. Work- and employment-related migration in Odisha seems largely male, with women taking care of the family at home.

Mazumdar et al. (2013) present a critical review of migration and gender in India and argue that it must not be seen from a mere labor and labor law perspective with capitalism, but also in terms of agrarian, caste, and patriarchy-based social relations embedded in migration-based wage work in industrial and service sectors. This is essential to connect the 'concepts, entitlement regimes, and empirical realities' (Mazumdar et al., 2013, p. 62). A concerted effort to study *specific* female migration streams from Odisha—of women live-in domestic workers in Mumbai and garment workers in Kerala (Mazumdar, 2024a, 2024b)—shows the intricate rural-urban nexus and the circularity of migration from deprived households in the source regions.

The contextual scenarios differ greatly based on the nature of female migration. During family migration, women are doubly burdened with productive (employment at destination sites) as well as reproductive (care in the household) activities. In cases of family migration, there is a 'care crisis' for those left behind, especially the elderly (Bhatt, 2009).

In cases of single women migrating, the possibility of exploitation is higher. Similarly, single-woman-headed households face more difficulties. In either case, gender disparity is generally high, particularly in the nature of assigned work and the scale of wages (Sansriti, 2007). The occupational roles are also stereotyped, indicating less diversification of female migrant occupations (Mazumdar et al., 2013).

When the workers migrate, especially through contractors to do precarious jobs, the families left behind—including the elderly—also face vulnerability. Sansriti (2007), in a study in Balangir and Nuapada, found that female-headed households at the source had to struggle for food, clothing, health, and educational expenses. In the OMS, too, female-headed households have poorer social and economic outcomes. Apart from these economic effects of migration on women, there are social (especially health-wise) as well as psychological consequences—some linked to violence and abuse of various kinds by employers, contractors, locals, and even within the household (ibid.).

In the coastal districts, the incidence of women migrating is found to be low, while in the western and KBK regions, the incidence of family migration is relatively higher (Ali & Sharma, 2014).

Fact-finding missions by civil society organizations (CSOs) and media reports have reported a huge number of women migrating to cities (Delhi, Mumbai, and Bengaluru) for domestic work. Since domestic work is not regularized and work via mediating agents/agencies is unprotected, the scope for acquiring decent work via this channel remains limited. Women provide cheap labor, and experience similar pressures of debt traps, health shocks, etc., making them vulnerable to unsafe migration and sexual exploitation.

Despite high mobility among the younger population, studies with a focus on youth migration are few. The average age of a migrant from coastal and western Odisha is 30 years, with over 90% migrants being younger than 46 (Ali & Sharma, 2014). The age range is the widest in western districts, with children below the age of 13 years comprising 10% of the migrant population, adolescents (14–18) 4%, and a considerable proportion above 46, pointing to longer migration cycles in this region. A recent study by NLUO (2020) in Nuapada and Balangir found that one-third of the migrant population was between 19 and 35 years of age; the group constituted half of the adult population. They noted that youth migrated due to limited local opportunities and declining interest in traditional work. OMS data further shows that the average age of migration has fallen, with people migrating at a younger age than before (see Chapter 3).

4.5 Climate-Induced Migration

As Odisha is significantly prone to natural disasters, climate- and weather-related events affect the livelihoods of people, especially in coastal areas. In terms of natural calamities, there have been only eight normal years without any occurrence of a natural calamity in the past 70 years. The first few decades since 1950 witnessed consistent floods and droughts, with some instances of cyclones. The past two decades also show similar trajectories but with higher instances of cyclonic storms (GoO, 2020). The regional terrain is such that the southern and western regions are prone to droughts, whereas coastal districts are affected by floods, winds, and cyclones. Changing climatic conditions, along with small size of the landholdings and exclusive dependence on natural water sources for irrigation adversely affect agriculture (Gram Vikas & CMID, 2024). Due to the disasters, the rural poor become more vulnerable and migrate for employment opportunities. Among the factors contributing to climate-led vulnerability, the highest risks are associated with health and agriculture. Migration hotspots and corridors are, therefore, also reinforced through climate-led events. It is usually climate variability, not climate change, which drives migration, largely due to either frequent extreme events or variance in climatic parameters (Panda, 2017).

In coastal areas, floods and cyclones can lead to salinization of agricultural fields, affecting paddy production. They cause damage to the nets and boats of fishermen and loss of livestock for marginal farmers. Studies have shown that the situation of poor women in coastal Odisha is particularly vulnerable, especially in the flood-prone districts of Ganjam, Jajpur, Kendrapara, and Jagatsinghpur (Patel & Giri, 2019). Primary studies indicate that such environmental factors force entire families to move to other destinations within Odisha, often permanently, for construction work, as opposed to inter-state migration, which is usually found to be single-male specific (ibid).

The western region witnesses drought-induced migration in the context of harvest losses (or very low yields). The environmental stress, as well as the lack of coping strategies for livelihoods locally, then becomes the key driver of migration (Jülich, 2011). Decreasing asset base and indebtedness are also found to be key drivers of temporary migration, which then becomes an adaptive response of the households to the climate event.

Using a historical narrative approach to study the impact of climate variability on migration in western Odisha (Nuapada and Balangir), Panda (2017) focuses on the mega-droughts of 1965 and 1974, which were a big blow to rural livelihoods and led people to sell or mortgage their assets for survival, entering cycles of indebtedness. He marks this as the first threshold of poverty. The second threshold was when the indebted households became more vulnerable due to droughts in the 1980s and 1990s, especially in 1985, 1996, and 1998. During this period, migration to Andhra Pradesh and other areas increased significantly. It turned into a pattern after the 2002 drought, which led to remittances becoming a major source of household income for the rural poor. However, low-paid work does not allow them to get out of the vicious cycle of poverty. Studies like this make an important contribution to mapping the impact of slow-onset disasters (such as droughts) on migration.

4.6 Unsafe Migration: Trafficking, Bondage, Unfreedom

The prevalence of bondage and trafficking in migration networks is significantly high. In 2021, as per official statistics, the highest number of human trafficking victims were from Odisha, with more than 80% trafficked for labor.[5] The official statistics tend to underreport, and therefore, the media and CSOs' reportage is richer and more reliable on this subject. Exploitation and unfreedoms of various kinds persist highly in brick kilns, where a big chunk of Odisha's migrants work.[6] After brick kilns, carpet factories in Uttar Pradesh, textile mills in Surat, and seafood companies are also primary destinations for trafficking.

Contractors are the key exploiters in this scenario, often acting as traffickers as well. Paying advances to migrants acts as a mechanism to control, as in the *Dadan* system. The prevalence of such labor contractors is intertwined with (trafficking) mafia groups that can maintain control over labor through coercion, especially because of the government's poorly endowed labor protection system (Raj & Axelby, 2019; Vidyarthi, 2014). The sub-contracting process allows recruitment of workers by labor contractors in the source states (Odisha) based on employers' demand in various parts of India. Such recruitment by unlicensed contractors is illegal. Often, the contractors further delegate the recruitment process to local petty contractors, thus increasing the distance between the worker and the principal employer and reducing the scope of accountability for the latter.

Dadan migrants suffer various kinds of injuries and disabilities at work, both due to accidents as well as physical violence and abuse. These incidents are reported in the media once in a while, but there's a dearth of systematic research. Acharya (2021)

---

[5] See: Highest number of human trafficking victims in 2021 from Odisha: NCRB, *The Print* (https://theprint.in/india/highest-number-of-human-trafficking-victims-in-2021-from-odisha-ncrb/1108228/).

[6] See: Why lakhs of people leave Odisha to work in distant, unsafe brick-kilns, *Scroll.in* (https://scroll.in/article/747416/why-lakhs-of-people-leave-odisha-to-work-in-distant-unsafe-brick-kilns)s

recently focused on the problems of *Dadan* migrants specifically and identified a few features of the migration process, such as: the preference for young migrants by contractors, wage contracts fixed by the contractor and not employers, employment on a temporary basis, and long working hours with low wages. The debt burden and lack of information about the work push migrants to remain in undesirable jobs where delays in payments, threats, and incidents of violence are very common. A majority of the workers who participated in Acharya's (2021) study reported having faced incidents such as slapping, kicking, pushing, pinching, being beaten up, and having an object thrown at them. Fewer but more dangerous incidents—threatening with a gun or knife, locking in a room, and sexual abuse—were also reported. The aggressors usually either worked as supervisors or contractors, rather than as the principal employer. Local people also acted as aggressors at times. Physical abuse and aggression acted as a deterrent for workers to resist/assert their concerns, leading to injuries and even disabilities. Language barriers also became a major hindrance to bargaining or negotiation of any kind (ibid.).

In a detailed study by the Tata Institute of Social Sciences (TISS, 2019), the various types of migration-trafficking processes in Odisha have been classified. The profile of the victims, the modus operandi of the traffickers, and even the economics behind the trafficking differ hugely for different forms such as labor, child bride, sex work, domestic work, organs, illegal adoption, and missing persons. The different modus operandi usually involve advance payments for labor trafficking, acquaintances convincing parents in cases of child trafficking, and the targeting of indebted poor households with young women for bride and sex trafficking, with established networks of intermediaries ensuring their transit across regions.

One of the biggest concerns for young girls and single women migrating, usually for domestic work, is exploitation—especially sexual violence. The Home Department data claims that around 3578 women (mostly minor and young girls) were missing or remained untraced between 2000 and 2005 (Daniel, 2014). Most of them belonged to Sundargarh, and it is feared that they were trafficked for domestic work or forced into the sex work industry.

In a study conducted in six villages across Nuapada, Kalahandi, and Balangir districts, Mishra (2016) collates several elements of unfreedom enforced, including lack of freedom to leave, and violence, among others. The extra-economic exploitation and the precarious nature of work are further compounded by hazardous working conditions, often devoid of protective gear and other safety measures. The illegal recruitment through unlicensed contractors allows employers to not cover any accidental damages. Ethnographic case studies of the workers fighting cases of bondage, trafficking, permanent disability, or even death identify the inefficacy of several labor laws (Factories Act, Wages Act, Contract Labor Act, ISMW Act, and Employees' Compensation Act), which will not be applicable in these scenarios (Vidyarthi, 2014).

Several CSOs in Odisha have consistently made efforts to bring these issues to the forefront, rescue and rehabilitate the survivors, and fight legally for justice (ibid). They provide a range of services, including building a thorough documentation process (database) to track migrant workers (and unlicensed contractors), ensuring delivery of government entitlements to workers, informally mediating between workers and contractors, organizing training and capacity-building for workers, and providing special attention to the issues of women and children (especially violence).

5 Legal and Policy Framework Addressing Migration

5.1 Legal Framework

Odisha was the first state to implement an act to protect the interests of migrant workers through the Orissa Dadan Labour (Control and Regulation) Act (ORLA), 1975. However, since the enactment of the ISMW Act, 1979, the former was repealed due to redundancy. The efficacy of the ISMW Act, however, has remained negligible in the country—and Odisha—due to the poor enforcement capacity of the government, compliance costs (for employers and contractors), and limitations of domicile restrictions (Daniel, 2014; Krishnan et al., 2020; Srivastava, 2020b).

In 2020, India underwent codification of labor laws, and the ISMW Act is now subsumed under the Occupational Safety, Health and Working Conditions Code, 2020 (OSH Code). It was expected that the central-level labor law reforms would now broaden the scope for inclusion of migrant workers. However, the Code has limited the applicability of the ISMW Act provisions to establishments employing 10 or more migrant workers. Only about 1.6% of establishments employ 10 or more workers, and the number of those employing 10 or more *migrant* (inter-state) workers would be even smaller, which defeats the purpose of the legislation (Munjal & Bamba, 2024). In addition, tools of accountability have been removed by the Code (such as maintenance of a passbook); the burden of accountability has been shifted from contractor to employer completely. The inspection mechanism has been diluted, with the inspector expected to play the role of a facilitator (ibid.). All these changes further reduce the scope of regulating work for migrant workers, thus pushing them (and the economy) toward informalization and precariousness.

Advance payment mechanisms by contractors—like Dadan—are not recognized by regulating authorities as a violation of any law and thus, do not prompt the state's intervention (Sengupta & Vijay, 2015).

The legal framework to prevent and protect the interests of migrant workers in the informal sector is also very limited. The Building and Other Construction Workers (Regulation of Employment and Conditions of Service) Act (BoCW Act) taxes the construction industry to collect funds for the welfare of construction workers. But it is truly effective only when registration by/of workers is properly completed, which is not the case in many regions. Srivastava (2012) argues that the Act does not consider locational or inter-sectoral mobility, thus imagining workers as immobile. Overall, the legal framework for labor is such that the conditions of migrant workers will be subject to the efficacy of relevant legislation in their destination states.

Anti-human trafficking units (AHTUs) are present in every state, but their functioning seems ineffective in controlling the large-scale, unsafe migration and trafficking phenomena in Odisha (TISS, 2019). The Railway Police Force (RPF) also has a key role to play in curbing trafficking during transit, but the traffickers have devised several ways to escape them.

5.2 Initiatives

The measures in place fall short of addressing broadly two types of problems in the source state: (i) illegal and exploitative recruitment and (ii) structural issues that lead to distress migration. To address these, the whole-of-government approach is required, implying inter-departmental as well as inter-regional coordination. One such initiative was a tripartite MoU between the labor departments of India, Odisha, and Andhra Pradesh to safeguard the interests of Odia migrants in the brick kilns of Andhra Pradesh (Daniel, 2014). This was achieved through ensuring their access to government entitlements (education and health insurance), food (PDS), and housing. However, it was a one-of-a-kind initiative that has neither been replicated nor scaled up.

Another initiative aimed at tapping the high number of migrants with a plumbing profile from Kendrapara prompted the state government to set up the State Institute of Plumbing Technology (SIPT) to facilitate upgrading of skills and offer improved employment prospects.

Seasonal hostels have also been set up for the children of seasonal migrant workers, starting in Nuapada, Balangir, and Bargarh districts and coming up in other places as well.

An action plan was prepared by the Department of Panchayati Raj, Odisha, in 2014 to address the migrant workers' concerns in 11 migration-prone districts. It requires convergence across several departments and involves: (i) a plan for periodic survey of migrants, (ii) voluntary registration, (iii) helpline to provide rescue support, (iv) signing of MoUs with departments of other states to create contact points to reach migrants, and (v) strengthening seasonal hostels for children of migrants (Srivastava, 2020a).

5.3 Schemes

The MGNREGA, as a progressive demand-driven public employment program that provides the *right to work,* has the potential to control distress migration and enhance retention in rural areas through local employment. Several primary studies across the districts of Mayurbhanj, Jajpur, Balangir, Kalahandi, and Nuapada have strongly indicated this (Nayak et al., 2023; Parida, 2016). In 2021, the Department of Panchayati Raj even extended the MGNREGA work days from 100 to 150. However, systemic failures, implementation hurdles, and in particular, pressures to digitize through the Aadhaar-Based Payment System (ABPS) have led to a decline in MGNREGA employment in Odisha, from 18.28 crore person days in 2023–24 to 11.92 crore person days in 2024–25 (LibTech India, 2025). Thus, despite strong grassroots demand and need for rural public employment, structural challenges seriously impede the functioning of the MGNREGA *(ibid).* The results of the Odisha Migration Study also show that sample households with the MGNREGA card in the rural areas had worked only for an average of 37 days in the past year.

5.4 Local Governance

In a survey of Panchayati Raj Institution (PRI) representatives on the issues of migration in Nuapada and Balangir, NLUO (2020) found that, at times, the contractors approach the sarpanches to facilitate the recruitment of migrants, against which service charges are paid. Most sarpanches were not aware of labor laws such as the ISMW, Contract Labor, BoCW, Child Labor, SC/ST Atrocities, and Trafficking Acts.

5.5 Civil Society Organizations

CSOs act as an important bridge between the government's effort to address migrant workers' concerns and the difficulties faced by migrants in reality. Over several years, to address and resolve issues, many CSOs have devised several points of intervention, such as:

> Village level registration and tracking, awareness on safe and protected migration, education of migrant children at source and destination, mobilization of migrants to access MGNREGA, social security, alternative livelihoods, imparting skill development to migrant youth, advocating for the rights of migrant laborers, remittance management, conducting rescue and facilitating rehabilitation of migrant bonded laborers. (Daniel, 2014, p. 113)

5.6 COVID-19, Reverse Migration, and the State's Response

Odisha's response to the COVID-19 lockdown-led reverse migration is known for having been one of the most supportive approaches by a state government at the time. The state had two immediate tasks at hand: (i) preventing the spread of the pandemic and (ii) handling reverse migration (logistically and economically).

Using its recently revamped disaster management experience, the Odisha government decentralized the response to the pandemic by involving frontline workers and local governance institutions (Sahoo & Kar, 2021). Several steps were undertaken on the health front, such as revamping health infrastructure, setting up COVID-19 hospitals to increase bed capacity, setting up intensive care units (ICUs) using the public-private partnership (PPP) model, and dedicating decentralized bureaucratic teams to ensure smooth coordination between district and village governance institutions (Behera et al., 2021; Pedi & Adabar, 2020). Mobilization of women's groups, especially via Accredited Social Health Activists (ASHAs) and self-help groups (SHGs), further contributed significantly (Sahoo & Kar, 2021).

In a large-scale reverse migration, almost six lakh migrants had returned to the state by the end of June 2020, when the lockdown was first eased. Reasons for reverse migration were loss of livelihoods, food insecurity, lack of access to general services, and fear of the virus spreading, among others. Labor supply in rural Odisha expanded significantly at the time. The returnees via Shramik special trains were more than two lakh people, the majority of whom were returning to the Ganjam, Baleshwar, Bhadrak, Khordha, Mayurbhanj, Cuttack, and Kendrapara districts. Their return journeys started mainly in Tamil Nadu, West Bengal, Telangana, Andhra Pradesh, Maharashtra, Karnataka, and Gujarat, among other states (Behera et al., 2021). Primary studies indicate a huge dip in the incomes of migrant workers across different occupational roles. For some of them, a total loss of employment and income was reported. This is corroborated by the OMS findings detailed in Chapter 3.

Logistical measures for returnee migrants included temporary shelter and food, a systematic way of ensuring the return journeys via registration, and paying incentives for quarantining (Rs 2000 per person). Some welfare measures were also announced to ensure livelihood opportunities for returnee migrants. Further, direct cash transfers to 22 lakh registered construction workers were announced for assistance (Meher & Nanda, 2020).

Later on, several waves of the pandemic and the larger-scale reverse migration affected the health system and made the cracks in it visible, impacting the lives of people in a detrimental way. Despite this, Odisha has paved the way for exemplary leadership, showcasing political will to support its migrant workers and frontline workers.

6 Migration, Livelihoods, and Gender: An Analytical Framework

Migration, rural livelihoods, and gender are concepts—and analytical categories—that underpin the themes and sub-themes discussed throughout this volume. An overview of how these three interact, overlap, and co-constitute each other provides a critical entry point into the analyses laid out in upcoming chapters, as well as the broader socio-economic landscapes and migration patterns within the state. In this section, we elaborate on the conceptual framework that enables us to examine how Odisha's development trajectory (discussed in the previous section), systemic agrarian distress, household strategies, and the unpaid, underrecognized, and undervalued labor of women intersect to shape migration pathways. It is also important to keep in view that embedded within the backdrop of migration-related decisions are intersectional experiences constructed through the structures of gender, caste, tribe, ethnicity, religion, and geographical disparity.

6.1 Migration and Livelihoods

Migration can be understood through the sustainable livelihood approach, which offers a nuanced explanation for livelihood diversification decisions.

> A livelihood comprises the capabilities, assets (stores, resources, claims and access) and activities required for a means of living: a living is sustainable which can cope with and recover from stress and shocks, maintain or enhance its capabilities and assets, and provide sustainable livelihood opportunities for the next generation; and which contributes net benefits to other livelihoods at the local and global levels and in the short and long term. (Chambers & Conway, 1991, p. 6).

Emerging from the capability, equity, and sustainability approaches (Chambers & Conway, 1991) and grounded in Sen's (1985) capability framework, the idea of sustainable livelihood centers on an individual, with a focus on their tangible and intangible resources. However, the capacities of individuals and households—especially with marginal landholdings—are increasingly constrained due to the pressures of ongoing deagrarianization (Datta, 2016; Jodhka, 2023). In Odisha, land continues to be the fulcrum of rural life and livelihoods, even more so in the absence of structurally transformative industrialization. With the predominance of subsistence agriculture, access to land is crucial to households' livelihoods and food security. The withdrawal of the state support for agriculture, coupled with climate and environmental changes, creates a scarcity of livelihood options, making households unable to meet their basic needs for survival (Bhandari & Grant, 2007; Hietala & Singh, 2014) and opt for livelihood diversification and a multi-locational livelihood strategy.

In the livelihoods framework, migration—and remittances—are seen as part of a diversified livelihood portfolio (Ellis, 2000). Conceptually, livelihood diversification is framed in terms of *distress* versus *opportunity*, *necessity* versus *choice*, but empirical reality does not fit into neat binaries, and can be more complex (Pritchard et al., 2013). In a similar vein, Deshingkar and Farrington (2009) contend that migration can be seen as *coping migration* or *accumulative migration.* In the former, migration is a mechanism through which households smooth consumption and manage risk, while the latter allows for the accumulation of assets, savings, and investments (Deshingkar & Farrington, 2009). At the same time, under favorable circumstances, coping migration streams may become *accumulative* over time (*ibid.*).

In the context of our study, livelihood diversification is less a choice than a necessity for a large proportion of the population. As is discussed in detail further in this volume (see Chapter 8), out-migration in Odisha is more likely to be distress-oriented—a response to livelihood insecurity and chronic poverty. Poor households engage in seasonal migration to supplement their inadequate incomes from local agricultural and non-agricultural sources (Sharma et al., 2014).

6.2 Gender

It must be noted, however, that livelihood diversification strategies are frequently gender-specific (Hussein & Nelson, 1998), and labor migration—especially seasonal—tends to be largely male-dominated, as we have discussed so far. Migration changes household configurations and leads to restructuring of households in tangible and intangible ways, influencing responsibilities, identities, and intra-household dynamics (Nguyen & Locke, 2014; Rao, 2014; Singh & Basu, 2019). Migrant households—especially, in the case of male migration—are characterized by both spatial mobility and immobility (Spiegel, 1986), the latter typically experienced by women. Even when women migrate along with their families, their relationship to livelihood diversification and contribution is markedly different from that of men, and so is the extent of their spatial mobility within the new location.

Women, who stay behind or are 'left behind' in their rural settings, bear the dual burden of contributing to livelihood diversification (through agriculture, livestock, and other home-based or local economic activities) and household responsibilities, including care work. The narratives of research participants from Odisha (see Chapter 11) speak volumes about women's experiences with extreme poverty and deprivation at home, managing large families with limited resources, and insufficient finances. These circumstances often translate to arduous routines, compromised health, isolation, and emotional strain. Additionally, while women are expected to provide—often single-handedly—the labor required to sustain the household, their role in shaping migration decisions—such as who migrates, who stays behind, the duration of migration, and terms—tends to be limited. This limited agency is not merely reflective of patriarchal norms but is also shaped by the structural pressures of survival, which leave little scope for deliberation and choice.

The framework of feminization of responsibility makes a valuable contribution to our conceptual framing here. It describes the increasing expectations placed on women to shoulder economic and caregiving burdens within households, often internalizing these roles as obligatory (Chant, 2008). This process is intensified due to male outmigration and does not necessarily lead to a corresponding feminization of power. While some research has found, women are likely to gain in authority and decision-making power following male out-migration (Findley & Williams, 1991), Kumar (2023) argues that these changes are contextual, as women's status within the patriarchy remains unchanged. On the other hand, some studies have indicated limited gains (Prati et al., 2022; Roy & Nangia, 2005) in autonomy and decision-making, and an analysis based on the NFHS-3 survey data reported that there was *no improvement* (Sinha et al., 2012) in women's status in migrant households.

Migration may alter household structures, but the process of transformation of women's status can be fractured and often transitory. Their active contribution to the livelihood portfolio, in terms of productive activity as well as facilitative activities (for instance, navigating the local governance systems, accessing government schemes by completing tedious procedures), does not establish them as economic actors. In patriarchal societies, women are often not recognized as owners of land, which impairs their ability to access non-land agricultural inputs (Food and Agriculture Organization, 2011) and, in turn, erodes their capacity to secure the household's livelihood. The autonomy and decision-making powers they might gain are also often short-lived, subject to the interventions of the extended family (De Haas & Van Rooij, 2010; Kaur, 2018) and the return of the men who have migrated. This systemic undermining of a key economic actor inevitably shapes the socio-economic landscape of the region and compounds household precarity through a distinct gendered dimension.

Building on this understanding, we contend that migration trajectories in Odisha cannot be understood in isolation without a focus on the agrarian distress as well as the fragility of livelihood base in the state. It would be equally futile to separate them from the gendered dynamics of livelihood diversification and the indispensability of women's paid and unpaid labor. The feminization of responsibility is both a consequence of chronic poverty and a condition that makes migration and remittance economies possible. Therefore, with this framework, we offer a critical conceptual foundation that engages meaningfully with the structural and intersectional dimensions of rural precarity and migration as a coping strategy—through our three-pronged approach—in order to inform future development interventions and policy reforms in Odisha.

7 Methodology

The Odisha Migration Study was carried out in two phases. The first phase of the study, the Odisha Migration Survey (OMS), consisted of a quantitative survey conducted across all 30 districts of Odisha (Map 1). The survey's primary goal was to determine the overall extent of migration from Odisha, including detailed breakdowns of intra-state (within the state), inter-state, and international migration flows. Additionally, the survey delved into several aspects of social and economic development, including work and employment, access to government programs, housing and amenities, asset ownership, land use and cropping patterns, household food consumption and security, and women's autonomy and mobility. The second phase comprised four studies in the areas of livelihoods and income, gender and well-being, women's autonomy and mobility, and youth aspirations and attitudes toward agriculture.

7.1 Phase I

A stratified multistage random sampling was used for selecting sample households for the OMS, with the primary sample unit being the household. The total sample size was fixed at 15,000 households to achieve a reasonably accurate estimate of the migrant population. Nonetheless, the determination of this sample size took into account a range of factors, including the desired confidence level, acceptable

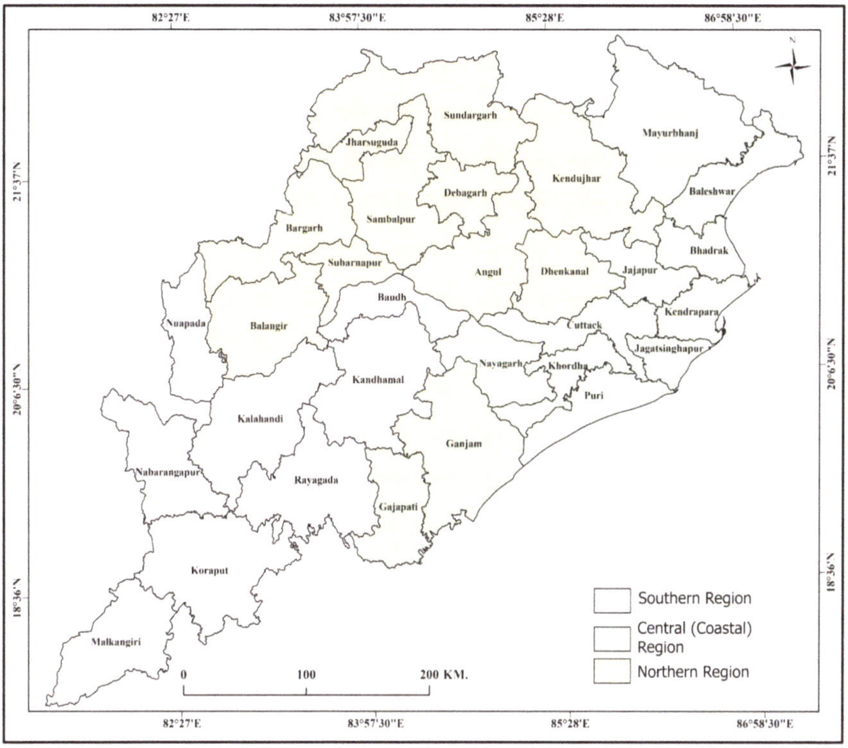

Map 1 The regions of Odisha

margin of error, the resources at hand (both in terms of finances and workforce), time limitations, and logistical complexities. Typically, a larger sample size tends to lead to more precise estimations and a reduction in sampling discrepancies. The resulting estimates also offer a higher degree of representativeness for the entire population, thereby enhancing the reliability of the findings. Striking a balance between the desired confidence level, margin of error, and practical considerations such as available resources and time was of utmost significance.

To achieve this, the distribution of sample households across districts was designed using a proportional allocation strategy. This entailed allocating sample households to both rural and urban strata within each district in accordance with the proportion of rural and urban households as documented in the 2011 Census. This approach ensured that the sample was representative of the overall demographic composition of each district, thereby enhancing the accuracy of the study's findings (Table 5).

Odisha consists of 30 districts, resulting in the establishment of 57 distinct strata, encompassing 30 rural and 27 urban sectors. For the selection of households within each segment, a precise and systematic approach was employed. Localities within each segment, known as gram panchayats (for rural areas) or municipal wards (for urban areas), were chosen using a proportional sampling methodology. Within these

Table 5 Households and sample localities by district, OMS 2023

District	Total households			Sample households			Sample localities		
	Total	Rural	Urban	Total	Rural	Urban	Total	Rural	Urban
Angul	297,050	249,733	47,317	450	390	60	15	13	2
Balangir	414,749	369,273	45,476	600	540	60	20	18	2
Baleshwar	533,001	477,434	55,567	840	750	90	28	25	3
Bargarh	370,308	336,130	34,178	570	510	60	19	17	2
Boudh	106,961	102,402	4559	240	240	0	8	8	0
Bhadrak	306,333	270,791	35,542	480	420	60	16	14	2
Cuttack	579,170	429,454	149,716	870	630	240	29	21	8
Debagarh	75,452	70,058	5394	240	240	0	8	8	0
Dhenkanal	279,364	253,446	25,918	450	420	30	15	14	1
Gajapati	128,523	112,365	16,158	240	210	30	8	7	1
Ganjam	758,267	596,062	162,205	1050	810	240	35	27	8
Jagatsinghpur	261,307	233,626	27,681	420	390	30	14	13	1
Jajpur	407,851	378,645	29,206	600	540	60	20	18	2
Jharsuguda	136,061	84,287	51,774	240	150	90	8	5	3
Kalahandi	401,251	373,304	27,947	600	570	30	20	19	1
Kandhamal	172,022	155,256	16,766	270	240	30	9	8	1
Kendrapara	321,934	305,868	16,066	510	480	30	17	16	1
Kendujhar	405,272	348,448	56,824	600	510	90	20	17	3
Khordha	494,212	247,304	246,908	780	390	390	26	13	13
Koraput	337,677	282,783	54,894	540	450	90	18	15	3
Malkangiri	137,599	126,225	11,374	240	210	30	8	7	1
Mayurbhanj	586,253	542,726	43,527	870	810	60	29	27	2
Nabarangpur	273,423	253,208	20,215	420	390	30	14	13	1
Nayagarh	228,315	210,850	17,465	360	330	30	12	11	1
Nuapada	152,210	144,299	7911	240	240	0	8	8	0
Puri	367,269	313,188	54,081	570	480	90	19	16	3
Rayagada	226,144	191,568	34,576	360	300	60	12	10	2
Sambalpur	249,597	179,411	70,186	360	270	90	12	9	3
Subarnapur	151,136	139,346	11,790	240	210	30	8	7	1
Sundargarh	479,109	312,497	166,612	750	480	270	25	16	9
Odisha	9,637,820	8,089,987	1,547,833	15,000	12,600	2400	500	420	80

Source Odisha migration survey 2023

selected localities, a method of systematic random sampling was implemented. This method ensured that every household within the chosen localities had an equal chance to be included in the research. Specifically, 30 households were selected from each chosen locality. This process was meticulously carried out across a total of 500 localities, spread throughout all 30 districts of Odisha. During this research phase, skilled field investigators undertook the task, utilizing the computer-assisted personal interviews (CAPI) technique to collect data. To pick households, district-level field supervisors collected household lists from Anganwadis and employed random sampling to choose 30 households from each area's total households. If a chosen household was inaccessible or declined to participate, the enumerator moved on to survey the next nearby household.

7.1.1 Raising Factor

In large-scale household surveys, a raising factor is referred to as a weighting factor or weight and is used to adjust sample data to match the population it represents. They are applied to adjust the influence of each sampled unit in the estimation of population parameters, making the results more representative of the target population. The raising factor is the reciprocal of the probability of selection for each unit in the sample. It is used to *raise* the sample observations to the level of the total population size.

In accordance with the sampling design utilized by the OMS, the raising factor at the district level was used as the sample weight. Since the probability of selecting a household in every locality was the same at 1/30, the raising factor for all the localities is identical. Thus, we only needed to focus on obtaining weights at the district level, where these raising factors may have varied from one district to another. The sample weights become accurate for analysis at the district level.

The number of households in each district in 2023 is estimated from Census 2001 and 2011 data. The raising factor based on households is calculated by dividing this number by the number of households sampled from each district. These raising factors are of utmost importance for our estimation process, ensuring the validity of our findings. Also, a similar approach can be taken to calculate raising factors for the entire population.

$$\textbf{The raising factor of Households(HHs)} = \frac{\textit{Total number of HHs}2023\ (\textit{Projected})}{\textit{Number of sample HHs}}$$

HHs 2023 (Projected): It represents the projected number of households in each district for the year 2023.

Sample HHs: It is the number of households sampled in each district.

$$\textbf{The raising factor of population} = \frac{\textit{Total population of}\ 2023(\textit{Projected})}{\textit{Total sample population}}$$

Population 2023 (Projected): This column provides the projected population for each district in 2023.

Sample Population: It represents the sampled population in each district (Table 6).

For example, the raising factor for the Bargarh district is as follows. The projected number of households in Bargarh for 2023 is 495,638. The sample households selected for the survey in Bargarh are 570. The raising factor applied to the sample households is 869.541, which is used to estimate the total number of households in Bargarh.

Meanwhile, the projected population for Bargarh in 2023 is 16,61,122. The sample population selected for the survey in Bargarh is 3434. The raising factor applied to the sample population is 516.789, which is used to estimate the total population in Bargarh.

The calculated raising factor on population fluctuates from the lowest, 544.276 for Rayagada, to the highest, 1032.796 for Nabarangpur district. Similarly, the raising factors based on households range between 438.888 and 1022.095, respectively, for the districts Debagarh and Balangir. Estimates from the sample at the state level are obtained as the weighted sum from district-level estimates using raising factors as weights.

The utilization of raising factors for sample households allows for an extrapolation of the total household count within each district while accounting for religious distribution. By applying these weights (raising factors), it becomes feasible to compute the population based on both religion and districts. The data presented in Table 7 outlines the households in Odisha, segmented by religion and districts, for the year 2023. Among these districts, Ganjam emerges with the most significant share of the population in comparison with Odisha's overall population. Conversely, Debagarh exhibits the lowest proportion of the population. When analyzing religious affiliations, the Hindu community constitutes the majority in Ganjam. In contrast, Sundargarh records the highest count of Christians, while Jajpur records the highest Muslim population.

In subsequent chapters, the results are analyzed by social group, district, region, locality, wealth status,[7] and household migration status. For social groups, we use the four-fold classification of SC, ST, upper caste, and OBC. We use the official classification of the 30 districts of Odisha and the administrative categorization of these

[7] At the household level, we construct the wealth index using Principal Component Analysis (PCA) on the ownership of 18 assets including tractor, agricultural machinery, non-agricultural machinery, four-wheeler vehicle, two-wheeler vehicle, bicycle or cycle rickshaw, basic mobile phone, smart mobile phone, color television, refrigerator, desktop computer, laptop, broadband internet connection, air conditioner, washing machine, microwave oven, radio, and bed. PCA is a multivariate statistical technique that transforms a large number of variables in a data set into a smaller set capturing most of the information of the large number of variables. The wealth index, based on the first principal component, is a linear index of the 18 assets accounting for the largest amount of information common to all variables included in this analysis. Following the Demographic and Health Survey approach, we further divide the wealth index into four quartiles after adjusting for sample weights and household size. Specifically, the households are categorized into poorest (quartile = 1), poor (quartile = 2), rich (quartile = 3), and richest (quartile = 4) households.

Table 6 Raising factor for households and population, OMS 2023

	District	No of households	Sample HH	HH raising factor	Total population	Sample pop	Pop raising factor
1	Bargarh	495,638	570	869.541	1,661,122	2007	827.664
2	Jharsuguda	185,449	240	772.703	675,977	732	923.466
3	Sambalpur	326,468	360	906.855	1,183,496	1335	886.514
4	Debagarh	105,333	240	438.888	365,784	632	578.773
5	Sundargarh	608,972	750	811.962	2,459,002	2881	853.524
6	Kendujhar	528,704	600	881.173	2,138,479	2238	955.531
7	Mayurbhanj	769,613	870	884.613	2,927,842	3077	951.525
8	Baleshwar	767,906	840	914.173	2,733,430	3260	838.476
9	Bhadrak	423,273	480	881.818	1,743,170	2289	761.542
10	Kendrapara	397,757	510	779.916	1,625,930	1911	850.827
11	Jagatsinghpur	322,107	420	766.920	1,240,077	1492	831.151
12	Cuttack	763,069	870	877.091	3,010,155	3864	779.026
13	Jajpur	539,906	600	899.844	2,104,324	2718	774.218
14	Dhenkanal	375,975	450	835.500	1,363,703	1924	708.785
15	Angul	415,252	450	922.782	1,455,296	1883	772.860
16	Nayagarh	316,950	360	880.417	1,095,572	1361	804.976
17	Khordha	699,248	780	896.472	2,800,560	3190	877.919
18	Puri	504,264	570	884.673	1,968,036	1911	1029.846
19	Ganjam	924,332	1050	880.317	4,028,217	4048	995.113
20	Gajapati	152,832	240	636.801	657,509	982	669.561
21	Kandhamal	210,543	270	779.790	849,807	1046	812.435
22	Boudh	145,990	240	608.292	538,947	901	598.165
23	Subarnapur	216,233	240	900.972	703,674	848	829.805
24	Balangir	613,257	600	1022.095	2,120,559	2395	885.411
25	Nuapada	198,999	240	829.162	721,963	1083	666.632
26	Kalahandi	527,714	600	879.523	1,924,775	2099	916.996
27	Rayagada	278,181	360	772.726	1,162,113	1527	761.043
28	Nabarangpur	341,843	420	813.912	1,504,784	1457	1032.796
29	Koraput	414,224	540	767.081	1,663,221	2093	794.659
30	Malkangiri	181,293	240	755.387	775,516	952	814.618
	Odisha	12,751,324	15,000		49,203,041	58,136	

Source Authors' calculation based on Census 2001 and 2011 figures

Table 7 Households of Odisha by religion and districts, 2023

	Sample households, OMS 2023					Estimated total households, Odisha, 2023				
District	Hindu	Christian	Muslim	Others	Total	Hindu	Christian	Muslim	Others	Total
Bargarh	567	2	1	0	570	493,030	1739	870	0	495,639
Jharsuguda	237	0	3	0	240	183,131	0	2318	0	185,449
Sambalpur	354	6	0	0	360	321,027	5441	0	0	326,468
Debagarh	239	1	0	0	240	104,894	439	0	0	105,333
Sundargarh	632	105	11	2	750	513,160	85,256	8932	1624	608,972
Kendujhar	600	0	0	0	600	528,704	0	0	0	528,704
Mayurbhanj	851	0	6	13	870	752,806	0	5308	11,500	769,614
Baleshwar	800	0	38	2	840	731,338	0	34,739	1828	767,905
Bhadrak	451	0	29	0	480	397,700	0	25,573	0	423,273
Kendrapara	503	0	7	0	510	392,298	0	5459	0	397,757
Jagatsinghpur	415	0	5	0	420	318,272	0	3835	0	322,107
Cuttack	825	2	43	0	870	723,600	1754	37,715	0	763,069
Jajpur	546	0	54	0	600	491,315	0	48,592	0	539,907
Dhenkanal	439	0	11	0	450	366,785	0	9191	0	375,976
Angul	447	1	1	1	450	412,484	923	923	923	415,253
Nayagarh	360	0	0	0	360	316,950	0	0	0	316,950
Khordha	707	3	66	4	780	633,806	2689	59,167	3585	699,247
Puri	558	0	10	2	570	493,648	0	8847	1770	504,265
Ganjam	1047	0	2	1	1050	921,692	0	1761	880	924,333
Gajapati	125	115	0	0	240	79,600	73,232	0	0	152,832
Kandhamal	208	61	0	1	270	162,196	47,567	0	780	210,543

(continued)

Table 7 (continued)

	Sample households, OMS 2023					Estimated total households, Odisha, 2023				
District	Hindu	Christian	Muslim	Others	Total	Hindu	Christian	Muslim	Others	Total
Boudh	240	0	0	0	240	145,990	0	0	0	145,990
Subarnapur	240	0	0	0	240	216,233	0	0	0	216,233
Balangir	597	3	0	0	600	610,191	3066	0	0	613,257
Nuapada	239	1	0	0	240	198,170	829	0	0	198,999
Kalahandi	592	0	6	2	600	520,678	0	5277	1759	527,714
Rayagada	354	6	0	0	360	273,545	4636	0	0	278,181
Nabarangpur	404	12	4	0	420	328,820	9767	3256	0	341,843
Koraput	452	83	5	0	540	346,721	63,668	3835	0	414,224
Malkangiri	238	1	1	0	240	179,782	755	755	0	181,292
Total	14,267	402	303	28	15,000	12,158,566	301,761	266,353	24,649	12,751,329

Source Authors' calculation

districts into three regions—Central/Coastal, Southern, and Northern regions[8]—to present a regional analysis. For locality, we use the census definition of rural and urban areas. For the categorization of household migration status, based on individual-level data on residential status, a three-fold classification of households: current migrant households, return migrant households, and resident households is used.[9,10] We now move to the methodology of Phase II of the Odisha Migration Study.

7.2 *Phase II*

The second phase of the Odisha Migration Study comprised four studies that were undertaken in 11 districts—Balangir, Bargarh, Kalahandi, Nuapada, Subarnapur, Ganjam, Gajapati, Rayagada, Koraput, Nabarangpur, and Khordha (Map 2). These districts were purposively selected as they had been identified as migration-prone by the government of Odisha (Srivastava, 2020a; The Telegraph, 2018). The first study (see Chapter 8) is a mixed-methods study on rural income and livelihoods. Detailed income and livelihood data was collected from 506 households in the 11 aforementioned districts. These households were a subset of a larger representative sample of 15,000 households that were interviewed in OMS Phase 1. In addition, 24 case studies were undertaken in two districts. The second study is a quantitative study that examines the impact of male migration on left-behind women. The data for this study was collected through a gender module administered to married women aged 18–49 in the same 506 households as the first study (see Chapter 10).

For the first two studies of Phase 2, the sample size of the study was predetermined at 500. In the 11 aforementioned districts, rural localities[11] with the highest migration rates in OMS Phase 1 were selected for data collection. Within each district, the number of localities (and households) was selected based on their probability proportionate to the sample in Phase 1. By this process, a total of 17 localities in 11 districts were selected. Locality- and district-wise details of the household sample are given in Table 8.

It may be noted that seven of the 11 study districts belong to the poorest and most deprived southern region of Odisha, while one district is part of the relatively

[8] The Central division or region includes Cuttack, Jagatsinghpur, Kendrapara, Jajpur, Balasore, Bhadrak, Puri, Khordha, Nayagarh, and Mayurbhanj districts. The Southern region includes Ganjam, Gajapati, Koraput, Nabarangpur, Rayagada, Malkangiri, Kalahandi, Nuapada, Kandhamal, and Boudh districts, and the Northern region includes Sambalpur, Deogarh, Jharsuguda, Bargarh, Balangir, Sonepur or Subarnapur, Sundargarh, Dhenkanal, Angul, and Keonjhar districts.

[9] See Sect. 8.3 for more details.

[10] We also use an alternate two-fold classification of migrant and non-migrant households. Here, migrant households include only current migrant households, and non-migrant households include resident households as well as return migration households, explained in the three-fold classification above. This schema is useful for some kinds of analysis that are concerned only with the current migration status of households.

[11] Localities here refer to the gram panchayat, as per the census classification.

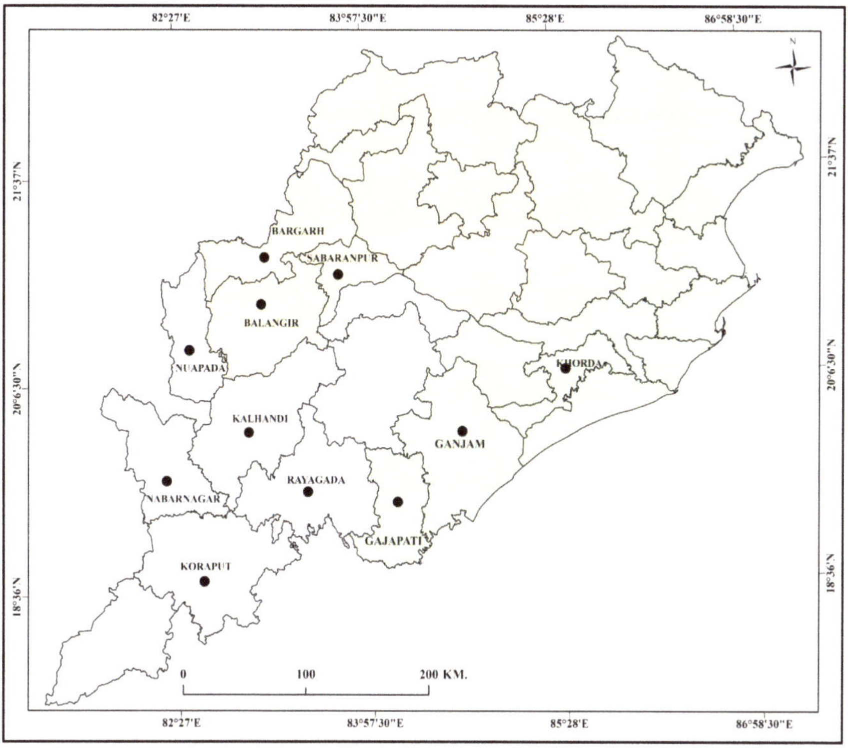

Map 2 Odisha migration study, phase II districts

backward northern region. The remaining three districts in the sample are from the relatively advanced coastal region. Overall, the sample is biased toward the relatively poor and backward regions of the state.

The third and fourth studies are qualitative studies. One conducted 44 in-depth interviews in two villages in Ganjam district to understand youth aspirations and attitudes toward agriculture in the context of high migration (see Chapter 9). The last study draws on semi-structured interviews and focus group discussions with migrant and non-migrant households in Kalahandi and Balangir to explore their experiences of work, livelihoods, health, and family dynamics (see Chapter 11).

Table 8 Distribution of sample households by districts and villages

District	Locality (Village)	Number of households
Balangir	Babejuri	30
	Dangapata	30
Bargarh	Agalpur	30
	Jujgaon	30
Gajapati	Kutama	30
Ganjam	Gangadahani	30
	Kandharanipada	28
	Paikapada	30
Kalahandi	Balagaon	29
	Jariguma	29
Khordha	Bhenkatarayapur	30
Koraput	Balel	30
	Konga	30
Nabarangpur	Gadabaguda	30
Nuapada	Ganiary	30
Rayagada	Beruguda	30
Subarnapur	Samarchipa	30
Total		506

Source Odisha Migration Study, Phase II, 2023. Household sample, Income and Livelihood Module

8 OMS Data Validation, Population Profile, and Household Migration

8.1 Data Validation

The average household size in Odisha, as per the OMS, is 3.9. This figure might appear lower than expected, especially when compared to the average household size from the previous census data. The average number of households can be lower than the average household size due to changes in living arrangements, family structures, and demographics over time (Table 9).

While the average household size has been decreasing over the years, indicating smaller families, the average number of households might not decrease at the same rate due to factors such as urbanization, migration, and changes in household composition.

According to the NFHS-5 (2019–2021), the TFR (the average number of children anticipated to be born to a woman during her reproductive years) of Odisha has declined from 2.1 in 2015–16 to 1.8 in 2019–21.

Table 9 Average household size

Districts	Average household size
Bargarh	3.5
Jharsuguda	3.1
Sambalpur	3.7
Debagarh	2.6
Sundargarh	3.8
Kendujhar	3.7
Mayurbhanj	3.5
Baleshwar	3.9
Bhadrak	4.8
Kendrapara	3.7
Jagatsinghpur	3.6
Cuttack	4.4
Jajpur	4.5
Dhenkanal	4.3
Angul	4.2
Nayagarh	3.8
Khordha	4.1
Puri	3.4
Ganjam	3.9
Gajapati	4.1
Kandhamal	3.9
Boudh	3.8
Subarnapur	3.5
Balangir	4.0
Nuapada	4.5
Kalahandi	3.5
Rayagada	4.2
Nabarangpur	3.5
Koraput	3.9
Malkangiri	4.0
Odisha	3.9
Average household size in Odisha as per Census	
2011	4.4
2001	4.8

Source Odisha Migration Survey 2023, Household sample; Census of India, various years

There are no significant differences across the major religious groups (Table 10). There has been a slight decrease in the share of the Hindu population, while the shares of the Christian and Muslim populations have remained constant. There has been a slight increase in the share of other religious groups functioning in Odisha. The religious composition has been, for the most part, observed to be unvaried across the 2011 Census and OMS.

The ST and SC composition has somewhat remained constant in both the 2011 Census and the OMS (Table 11). A slight increase can be noted in the ST population in the OMS when compared to the 2011 Census.

The sex ratio favors the male population and has subsequently worsened (Table 12). It has seen a negative trend, with the number of females per 1,000 males decreasing to 926 in the OMS compared to 979 females per 1000 males in the 2011 Census. This is not a favorable indicator of social development and fertility trends. This apparent decline in the sex ratio may also be on account of the underestimation of male-dominated outmigration, which is not adequately captured in the Census, but has been done in the OMS.

Table 10 Distribution of households by religion, OMS 2023 and Census 2011

Religion	OMS (% of households)	2011 Census (% of households)
Hindu	95.4	93.6
Christian	2.4	2.8
Muslim	2.1	2.3
Others	0.1	1.4
Total	100.0	100.0

Source Odisha Migration Survey 2023, Household sample; Census of India, 2011

Table 11 Proportion of SC and ST in the population, OMS 2023 and Census 2011

	OMS (% of households)	2011 Census (% of households)
SC	17.8	17.1
ST	23.6	22.8

Source Odisha Migration Survey, 2023. Household sample; Census of India, 2011

Table 12 Sex ratio of the population, OMS 2023 and Census 2011

Study	Sex ratio (number of females per 1000 males)
OMS 2023	926
Census 2011	979

Source Odisha Migration Survey 2023, Household sample; Census of India, 2011

8.2 *Background Profile of the Sample Population*

While conducting the survey, there was a notable instance of population under-reporting for individuals below the age of 18 years. Nevertheless, data from both the United Nations Population Fund (UNPF) and the NFHS-5 indicates a declining trend in total fertility rates within Odisha (Table 13). This pattern is further evident in the age pyramid constructed from the UNPF report, revealing a contraction in the 0–4 age group between 2021 and the 2011 Census. This trend is mirrored in the sample population studied by the Odisha Migration Study, despite some instances of under-reporting. Regarding the population aged 60 years and above, parity is observed between males and females in both the Census and UNPF data. However, the OMS study shows a marginal increase among males, compared to their female counterparts (Figs. 2 and 3).

The median age of the sample population is 31 years, with a wide age range spanning from 0 to 103 years. This median age suggests that the sample population is evenly split, with half of the individuals being older and the other half being younger than 31. The median age of non-residents, or migrants, is lower than that of the overall sample, at 30 years. Upon examining Fig. 4, it becomes evident that over 60% of both male and female individuals who have experienced migration can be categorized within the age range of 20 to 39 years. This phenomenon could be indicative of various factors influencing migration decisions, such as educational

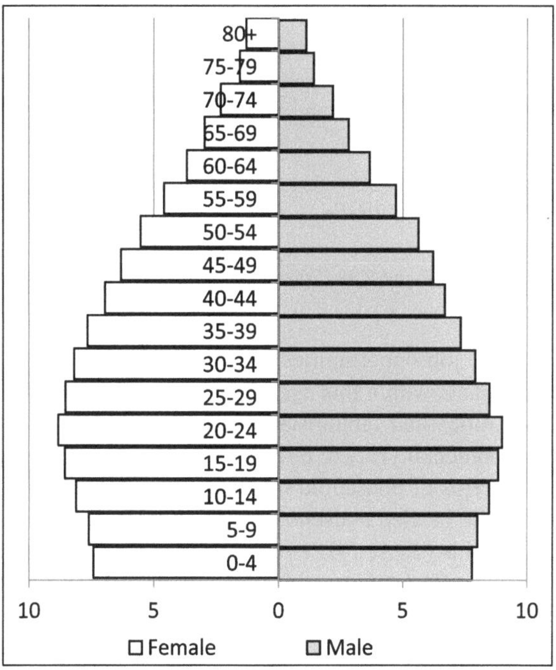

Fig. 2 Age pyramid of Odisha, 2021 (UNPF). *Source* UNPF, *India: district level population projections in selected states of India 2021 and 2026*

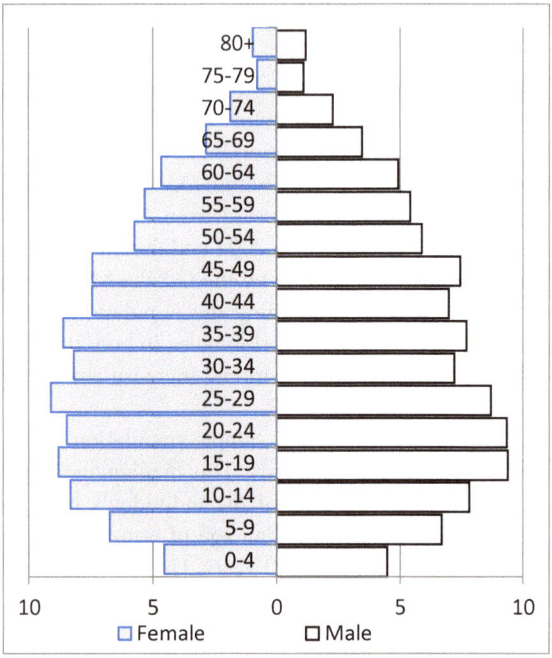

Fig. 3 Age pyramid, Odisha Migration Study, 2023. *Source* Odisha migration survey 2023, household sample

Table 13 Broad age group of sample population, OMS 2023, Census 2011, and UNPF 2021

	OMS 2023			Census 2011			UNPF, 2021		
	Male	Female	Total	Male	Female	Total	Male	Female	Total
0–14	19.0	19.6	19.3	29.2	28.5	28.9	23.6	24.2	23.1
15–59	68.1	69.2	68.6	61.7	62.1	61.9	64.9	64.7	65.1
60 +	12.9	11.1	12.1	9.2	9.4	9.3	11.5	11.1	11.8
Total	100.0	100.0	100.0	100.0	100.0	100.0	100.0	100.0	100.0

Source Odisha migration survey 2023, Household sample; Census of India, 2011; UNPF, *India: District Level Population Projections in Selected States of India 2021 and 2026*

pursuits, job opportunities, or seeking better living conditions. The concentration of migrants within this age group underscores the importance of understanding the motivations and circumstances that drive individuals in their prime working and developmental years to move from one location to another.

In terms of household headship, approximately 15.2% of the total population is in female-headed households, while the majority, about 84.8%, are in male-headed households (Table 14). This data indicates the distribution of household leadership within the population, with a notable proportion being led by females.

About 23,361 individuals have never been married. Of these, 13,527 are males (44.8% of the total population) and 9834 are females (35.2% of the total population). However, among the never-married population, 14,214 individuals are above the age

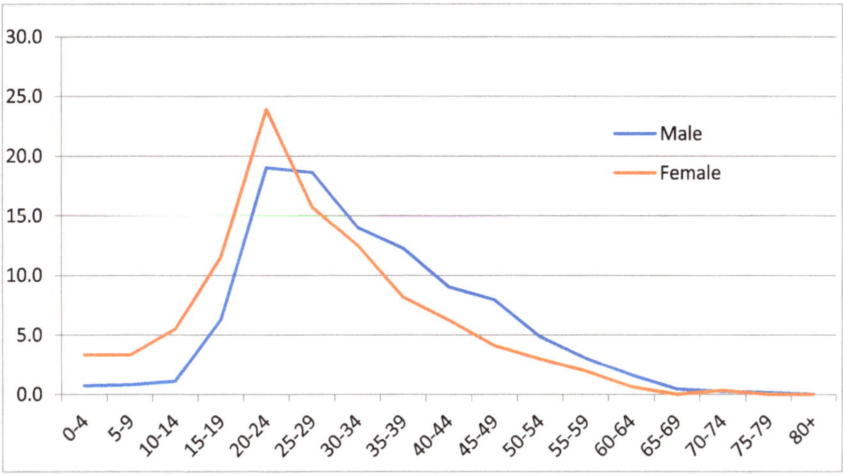

Fig. 4 Age distribution of the non-residents among the sample population. *Source* Odisha migration survey 2023, household sample

Table 14 Household headship

	Household headship
Male	84.8
Female	15.2
Total	100.0

Source Odisha migration survey 2023, household sample

of 18 years (20.5% of males and 10.6% of females are above the age of 18 years). A larger proportion of females is widowed compared to males. The 'Divorced' and 'Separated' categories have a very small representation in the population (Table 15).

Table 15 Marital status of the sample population

	Number			Per centage		
Number	Male	Female	Total	Male	Female	Total
Never Married	13,527	9834	23,361	44.8	35.2	40.2
Married	15,761	15,485	31,246	52.2	55.4	53.7
Widow/ Widower	825	2458	3283	2.7	8.8	5.6
Divorced	22	57	79	0.1	0.2	0.1
Separated	55	112	167	0.2	0.4	0.3
Total	30,190	27,946	58,136	100.0	100.0	100.0

Source Odisha migration survey 2023, household sample

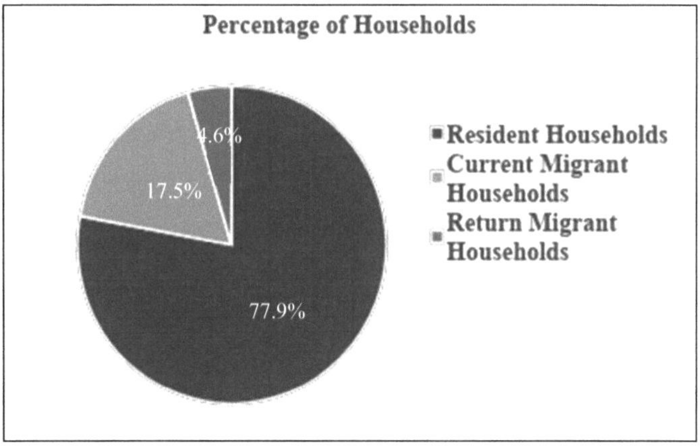

Fig. 5 Distribution of sample households by residential status. *Source* Odisha migration survey 2023, household sample

8.3 Household Migration

As discussed in Sect. 7, the OMS collected data on the residential status of each member of the sample households. At the time of the survey, household members were recorded as residents, current migrants, or return migrants. Based on this individual-level data on residential status, a three-fold classification of households is used: (i) current migrant households, (ii) return migrant households, and (iii) resident households. Current migrant households are households that include at least one migrant member at the time of the survey; return migrant households are households where members had migrated in the past but did not migrate at the time of the survey; and resident households are households where no member had ever migrated, i.e., resident households did not have any current or return migrants.

Based on this classification, about 18% of the sample households had at least one current migrant member at the time of the survey, and nearly 5% of households had return migrants—members who had migrated at some time in the past (Fig. 5). Thus, migration is a critical phenomenon and—we will see in the subsequent chapters—it is closely associated with living standards and well-being in Odisha.

9 Chapterization

This book is divided into 12 chapters, each exploring distinct but interconnected aspects of the migration and development processes in Odisha. Chapter 1 sets up the broader context and traces the development trajectory of the state by outlining its political economy and its evolution in response to the structural changes over the past several decades—with a specific focus on agriculture and industrialization. It presents a socio-economic profile of the state and brings to the fore the persistent and emerging challenges faced by the population, including but not limited to agrarian distress and poverty; regional, gender, and social disparities; health, education, and food insecurity; and the patterns, magnitude, and precarity of migration. It foregrounds the rest of the chapters through the analytical framework anchored in migration, livelihoods, and gender, followed by a detailed methodology section covering the two phases of the Odisha Migration Study.

Chapter 2 examines housing conditions, access to basic amenities, and participation in government schemes, with a focus on the PDS and MGNREGA. It also analyzes household asset ownership and changes in income levels since the COVID-19 pandemic. Chapters 3 and 4 unpack the migration story of the state. Chapter 3 starts with district-wise estimates of current and return migrants from Odisha and then dives deeper into the characteristics of migrant households. This is followed by a discussion on migration streams, destinations, work and occupations before and after migration, sources of information on migration, reasons for migration, and reasons for return. In Chapter 4, we turn to the size of remittances and the role they play in supporting households and local economies. Chapters 5 and 6 present an analysis of household-level food consumption and dietary practices and an overview of educational attainments, respectively, offering crucial insights into how livelihoods shape, and are in turn shaped by, these aspects in the short and long term.

Chapter 7 dives deeper into the work and employment scenario and estimates the overall Workforce Participation Rate (WPR), as well as its variation across gender, social group, age, and other categories. Chapter 8, drawing on the primary survey and qualitative case studies, shifts the lens to household income distribution and develops livelihood- and income-based typologies to analyze the contributions of agriculture, non-agriculture, and remittances to rural livelihoods. Continuing the discussion—particularly centered on agriculture—Chapter 9 explores youth aspirations and attitudes toward agriculture against the backdrop of smallholder rainfed cultivation in a high-migration region of Odisha.

Chapters 10 and 11 focus on the impact of male migration on women who stay behind or are 'left behind'. The former undertakes a quantitative analysis to understand the association, if any, between male migration and left-behind women's employment and autonomy outcomes. Based on a qualitative study, Chapter 11 delves into left-behind women's experiences pertaining to work, livelihood, family dynamics, health, and emotional stress and isolation. It also brings to the fore the direct connection between male migration and the increased burden of care responsibilities on women. Chapter 12 discusses policy implications and concludes.

References

Acharya, A. K. (2021). Caste-based migration and exposure to abuse and exploitation: Dadan labour migration in India. *Contemporary Social Science, 16*(3), 371–383.

Acharya, S. S., Mukherjee, M., & Patro, G. (2021). Correlates of healthcare among women and children in Odisha: Understanding barriers in access. In A. Hans, A. Patel, B. Mohanty, & S. Tripathy (Eds.), *Women reinventing development* (pp. 95–126). Routledge.

Adduci, M. (2011). Neoliberalism and class reproduction in India: The political economy of privatisation in the mineral sector in the Indian state of Orissa. *Forum for Social Economics, 41*(1), 68–96. https://doi.org/10.1007/s12143-011-9091-z

Ali, Z., & Sharma, A. (2014). Migration trends from coastal and western Odisha: A study of migration, incidence, and issues. In A. Sharma, R. Kulkarni, & R. Khandelwal (Eds.), *Studies, stories and canvas: Seasonal labor migration and migrant workers from Odisha* (pp. 1–33). Centre for Migration and Labor Solutions, Aajeevika Bureau. https://www.humandignity.foundation/wp-content/uploads/2018/11/Odisha-State-Migration-Profile-Report.pdf

Ambagudia, J. (2010). Tribal rights, dispossession and the state in Orissa. *Economic and Political Weekly, 45*(33). https://www.epw.in/journal/2010/33/special-articles/tribal-rights-dispossession-and-state-orissa.html

Bal, C., Das, A., & Kumar, S. C. (2015). Silver lining in Odisha's organised manufacturing sector. *Economic and Political Weekly, 50*(15), 69–79.

Barik, S. (2023, March 15). Land held by tribals in Odisha is shrinking, says a draft CAG report. *The Hindu*. https://www.thehindu.com/news/national/other-states/land-held-by-tribals-in-odisha-is-shrinking-says-a-draft-cag-report/article66997133.ece

Behera, M., Mishra, S., & Behera, A. R. (2021). The COVID-19-led reverse migration on labour supply in rural economy: Challenges, opportunities, and road ahead in Odisha. *The Indian Economic Journal, 69*(3), 392–409.

Bhandari, B. S., & Grant, M. (2007). Analysis of livelihood security: A case study in the Kali-Khola watershed of Nepal. *Journal of Environmental Management, 85*(1), 17–26.

Bhatt, W. (2009). The gender dimension of migration in India: The politics of contemporary space in Orissa and Rajasthan. *Development in Practice, 19*(1), 87–93.

Bhowmik, S. (1981). *Class formation in the plantation system*. People's Publishing House.

Breman, J. (2019). Capitalism, labour bondage and the social question. In *Cambridge University Press eBooks* (pp. 237–265). https://doi.org/10.1017/9781108687485.009

Chambers, R., & Conway, G. (1991). *Sustainable rural livelihoods: Practical concepts for the 21st century* (IDS Discussion Paper No. 296). Institute of Development Studies.

Chandrasekhar, S., & Naidu, D. (2021). *Changes in utilization trends of services at public hospitals after the launch of Biju Swasthya Kalyan Yojana & other health initiatives in Odisha* (Working Paper HSTP 2021/HCF1). Health Systems Transformation Platform.

Chant, S. (2008). The 'feminisation of poverty' and the 'feminisation' of anti-poverty programmes: Room for revision? *The Journal of Development Studies, 44*(2), 165–197. https://doi.org/10.1080/00220380701789810

Centre for Youth and Social Development. (2024). *Emergent Odisha: Demography and development*. Centre for Youth and Social Development.

Dandekar, A., & Ghai, R. (2020). Migration and reverse migration in the age of COVID-19. *Economic and Political Weekly, 55*(19), 28–31.

Daniel, U. (2014). Analytical review of market, state and civil society response to seasonal migration from Odisha. In A. Sharma, R. Kulkarni, & R. Khandelwal (Eds.), *Studies, stories and canvas: Seasonal labor migration and migrant workers from Odisha* (pp. 106–115). Centre for Migration and Labor Solutions, Aajeevika Bureau. https://www.humandignity.foundation/wp-content/uploads/2018/11/Odisha-State-Migration-Profile-Report.pdf

Das, A., & Acharya, S. (2016). Mining and Odisha's economy. In P. B. Nayak, S. C. Panda, & P. K. Pattanaik (Eds.), *The economy of Odisha: A profile* (pp. 141–173). Oxford University Press.

Das, S. (2016). Economics of natural disasters in Odisha. In P. B. Nayak, S. C. Panda, & P. K. Pattanaik (Eds.), *The economy of Odisha: A profile* (pp. 266–300). Oxford University Press.

Das, S. P. (2016). Transportation and power. In P. B. Nayak, S. C. Panda, & P. K. Pattanaik (Eds.), *The economy of Odisha: A profile* (pp. 174–230). Oxford University Press.

Datta, A. (2016). Migration, remittances, and changing sources of income in rural Bihar (1999–2011): Some findings from a longitudinal study. *Economic and Political Weekly, 51*(31), 85–93.

Datta, A. (2022). *Migration and development in India: The Bihar experience.* Routledge.

De Haas, H., & Van Rooij, A. (2010). Migration as emancipation? The impact of internal and international migration on the position of women left behind in rural Morocco. *Oxford Development Studies, 38*(1), 43–62. https://doi.org/10.1080/13600810903551603

Deshingkar, P., & Farrington, J. (2009). A framework of understanding circular migration. In P. Deshingkar & J. Farrington (Eds.), *Circular migration and multilocational livelihood strategies in rural India.* Oxford University Press.

Deshingkar, P., & Akter, S. (2009). *Migration and human development in India* (Human Development Research Paper No. 13). United Nations Development Programme, Human Development Report Office.

Ellis, F. (2000). *Rural livelihoods and diversity in developing countries.* Oxford University Press.

Findley, S. E., & Williams, L. (1991). Women who go and women who stay: Reflections of family migration processes in a changing world. *World Population and Labor Policies Working Paper, 176*, ILO. http://www.ilo.org/public/libdoc/ilo/1991/91B09_196_engl.pdf

Food and Agriculture Organization. (2011). *The state of food and agriculture: Women in agriculture, closing the gender gap for development* (ISBN 978-92-5-106768-0). http://www.fao.org/3/a-i2050e.pdf

Gaurav, S. (2023). The thorny road to evaluating direct benefit transfers for agricultural households: Insights from KALIA in Odisha. *Economics and Political Weekly., 58*(25–26), 13–21.

Gaurav, S., & Mishra, S. (2016). Land ownership and tenancy in Odisha. In P. B. Nayak, S. C. Panda, & P. K. Pattanaik (Eds.), *The economy of Odisha: A profile* (pp. 54–86). Oxford University Press.

Ghosh, S., Verma, H. C., Panda, D. K., Nanda, P., & Kumar, A. G. (2012). Irrigation, agriculture, livelihood, and poverty linkages in Odisha. *Agricultural Economics Research Review, 25*(1), 99–105.

Government of India. (2000). *Report of the eleventh finance commission.* Ministry of Finance, Government of India. https://fincomindia.nic.in/asset/doc/commission-reports/11th-FC/11threport.pdf

Government of India. (2010). *Migration in India 2007–2008.* National Sample Survey Office, Ministry of Statistics & Programme Implementation, Government of India.

Government of India. (2023). *National multidimensional poverty index: A progress review 2023.* NITI Aayog. https://www.niti.gov.in/sites/default/files/2023-08/India-National-Multidimentional-Poverty-Index-2023.pdf

Government of India. (2024). *Implementation of Beti Bachao Beti Padhao scheme in Odisha* [Rajya Sabha report]. Ministry of Women and Child Development.

Government of Odisha. (2001). *Industrial policy resolution, 2001.* Directorate of Industries, Department of Industries, Government of Odisha. https://diodisha.nic.in/Doc/IPR/ipr_2001.pdf

Government of Odisha. (2020). *Five decades of Odisha agricultural statistics.* Directorate of Agriculture and Food Production, Government of Odisha.

Government of Odisha. (2023). *Economic survey 2021–22.* Planning and Convergence Department, Directorate of Economics and Statistics, Government of Odisha. https://pc.odisha.gov.in/publication/economic-survey-report

Government of Odisha. (2025). *Economic survey 2021–22.* Planning and Convergence Department, Directorate of Economics and Statistics, Government of Odisha. https://pc.odisha.gov.in/publication/economic-survey-report

Gram Vikas & CMID (Centre for Migration and Inclusive Development) (2024). *Labour Migration from Rural Odisha Daringbadi Block, Kandhamal.* https://www.gramvikas.org/wp-content/uploads/2025/01/Migration-Profile-Daringbadi-Final-Web-Gram-Vikas-CMID.pdf

Hans, A., Patel, A., Mohanty, B., & Tripathy, S. (Eds.). (2021). Introduction. In *Women reinventing development: The Odisha experience.* Routledge.

Hietala, R., & Singh, R. B. (2014). Livelihood security in changing socio-economic environment: Summary and policy recommendations. In *Livelihood security in Northwestern Himalaya: Case studies from changing socio-economic environments in Himachal Pradesh, India* (pp. 249–257), Springer.

Hoda, A., Gulati, A., Wardhan, H., & Rajkhowa, P. (2021). Drivers of agricultural growth in Odisha. In A. Gulati, R. Roy, & S. Saini (Eds.), *Revitalizing Indian agriculture and boosting farmer incomes. India studies in business and economics* (pp. 247–278). Springer.

Hussein, K., & Nelson, J. (1998). *Sustainable livelihood and livelihood diversification* (IDS Working Paper No. 69). Institute of Development Studies.

Indian Employment Report (IER). (2024). *India employment report 2024: Youth employment, education, and skill.* International Labour Organization & Institute for Human Development. https://www.ilo.org/publications/india-employment-report-2024-youth-employment-education-and-skills

Jodhka, S. S. (2023). *The Indian village: Rural lives in the 21st century.* Aleph.

Jülich, S. (2011). Drought-triggered temporary migration in an East Indian village. *International Migration, 49*, e189–e199.

Kaur, A. P. (2018). International migration and impact of remittances on left-behind wives: A case study of the Doaba region of Punjab. In S. I. Rajan & N. Neetha (Eds.), *Migration, gender and care economy* (pp. 113–127). Routledge India. https://www.taylorfrancis.com/chapters/edit/10.4324/9780429426704-7/international-migration-impact-remittances-left-behind-wives-atinder-pal-kaur

Khan, M. F., Chandra, H., Mohanty, B. N., & Sahoo, S. (2021). District-level estimates of unemployment rates in Odisha. *Economic and Political Weekly, 56*(38).

Krishnan, K., Burman, A., & Rai, S. (2020, May 9). Migrant Workmen Act, 1979, must be rationalised to remove requirements that disincentivise formalisation. *The Indian Express.* https://indianexpress.com/article/opinion/columns/india-lockdown-inter-state-migrant-workmen-act-6400710/

Kumar, K. (2014). Confronting extractive capital: Social and environmental movements in Odisha. *Economic and Political Weekly, 49*(14), 66–73.

Kumar, R. (2023, March 23). *Left behind or left ahead? Implications of male migration on female political engagement*. Ideas for India. Retrieved May 11, 2024 from https://www.ideasforindia.in/topics/social-identity/left-behind-or-left-ahead-implications-of-male-migration-on-female-political-engagement.html

Kurian, N. J. (2000). Widening regional disparities in India: Some indicators. *Economic and Political Weekly, 35*(7), 538–550.

Lerche, J., & Shah, A. (2018). Conjugated oppression within contemporary capitalism: Class, caste, tribe and agrarian change in India. *Journal of Peasant Studies, 45*(5–6), 927–949.

LibTech India. (2025). *The missing work: A national review of MGNREGA implementation (FY 2024–25).* LibTech India.

Mazumdar, I. (2024a). *Placement agencies and migrant live-in domestic workers in an Indian metro city: A view from below into the evolving practices of intermediaries in Mumbai.* International Labour Organization.

Mazumdar, I. (2024b). *Gendering internal labour migration corridors. Migrant women workers in southern India's garment industry.* International Labour Organization.

Mazumdar, I., Neetha, N., & Agnihotri, I. (2013). Migration and gender in India. *Economic and Political Weekly, 48*(10), 54–64.

Meher, S. K. (2019). Impact of distress seasonal migration from a socio-economic perspective: A case study of Nuapada District in Kalahandi Balangir Koraput Region of Odisha. *The Indian Journal of Labour Economics, 62*(4), 763–782.

Meher, S., & Nanda, J. (2020). *COVID-19 and migrant workers: Challenges and opportunities for Odisha* (Working Paper No. 79). Nabakrushna Choudhury Centre for Development Studies.

Mishra, D. K. (2016). Seasonal migration from Odisha: A view from the field. In D. K. Mishra (Ed.), *Internal migration in contemporary India* (pp. 263–290). Sage Publications.

Mishra, S. (2009). Poverty and agrarian distress in Orissa. In *Proceedings of the 92nd Annual Conference of the Indian Economic Association* (Vol. 2, pp. 309–316).

Misra, B. (2016). Dimensions of poverty and prospects of economic change in Odisha. In P. B. Nayak, S. C. Panda, & P. K. Pattanaik (Eds.), *The economy of Odisha: A profile* (pp. 382–414). Oxford University Press.

Mitra, A., & Pradhan, B. K. (2016). *Migration, remittances, and changing patterns of livelihood: Evidence from western Odisha villages* (Working Paper No. 363). Institute of Economic Growth.

Mohanty, A. (2016). Industry in Odisha: Evolution, policy, and performance. In P. B. Nayak, S. C. Panda, & P. K. Pattanaik (Eds.), *The economy of Odisha: A profile* (pp. 111–140). Oxford University Press.

Mohanty, A. K., Nayak, N. C., & Chatterjee, B. (2016). Does infrastructure affect human development? Evidences from Odisha, India. *Journal of Infrastructure Development, 8*(1), 1–26.

Mohanty, B. B., & Lenka, P. K. (2019). Small farmers' suicide in Odisha. *Economic and Political Weekly, 54*(22), 51–59.

Mohanty, M. (2014). Persisting dominance: Crisis of democracy in a resource-rich region. *Economic and Political Weekly, 49*(14), 39–47.

Munjal, K. (2021, October 29). Changes in income structure of agricultural households: Insights from the Situation Assessment Surveys. *Foundation for Agrarian Studies (FAS) Blog*. http://fas.org.in/changes-in-income-structure-of-agricultural-households-insights-from-the-situation-assessment-surveys/

Munjal, K., & Bamba, I. (2024). Migration, vulnerability, and protection: Changing labour law regime in contemporary India. *Asian Studies Review, 48*(3), 617–635.

Nag, M., Peter, B., & Verma, D. (2023). Surat or Kerala: Exploring caste dynamics in labour migration across two key interstate labour migration corridors from Odisha's Ganjam district. *Odisha Economic Journal, 55*(1), 113–130.

Nayak, C., & Kumar, C. R. (2019). Crop diversification in Odisha: An analysis based on panel data. *Agricultural Economics Research Review, 32*(1), 67–80.

Nayak, N. C., Sahoo, B. K., & Mohanty, A. R. (2023). Do Mahatma Gandhi NREGA and convergence measures arrest distress migration? An empirical assessment of the migration-prone regions of Odisha, India. *Letters in Spatial and Resource Sciences, 16*(1), 7.

Nayak, N. C., Dhar, S., & Mahakur, P. K. (2016a). Educational outcomes in Odisha. In P. B. Nayak, S. C. Panda, & P. K. Pattanaik (Eds.), *The economy of Odisha: A profile* (pp. 303–349). Oxford University Press.

Nayak, P. B., Panda, S. C., & Pattanaik, P. K. (2016b). Introduction. In P. B. Nayak, S. C. Panda, & P. K. Pattanaik (Eds.), *The economy of Odisha: A profile* (pp. 1–26). Oxford University Press.

Nayak, P. B., Panda, S. C., & Pattanaik, P. K. (2016c). Some political constraints on economic development. In P. B. Nayak, S. C. Panda, & P. K. Pattanaik (Eds.), *The economy of Odisha: A profile*. Oxford University Press.

Nayyar, G., & Kim, K. Y. (2018). India's internal labor migration paradox: The statistical and the real. *World Bank Policy Research Working Paper* (No. 8356). World Bank.

Nguyen, M. T., & Locke, C. (2014). Rural-urban migration in Vietnam and China: Gendered house holding, production of space and the state. *The Journal of Peasant Studies, 41*, 855–876.

National Law University Odisha (NLUO). (2020). *Social mapping of migrant workers in Odisha.* Labour and ESI Department, Government of Odisha.

NSO (2020). *Annual Report, Periodic Labour Force Survey 2018–19.* National Statistical Office, Ministry of Statistics and Programme Implementation, Government of India.

Padhi, B., & Panda, S. (2021). Employment and economic growth dynamics in Odisha, India. *Journal of Public Affairs, 21*(2), Article e2168.

Padhi, R., & Sadangi, N. (2020). *Resisting dispossession: The Odisha story.* Aakar Books.

Padhi, S., & Panigrahi, N. (2016). Tribal movements and livelihoods: Recent developments in Odisha. In P. B. Nayak, S. C. Panda, & P. K. Pattanaik (Eds.), *The economy of Odisha: A profile* (pp. 448–478). Oxford University Press.

Panda, A. (2017). Climate change, drought and vulnerability: A historical narrative approach to migration from Western Odisha, India. In *Climate change, vulnerability and migration* (pp. 193–211). Routledge India.

Panda, M. (2008). Economic development in Orissa: Growth without inclusion (Working Paper No. 2008–025). Indira Gandhi Institute of Development Research.

Panda, M. (2016). Malnutrition and food insecurity in Odisha. In P. B. Nayak, S. C. Panda, & P. K. Pattanaik (Eds.), *The economy of Odisha: A profile* (pp. 415–447). Oxford University Press.

Panda, R. K. (2016). Rural unemployment and agricultural wages in Odisha: Analysis of major trends and policy options. In P. B. Nayak, S. C. Panda, & P. K. Pattanaik (Eds.), *The economy of Odisha: A profile* (pp. 87–108). Oxford University Press.

Parida, J. K. (2016). MGNREGS, distress migration and livelihood conditions: A study in Odisha. *Journal of Social and Economic Development, 18*(1), 17–39.

Patel, A., & Giri, J. (2019). Climate change, migration and women: Analysing construction workers in Odisha. *Social Change, 49*(1), 97–113.

Patnaik, P. (2016). A perspective on Odisha's recent development paradigm. In P. B. Nayak, S. C. Panda, & P. K. Pattanaik (Eds.), *The economy of Odisha: A profile* (pp. 497–517). Oxford University Press.

Patra, R. (2014). Agricultural development in Odisha: Are the disparities growing? *International Journal of Food and Agricultural Economics, 2*(1128-2016-92052), 129–144.

Pedi, M., & Adabar, K. (2020). Out-migration from Odisha: An analysis in the wake of the COVID-19 crisis. *Orissa Economic Journal, 52*(3), 137–153.

Planning Commission. (2012). *Databook for DCH 10 April 2012.* Government of India.

Prati, G., Cazcarro, I., & Hazra, S. (2022). Gender dimensions of the migration, sustainability, and care nexus: The case study of the Mahanadi delta, India. *Current Research in Environmental Sustainability, 4*, Article 100104. https://doi.org/10.1016/j.crsust.2021.100104

Pritchard, B., Rammohan, A., Sekher, M., Parasuraman, S., & Choithani, C. (2013). *Feeding India.* Routledge. https://doi.org/10.4324/9780203117620

Raj, J., & Axelby, R. (2019). From labour contractors to worker-agents: Transformations in the recruitment of migrant labourers in India. *Contributions to Indian Sociology, 53*(2), 272–298.

Rajan, S. I., & Retnakumar, J. (2025). Unravelling India's demographic future: Population projections for states and union territories, 2021–2051. *International Institute for Migration and Development, Thiruvananthapuram, and Population Foundation of India.*

Rajan, S. I., Sami, B. D., Raj, S. A., & Sivakumar, P. (2021). *Tamil migrants: A demographic, social and economic analysis.* Orient Blackswan.

Rao, N. (2014). Migration, mobility and changing power relations: Aspirations and praxis of Bangladeshi migrants. *Gender, Place & Culture, 21*, 872–887.

Rawal, V. (2008). Ownership holdings of land in rural India: Putting the record straight. *Economic & Political Weekly, 43*(10), 43–47.

Rodgers, G., Datta, A., Rodgers, J., Mishra, S. K., & Sharma, A. N. (2013). *The challenge of inclusive development in rural Bihar.* Institute for Human Development & Manak Publications.

Rogaly, B., Coppard, D., Safique, A., Rana, K., Sengupta, A., & Biswas, J. (2002). Seasonal migration and welfare/illfare in eastern India: A social analysis. *Journal of Development Studies, 38*(5), 89–114.

Rout, H. S., & Hota, A. K. (2016). Health and healthcare in Odisha. In P. B. Nayak, S. C. Panda, & P. K. Pattanaik (Eds.), *The economy of Odisha: A profile* (pp. 350–381). Oxford University Press.

Roy, A. K., & Nangia, P. (2005). Impact of male out-migration on health status of left behind wives: A study of Bihar, India [Paper presentation]. *XXV International Population Conference,*

International Union for the Scientific Study of Population, Tours, France. https://iussp2005.princeton.edu/papers/51906
Sahoo, N., & Kar, M. R. (2021). Evaluating Odisha's COVID-19 response: From quiet confidence to a slippery road. *Journal of Social and Economic Development, 23*(Suppl 2), 373–387.
Sahoo, P., & Nayak, R. K. (2023). Impact of public distribution system on poverty in Odisha. *Economic and Political Weekly, 58*(1).
Sahoo, P., & Senapati, A. K. (2022). Poverty alleviation and pro-poor growth in Odisha. *Economic and Political Weekly, 57*(46), 45–52.
Sahu, B. (2018). Household drought coping, food insecurity, and women in Odisha. *Economic and Political Weekly, 53*(17), 70–78.
Samal, J. K. (2000). *Economy of colonial Odisha, 1866–1947*. Munshiram Manoharlal Publishers.
Samantaraya, A., Sahoo, A. K., Mallick, A., & Bhuyna, B. (2014). Has Odisha become less poor in the last decade? *Economic and Political Weekly, 49*(46), 62–67.
Sansriti. (2007). *Impact of increasing migration on women in Orissa: Study in the districts of Bolangir and Nuapada.* https://ncwapps.nic.in/pdfReports/NCWMigrationReportOrissa.pdf
Sarap, K., & Sahu, P. P. (2016). Emerging trends in cropping pattern, crop diversification, and agricultural productivity. In P. B. Nayak, S. C. Panda, & P. K. Pattanaik (Eds.), *The economy of Odisha: A profile* (pp. 27–53). Oxford University Press.
Sarkar, A., & Mukherji, A. (2025). Perspectives from historical analyses of agri-food system transformations: A case study of Odisha, India. *World Development Perspectives, 38*, Article 100686.
Sen, A. (1985). A sociological approach to the measurement of poverty: A reply to Professor Peter Townsend. *Oxford Economic Papers, 37*(4), 669–676.
Sen, T. K., & Rout, S. K. (2016). The impact of fiscal adjustments in Odisha. In P. B. Nayak, S. C. Panda, & P. K. Pattanaik (Eds.), *The economy of Odisha: A profile* (pp. 481–498). Oxford University Press.
Sengupta, T., & Vijay, G. (2015). *A survey of migration from western Orissa to Telangana* [Report submitted to SR Sankaran, Chair (Rural Labour)], National Institute of Rural Development (NIRD), Hyderabad.
Sharma, A., Kulkarni, R., & Khandelwal, R. (2014). *Studies, stories and a canvas: Seasonal labour migration and migrant workers from Odisha.* Centre for Migration and Labour Solutions.
Singh, C., & Basu, R. (2019). Moving in and out of vulnerability: Interrogating migration as an adaptation strategy along a rural–urban continuum in India. *Geographical Journal, 186*(1), 87–102.
Sinha, B., Jha, S., & Negi, N. S. (2012). Migration and empowerment: The experience of women in households in India where migration of a husband has occurred. *Journal of Gender Studies, 21*(1), 61–76. https://doi.org/10.1080/09589236.2012.639551
Skillshare International India (SII). (2014). *The state of the Adivasis in Odisha 2014: A human development analysis.* SAGE Publications India.
Spiegel, A. D. (1986). The fluidity of household composition in Matatiele, Transkei: A methodological problem. *African Studies, 45*, 17–35.
Srivastava, R. (2020a). *Integrating migration and development policy in India: A case study of three Indian states* (WP 03/2020, Centre for Employment Studies Working Paper Series). Institute for Human Development.
Srivastava, R. (2020b). *Vulnerable internal migrants in India and portability of social security and entitlements* (WP 02/2020). Institute for Human Development. http://www.ihdindia.org/working-papers/2020/IHD-CES_WP_02_2020.pdf
Srivastava, R. (2012). Internal migration and social protection in India: The missing links. In *National workshop on internal migration and human development in India: Workshop compendium* (Vol. II, pp. 167–193). United Nations Educational, Scientific and Cultural Organization & UNICEF India Country Office.
Swain, M. (2017). Transition in agrarian structure in Odisha. *Review of Development and Change, 22*(1), 81–107.

Tata Institute of Social Sciences (TISS). (2019). Human trafficking in vulnerable districts of Odisha: State report. In *A study on human trafficking in vulnerable districts in India*. Tata Institute of Social Sciences.

The Telegraph. (2018). *11 districts migration-prone*. The Telegraph, April 10. https://www.telegraphindia.com/odisha/11-districts-migrationprone/cid/1412164

Tumbe, C. (2011). *Remittances in India: Facts & issues* (IIM Bangalore Research Paper No. 331). Indian Institute of Management Bangalore.

Vidyarthi, A. (2014). In pursuit of inverted dreams: Ethnographic engagement with legal disputes faced by migrant workers of Odisha. In A. Sharma, R. Kulkarni, & R. Khandelwal (Eds.), *Studies, stories and canvas: Seasonal labor migration and migrant workers from Odisha*. Centre for Migration and Labor Solutions, Aajeevika Bureau.

Xaxa, V. (2012). Identity, power, and development: The Kondhs in Orissa, India. In S. Sawyer & E. T. Gomez (Eds.), *The politics of resource extraction* (International Political Economy Series). Palgrave Macmillan. https://doi.org/10.1057/9780230368798_9

Zachariah, K. C., & Rajan, S. I. (2016). Kerala migration study 2014. *Economic and Political Weekly, 51*(6), 66–71.

Chapter 2
Household Characteristics and Living Conditions

Amrita Datta, Rohit Irudayarajan, and Haripriya Narasimhan

Abstract Based on the Odisha Migration Survey, this chapter presents household characteristics related to housing status and amenities, viz., lighting sources, cooking fuel, drinking water, and toilet facilities, disaggregated by social group, region, locality (rural/urban), and migration status. It examines access to government programs and schemes, with an emphasis on the Public Distribution System and the Mahatma Gandhi National Rural Employment Guarantee Program. This is followed by an analysis of asset ownership, landownership, irrigation, and cropping patterns. The chapter then discusses changes in the income levels of households since the COVID-19 pandemic, focusing on the reasons and magnitude of the decline among households that experienced a fall in income levels. It emerges that relatively better-off upper-caste households were less adversely impacted by the pandemic and could bounce back more quickly than other social groups, particularly the Scheduled Tribes, who reported the worst income outcomes among all social groups. Overall, the chapter shows that development outcomes varied significantly by caste, region, and migration status.

Keywords Housing · Amenities · Sanitation · MGNREGA · COVID-19 · Odisha Migration Survey

1 Introduction

Based on household data of the Odisha Migration Survey (OMS), this chapter first presents results on housing status and amenities, viz., lighting sources, cooking fuel, drinking water, and toilet facilities. It then examines access to government programs and schemes, with an emphasis on the Public Distribution System (PDS) and the

A. Datta (✉) · H. Narasimhan
Indian Institute of Technology, Hyderabad, India
e-mail: amritadatta@la.iith.ac.in

R. Irudayarajan
The International Institute of Migration and Development, Thiruvananthapuram, India

A. Datta and S. I. Rajan (eds.), *Migration, Livelihoods and Gender*, International Perspectives on Migration, https://doi.org/10.1007/978-981-95-5465-2_2

program under the Mahatma Gandhi National Rural Employment Guarantee Act (MGNREGA). This is followed by an analysis of the asset ownership of survey households. Last, the chapter discusses changes in the income levels of households since the COVID-19 pandemic, focusing on the reasons and magnitude of the decline among households that experienced a fall in income levels.

The results of the survey are analyzed by social group, district, region, locality, wealth quartile,[1] and household migration status.

2 Housing Status

2.1 Home Ownership

The survey asked questions related to home ownership and housing quality. Survey results show that home ownership is near-universal in Odisha, as 97.3% of the survey households reported living in their own homes. The remaining households reported—their current housing status as—living in rented housing (1.4%), leased housing (0.1%), government quarters (0.2%), or other housing (0.9%). A majority of the households in the category "other" housing reported that they lived on encroached government land. While there was little variation in current housing status by social group or region, location (rural or urban) mattered; compared to rural households, sample households in the urban areas were nearly 10 percentage points less likely to live in their own homes, and nearly six percentage points more likely to live in rental or leased housing.

In 94% of the cases, titles existed for the house or homestead land owned by the households. Interestingly, here, variation by location (rural/urban) or social group was relatively low, but this was not so by region. 99% of the sample households in the northern region reported house and/or land titles, while the coastal and southern regions lagged at 94% and 87%, respectively. In terms of districts, all sample households in Jajpur, Puri, Boudh, and Nuapada had land or house titles, while these were most lacking in Nayagarh (67.5%), Ganjam (73.6%), and Nabarangpur (77.6%) districts.

2.2 Housing Quality

The survey used a five-fold categorization of the type of housing to determine housing quality, as follows: (i) Luxurious—a house with three or more bedrooms with attached bathrooms, concrete roof, mosaic floor; (ii) Very good—a house with two bedrooms with attached bathrooms, concrete roof, mosaic floor; (iii) Good—a house with one

[1] See Chap. 1 (Endnote 7) for details on the household level wealth index constructed using Principal Component Analysis (PCA) on the ownership of 18 assets.

bedroom, brick, and cement walls, concrete or tile roof; (iv) Poor—house with brick walls, cement floor, tin, or asbestos roof; (v) Kutcha—house with mud walls, mud floor and/or thatched roof.

At the aggregate level, survey results show that about half the survey households (50.6%) lived in luxurious, good, or very good housing. However, housing quality for the remaining 49.4% of households is a matter of serious concern. In particular, more than one in five sample households lived in kutcha dwellings. Social group and region emerged as important markers of housing quality. The worst-off were the Scheduled Tribes (STs) and Scheduled Castes (SCs), with 72% and 58% of households living in poor or kutcha housing, respectively. On the other hand, the upper castes were least likely to live in poor or kutcha housing and most likely to live in luxurious or very good housing categories (Table 1).

Survey results also show regional variations in housing quality, with the coastal region faring far better than the northern and southern regions, respectively (see Table 2). By districts, Nabarangpur, Kalahandi, Gajapati, and Malkangiri ranked the worst in housing quality, while Jajpur, Cuttack, and Khordha ranked the best.

Migration status also emerged as an important indicator of housing quality. The survey results show that the migrant households report better housing quality, with 58% living in luxurious, good, or very good housing. On the other hand, 51% of the non-migrant households and 54% of return migrant households lived in poor or kutcha houses (see Appendix Table 37).

Table 1 Housing quality by social group (% of households)

Social group	Type of housing					
	Luxurious	Very good	Good	Poor	Kutcha	Total
Scheduled caste	1.5	8.3	32.3	32.5	25.4	100.0
Scheduled tribe	0.2	2.5	25.3	36.2	35.8	100.0
Other backward class	3.1	16.9	39.3	25.1	15.6	100.0
Upper caste	6.7	26.5	37.2	18.1	11.5	100.0
Total	2.7	13.5	34.4	27.9	21.5	100.0

Source Odisha migration survey 2023, Household sample

Table 2 Housing quality by region (% of households)

Region	Type of housing					
	Luxurious	Very good	Good	Poor	Kutcha	Total
Coastal/central	4.8	19.9	32.3	20.9	22.1	100.0
Southern	1.8	11.1	32.4	32.4	22.3	100.0
Northern	0.5	6.4	39.2	34.1	19.8	100.0
Total	2.7	13.5	34.4	27.9	21.5	100.0

Source Odisha migration survey 2023, Household sample

3 Amenities

3.1 Source of Lighting

The survey asked questions related to the source of lighting used by households. The survey used a five-fold categorization of the source of lighting: (i) wood, (ii) electricity, (iii) kerosene, (iv) LPG gas, and (v) others. The most common source of lighting was electricity, making up a significant majority of 91% of the sample households (Fig. 1). Wood was the next most-used lighting source, with 6.5% of households reporting it as their source of lighting. Kerosene and Liquefied Petroleum Gas (LPG), which account for nearly 1% and 1.7%, respectively, are less commonly used sources of lighting (Fig. 1). There has been rapid electrification in the state, particularly rural electrification in the post-2000 period (Government of Odisha, 2021). This reflects in the survey data, which shows that a vast majority of households in Odisha use electric-powered lighting.

In both rural and urban areas, electricity continues to be the main source of lighting, indicating the prevalence of electrification in Odisha (Table 3). More than 90% of rural households and about 93% of urban households reported electricity as their main source of household lighting. In rural areas, a higher percentage of people rely on traditional wood-based sources for lighting than in urban areas (7.3 and 2.9%, respectively). Kerosene also seems to be a source consumed more often by rural households than urban ones. On the other hand, LPG was a more prevalent source in urban areas than in rural areas.

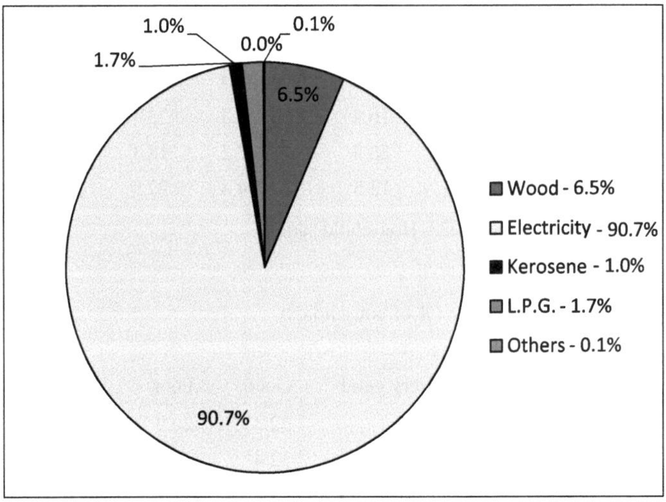

Fig. 1 Source of lighting in sample households (% of households). *Source* Odisha migration survey 2023, Household sample

Table 3 Source of lighting by locality (% of households)

	Wood	Electricity	Kerosene	LPG	Others	Total
Rural	7.3	90.2	1.0	1.4	0.1	100.0
Urban	2.9	93.2	0.7	3.2	0.0	100.0
Total	6.5	90.7	1.0	1.7	0.1	100.0

Source Odisha migration survey 2023, Household sample

Table 4 Source of lighting by social group (% of households)

	Wood	Electricity	Kerosene	LPG	Others	Total
Scheduled caste	8.0	90.4	0.8	0.6	0.2	100.0
Scheduled tribe	10.6	86.1	1.9	1.3	0.1	100.0
Other backward class	3.4	94.5	0.7	1.3	0.1	100.0
Upper caste	7.3	87.6	0.6	4.6	0.0	100.0
Total	6.5	90.7	1.0	1.7	0.1	100.0

Source Odisha migration survey 2023, Household sample

Table 4 shows the breakdown of sources of lighting by social group, namely, SC, ST, Other Backward Class (OBC), and upper caste. More than 90% of SCs and nearly 95% of OBCs reported having electricity as their primary source of lighting. Among the SCs, STs, and OBCs, wood was the second most common source, followed by kerosene and LPG. Among all, the upper caste category accounted for the highest usage of LPG gas, indicating how social stratification affects standards of consumption.

Survey results also show that migrant households are more likely to use electricity compared to non-migrant households (Table 5). Table 5 classifies sources of lighting based on migration status in Odisha, comprising non-migrants, current migrants, and return migrants, as well as the overall distribution. We observe similar patterns and find that electricity accounts for the most common source for all categories (more than 90% among all subgroups). In the resident/non-migrant category, wood accounted for the next best source, followed by LPG and kerosene. Both current and return migrants also follow the same pattern. Kerosene and LPG are most commonly used by non-migrants (1.0% and 1.8%, respectively) than the others.

3.2 *Cooking Fuel*

Figure 2 represents the types of fuel used for cooking in the sample households in Odisha. The survey used a five-fold categorization of the type of cooking fuel used most often: (i) wood, (ii) electricity, (iii) kerosene, (iv) LPG, and (v) others. The majority of the sample households rely on wood as the primary fuel for cooking

Table 5 Source of lighting by residential status (% of households)

	Wood	Electricity	Kerosene	LPG	Others	Total
Resident/non-migrant	6.8	90.2	1.0	1.8	0.1	100.0
Current migrant	6.3	91.4	0.8	1.4	0.0	100.0
Return migrant	2.4	96.5	0.7	0.1	0.2	100.0
Total	6.5	90.7	1.0	1.7	0.1	100.0

Source Odisha migration survey 2023, Household sample

(71.4%). This may be due to a lack of both access and affordability of modern energy sources. LPG is the next best alternative and has accounted for about 22.1%. A relatively small percentage of the sample uses electricity for cooking (6.0%). Kerosene is the least-used type of fuel (about 0.5%).

Table 6 disaggregates the types of fuel used for cooking based on the location (rural or urban). A vast majority of the rural population relies on wood as the primary fuel for cooking (78.1%). LPG is the second most important source for rural households, accounting for about 17.1%. A relatively small percentage (4.4%) of the rural population uses electricity for cooking, likely due to the limited infrastructure or availability. On the other hand, in urban areas, LPG was the most-used source of fuel (51.0%), followed by wood (35.0%) and electricity (13.0%). As expected, urban areas constituted a higher proportion of consumption when it comes to electricity, kerosene, and LPG when compared to the rural households.

Table 7 provides a breakdown of the types of fuel used for cooking based on different social categories, such as SC, ST, OBC, and upper caste. Among the SCs, a significant majority (77.3%) of the population relies on wood as the primary fuel for cooking. LPG is the second most common source for about 17.4% of the sample SC households. Electricity and kerosene form the least-used sources for SCs. Among the STs, wood, again, accounted for the major source (about 87.2%), followed by LPG and electricity. Even for the OBCs, the majority of the households reported

Fig. 2 Primary fuel source for cooking (% of households). *Source* Odisha migration survey 2023, Household sample

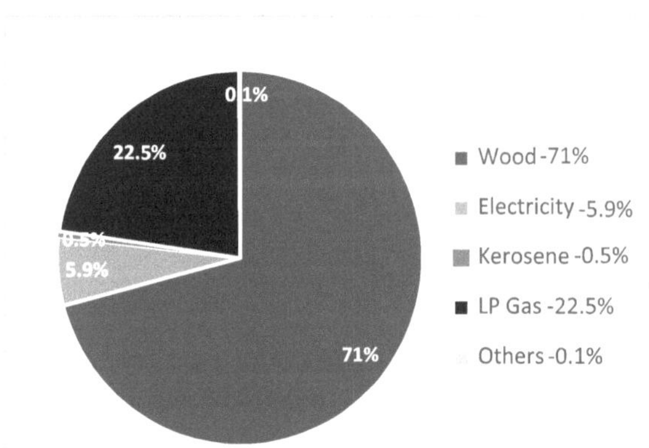

Table 6 Primary fuel source for cooking by locality (% of households)

	Wood	Electricity	Kerosene	LPG	Others	Total
Rural	78.1	4.4	0.4	17.0	0.1	100.0
Urban	35.1	13.4	0.9	50.6	0.0	100.0
Total	71.0	5.9	0.5	22.5	0.1	100.0

Source Odisha migration survey 2023, Household sample

Table 7 Primary fuel source for cooking by social group (% of households)

	Wood	Electricity	Kerosene	LPG	Others	Total
Scheduled caste	77.3	5.0	0.3	17.4	0.0	100.0
Scheduled tribe	87.2	4.1	0.7	8.0	0.0	100.0
Other backward class	66.6	7.0	0.5	25.8	0.1	100.0
Upper caste	51.4	6.4	0.4	41.8	0.0	100.0
Total	71.0	5.9	0.5	22.5	0.1	100.0

Source Odisha migration survey 2023, Household sample

wood (66.6%), followed by LPG and electricity. When it comes to OBCs, a higher proportion (about 25.8%) of households use LPG than SCs and STs. Among the upper castes, again, wood was the common source (51%), followed by LPG and kerosene. From Table 7, we can observe that ST households were most likely to use wood as their primary source compared to other social groups, whereas the upper-caste households were least likely to use wood (51%). On the other hand, when it comes to LPG use, upper castes accounted for the highest number of households, while STs had the lowest (8.0%). Kerosene accounted for the least-used source of fuel in all the categories (less than 1%).

Table 8 provides a breakdown of the most commonly used fuel for cooking based on migration status, including non-migrants, current migrants, and return migrants. About 70.0% of the non-migrant households rely on wood as a major source of cooking fuel. Whereas, this accounts for an even higher proportion when it comes to current migrants (72.6%) and return migrants (82.3%). Electricity is more common as a source for non-migrants (6.5%) than the current or return migrants. LPG has the highest number of user households under the current migrant category (24.0%), followed by non-migrants and return migrants. Kerosene, on the other hand, is the least consumed fuel among all categories (less than 0.5%) (Table 8).

3.3 *Drinking Water*

Odisha has extensive water bodies with lakes like Chilika and Ansupa, rivers including the Mahanadi, Baitarani, Brahmani, Salandi, Subarnarekha, etc., as well

Table 8 Primary fuel source for cooking by residential status (% of households)

	Wood	Electricity	Kerosene	LPG	Others	Total
Non-migrants	70.0	6.5	0.5	22.9	0.1	100.0
Current migrants	72.6	3.0	0.5	23.9	0.0	100.0
Return migrants	82.3	5.4	0.0	12.3	0.0	100.0
Total	71.0	5.9	0.5	22.5	0.1	100.0

Source Odisha migration survey 2023, Household sample

as numerous rivulets, as its source of water. However, due to industrial development, many water bodies are polluted. A recent study in 15 districts of Odisha found that 40% of the households lack access to safe drinking water (Atmashakti Trust, 2024). To analyze this scenario in detail, the OMS 2023 inquired regarding the primary source of drinking water in survey households.

The survey classified the known sources of drinking water into six categories: (i) piped into dwelling, (ii) piped into plot/yard, (iii) own hand pump or own well, (iv) community tap or community tank or community hand pump or community well, (v) tanker truck, and (vi) surface water. Above 50% of the households use a community tap or community tank or community hand pump or community well as their primary source of drinking water (Fig. 3). Nearly 19% of the households rely on a source that is piped into either their dwelling or their plot, or yard for drinking water. The least utilized source of drinking water is the tanker truck (0.3%). Only a small percentage of households (2.3%) use natural sources of water for drinking.

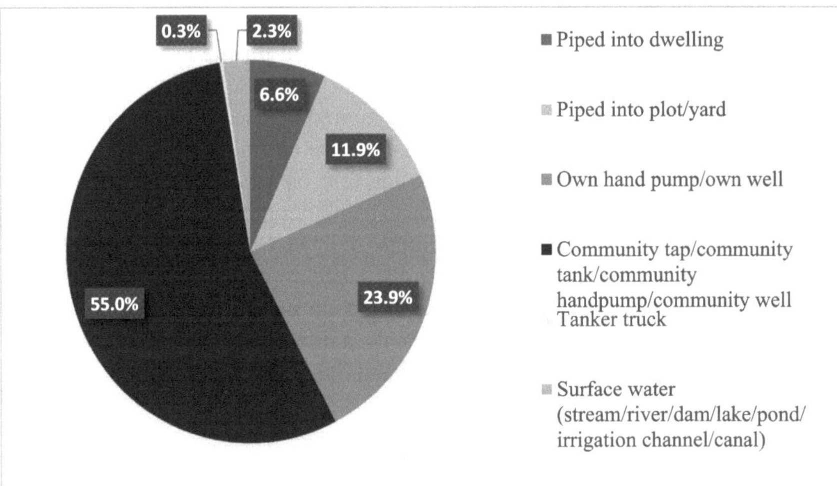

Fig. 3 Primary source of drinking water (% of households). *Source* Odisha migration survey 2023, Household sample

By locality, rural areas rely more (59.1% sample households) on community sources for drinking water—a community tap or community tank or community hand pump or community well—as compared to urban areas (33.9%). 47.5% of urban households have a drinking water source piped into their dwelling or their plot/yard, compared to 12.8% in rural localities. Overall, surface water usage remains low across rural and urban localities. Thus, rural areas rely more on public and community sites to access water, while access in urban areas is predominantly inside private residences.

Disaggregated by social group, reliance on community sources follows a clear caste pattern (Table 10). The STs disproportionately rely on public sources of drinking water, followed by SCs. On the other hand, a majority of upper-caste households use private sources of drinking water. The SC and ST households are more likely to utilize surface water as a source of drinking water when compared to other social groups. Typically, households resort to using surface water for drinking when they are unable to access other safer water sources. This water precarity is disproportionately experienced by ST households, as nearly half of the total households using surface water are ST households.

Regional patterns persist in access to drinking water (Table 11). Sample households in the relatively better-off coastal region are more likely to rely on private sources of water, while the poorer northern region and the most deprived southern region are more likely to rely on community and public sources of water. Households in the southern region also have a greater likelihood of using surface water, the most precarious source of drinking water (Table 11).

By migration status, current migrant households (32.7%) rely more on their hand pumps or wells compared to non-migrants (22.1%) and return migrants (15.7%) (Table 12). Drinking water source "piped into dwelling or into plot/yard" has been utilized widely by the non-migrant households (nearly 20%). The return migrant households are the worst-off when it comes to the source of drinking water; they mostly utilize the community sources as their primary source of drinking water (Table 12).

Table 9 Primary source of drinking water by locality (% of households)

	Piped into dwelling	Piped into plot/yard	Own hand pump/own well	Community tap/ community tank/community handpump/ community well	Tanker truck	Surface water	Total
Rural	5.1	7.8	25.4	59.1	0.3	2.3	100.0
Urban	14.8	32.7	16.4	33.9	0.0	2.2	100.0
Total	6.6	11.9	23.9	55.0	0.3	2.3	100.0

Source Odisha migration survey 2023, Household sample

Table 10 Primary source of drinking water by social group (% of households)

	Piped into dwelling	Piped into plot/yard	Own hand pump/own well	Community tap/ community tank/ community handpump/ community well	Tanker truck	Surface water	Total
Scheduled caste	6.9	9.6	22.2	58.2	0.2	2.9	100.0
Scheduled tribe	3.1	8.7	7.6	76.2	0.2	4.2	100.0
Other backward class	7.2	14.0	28.0	48.8	0.4	1.6	100.0
Upper caste	10.1	13.9	39.5	35.6	0.4	0.5	100.0
Total	6.6	11.9	23.9	55.0	0.3	2.3	100.0

Source Odisha migration survey 2023, Household sample

Table 11 Primary source of drinking water by region (% of households)

	Piped into dwelling	Piped into plot/ yard	Own hand pump/own well	Community tap/ community tank/ community handpump/ community well	Tanker truck	Surface water	Total
Coastal/ Central	8.3	10.8	35.6	44.9	0.1	0.3	100.0
Southern	4.7	17.3	12.3	58.9	0.2	6.6	100.0
Northern	5.7	8.9	17.6	65.9	0.6	1.3	100.0
Total	6.6	11.9	23.9	55.0	0.3	2.3	100.0

Source Odisha migration survey 2023, Household sample

3.4 Sanitation and Toilet Facilities

Facilitating hygienic and basic sanitation facilities is an essential social development goal. Provision of clean drinking water and clean sanitation facilities come under the United Nations Sustainable Development Goals (Goal number six). Odisha was declared Open Defecation Free in 2019 and adopted rural and urban sanitation policies in 2020 and 2024, respectively. Both policies aim to not only improve sanitation but also make it inclusive (Government of Odisha, 2020; Government of Odisha,

Table 12 Primary source of drinking water by migration status (% of households)

	Piped into dwelling	Piped into plot/yard	Own hand pump/own well	Community tap/community tank/community handpump/community well	Tanker truck	Surface water	Total
Resident	7.0	12.7	22.4	55.0	0.3	2.6	100.0
Current migrant	4.9	10.0	32.9	50.7	0.4	1.1	100.0
Return migrant	5.0	5.8	15.8	71.2	0.0	2.2	100.0
Total	6.6	11.9	23.9	55.0	0.3	2.3	100.0

Source Odisha migration survey 2023, Household sample

2024). To understand the scenario on the ground, the OMS inquired about the toilet facilities in the household.

The survey classified the type of toilet facilities into nine categories: (i) flush to piped sewer system, (ii) flush to septic tank, (iii) flush/pour flush to pit latrine, (iv) flush/pour flush to elsewhere, (v) ventilated improved pit latrine, (vi) composting toilet, (vii) pit latrine with slab, (viii) pit latrine without slab, and (ix) no facilities/bush/field. Survey results show that nearly 30% of the households had no facilities of sanitation. The least-used type of facility is the flush to piped sewer system. More than 20% of the households utilize pit latrines, and more than 15% utilize flush or pour flush type of toilets (Fig. 4).

By location, flush to septic tank (30.7%) for private sanitation is the most common sanitation facility reported by urban households, while the least utilized facility is the pit latrine without slab (3.7%). But it is a contrasting scenario in the case of the rural households, where nearly one-third—a substantial proportion of rural households—did not have any toilet facility and reported using open fields and bushes for sanitation (Table 13).

Disaggregated by social group, survey results show that SC and ST groups account for the majority of the households using bushes and open spaces as an avenue for private sanitation. In contrast, the incidence of open defecation was lower among upper castes and OBCs. The use of flush to piped sewer system was low across all social groups. A feasible and reasonably hygienic sanitation option of flush to septic tank facility was found to be higher, but with significant variations across social groups—the highest among the upper castes, followed by the OBC, SC, and ST households (Table 14). The SC and ST households lacked adequate sanitation facilities, while the upper-caste and OBC households had relatively better access to hygienic and adequate sanitation facilities. By district, Bhadrak, Khordha, and

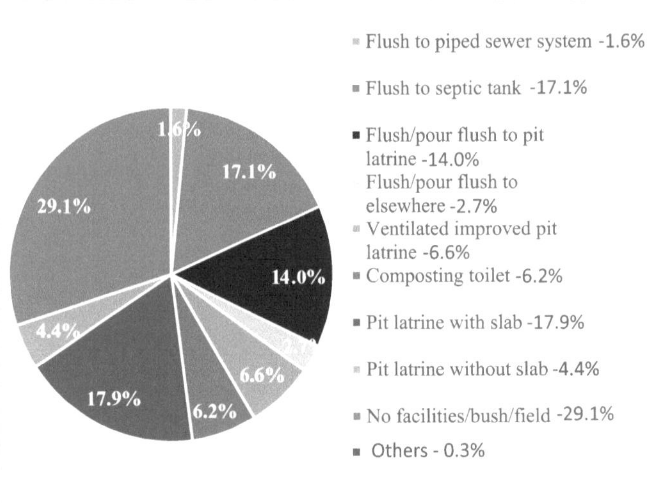

Fig. 4 Type of toilet facility (% of households). *Source* Odisha migration survey 2023, Household sample

Baleshwar—at 8%, 8%, and 4%, respectively—have the lowest rates of open defecation. In contrast, Nuapada, Boudh, and Rayagada have the highest rates of open defecation at 84%, 76%, and 73%, respectively.

A basic overview across current migrant, return migrant, and non-migrant households shows that current migrant households have better sanitation facilities than the other household categories. Their likelihood of open defecation was the lowest, and these households had better toilet facilities compared to other households across all types of toilet facilities other than composting toilets. Interestingly, non-migrant households are better-off than return migrant households in terms of sanitation facilities. This may be the case as return migrant households include the most precarious streams of short-term and seasonal migrants that are among the poorest households. It could also be due to a lack of remittances post-return, which stunts their income, which could be a reason affecting their household's development (Table 15).

3.5 *Government Schemes and Programs*

Government programs in food security, health, and employment play a critical role in enhancing development outcomes, particularly among poor and marginalized households. To access some state entitlements—and schemes—a plethora of official documents may be required at the individual and household levels. In this section, we gauge the participation of sample households in key development programs operational in Odisha.

Table 13 Type of toilet facility by location (% of households)

	Flush to piped sewer system	Flush to septic tank	Flush/pour flush to pit latrine	Flush/pour flush to elsewhere	Ventilated improved pit latrine	Composting toilet	Pit latrine with slab	Pit latrine without slab	No facilities/ bush/ field	Others	Total
Rural	1.1	14.5	14.6	3.1	6.7	6.5	17.3	4.6	31.4	0.3	100.0
Urban	4.2	30.7	11.0	1.0	5.8	5.0	21.0	3.9	17.6	0.0	100.0
Total	1.6	17.1	14.0	2.7	6.6	6.2	17.9	4.4	29.1	0.3	100.0

Source Odisha migration survey 2023, Household sample

Table 14 Type of toilet facility by social group (% of households)

	Flush to piped sewer system	Flush to septic tank	Flush/ pour flush to pit latrine	Flush/pour flush to elsewhere	Ventilated improved pit latrine	Composting toilet	Pit latrine with slab	Pit latrine without slab	No facilities/ bush/ field	Others	Total
Scheduled caste	0.7	13.8	12.5	2.1	5.1	3.5	17.0	6.1	39.1	0.2	100.0
Scheduled tribe	0.6	5.2	14.0	2.8	5.1	13.7	10.1	5.1	43.1	0.4	100.0
Other backward class	1.8	20.5	13.5	3.2	7.6	4.2	20.4	4.2	24.3	0.2	100.0
Upper caste	3.5	29.8	17.0	1.9	7.7	3.5	24.3	2.3	9.7	0.4	100.0
Total	1.6	17.1	14.0	2.7	6.6	6.2	17.9	4.4	29.1	0.3	100.0

Source Odisha migration survey 2023, Household sample

Table 15 Type of toilet facility by residential status (% of households)

	Flush to piped sewer system	Flush to septic tank	Flush/pour flush to pit latrine	Flush/pour flush to elsewhere	Ventilated improved pit latrine	Composting toilet	Pit latrine with slab	Pit latrine without slab	No facilities/ bush/ field	Others	Total
Non-migrants	1.6	16.1	13.4	3.0	6.4	7.1	18.0	4.6	29.5	0.3	100.0
Current migrants	1.6	22.7	17.1	2.0	7.7	2.6	18.4	3.5	24.2	0.2	100.0
Return migrants	1.2	14.2	12.3	0.3	5.7	5.3	14.2	5.0	41.8	0.0	100.0
Total	1.6	17.1	14.0	2.7	6.6	6.2	17.9	4.4	29.1	0.3	100.0

Source Odisha migration survey 2023, Household sample

It can be seen in Table 16 that nearly all households have at least one member with a voter identification (ID) card issued by the Election Commission of India. The prevalence of the voter ID card is higher in rural areas (98.8%) compared to urban areas (97.8%). Interestingly, the penetration of Aadhaar is even higher than that of the Voter ID card in survey households. Aadhaar, a 12-digit individual identification number issued by the Unique Identification Authority of India on behalf of the Government of India (GOI), albeit being voluntary, is required to access most government schemes and programs. Its reach was all-pervasive in both rural and urban areas, across social groups, and across regions.

The Permanent Account Number (PAN) card, on the other hand, issued by the Income Tax Department, is necessary to file income tax returns, and its number needs to be reported in case of large financial transactions. While more than two-thirds of the sample households had member(s) with the PAN card, its ownership varied substantially by location, social group, region, and migration status. As expected, households in the urban areas (78.5%), coastal region (70.8%), and upper-caste (81.4%) and current migrant households (79.2%) were more likely to report ownership of PAN card while households in the rural areas (64.9%), northern region (62.2%), STs (54.3%), and return migrant households (60.4%) were less likely to do so.

The ration card facilitates access to entitlements through the PDS and is critical in ensuring food security. Survey results show that nearly nine in 10 households had a ration card. This is discussed in detail, along with the MGNREGA, in the next subsection.

In August 2021, the GOI launched the e-Shram registration portal to create a national database of unorganized workers to be seeded to Aadhaar. At the time of the survey in 2023, nearly 60% of the households had members who had registered in the e-Shram portal. This is indeed quite high. Households in the backward southern region (63.5%), rural localities (64.1%), SC (62.4%), ST (61.2%), and return migrant households (75.3%) were more likely to have registered under e-Shram than households in the better-off coastal regions (55.7%), resident households (57.6%), upper-caste households (54.6%), and urban households (38.6%).

The Prime Minister Employment Generation Programme is a credit-linked subsidy scheme launched in 2008 under the Ministry of Micro, Small, and Medium Enterprises. The overall penetration of this program is quite low. Still, households in the more backward southern regions (5.6%), rural areas (4.1%), SC households (5.4%), and resident households (4.2%) are more likely to participate. Nearly 10% of the sample households reported having the "labor card" issued by Odisha's Building and Other Construction Workers Welfare Board. This helps them access several benefits. Ironically, ST household members, who are more likely to work in the building and construction sectors, are least likely to report having a labor card. (5.2%). In contrast, the upper castes, less likely to work in construction, are more likely to own it. Similarly, the more advanced coastal region households (15.8%) have this card, as do current and return migrant households (12.8% and 14.2%, respectively).

Mission Shakti, Odisha government's flagship self-help group (SHG) program for the economic empowerment of women since 2001, has been widely accessed by 45% of survey households. The program's penetration is deeper among households in

Table 16 Ownership of documents for government schemes and programs (% of households)

Election/ voter ID	Aadhar card	Pan card	Ration card	Biju swasthya kalyan yojana card	E-Shram portal registration	MGNREGA (job card)	PM employment generation programme	CM employment generation programme	BOCWWBE*(labor card)	Membership in mission shakti SHG	Membership in SHG	Skill training program
98.7	99.9	67.2	88.1	87.6	59.9	40.5	3.9	1.1	9.8	44.8	13.5	0.6

*Building and other construction workers welfare board enrolment card
Source Odisha migration survey 2023, Household sample

coastal regions, migrant households, and households across all social groups except ST households. This is in line with empirical studies that find that microfinance organizations and microcredit are more likely to reach better-off regions and social groups, rather than the poorest and most marginalized (Kaur, 2016; Datta, 2004). Survey households report a lower incidence in SHG programs other than Mission Shakti; however, participation in other SHG programs is more widely spread across regions and social groups.

Last, participation in skill training programs is very low. That said, members of upper-caste and current migrant households are more likely to participate in such programs. Among these, the Pradhan Mantri Kaushal Vikash Yojana was most widely reported (36.7%), followed by Deen Dayal Upadhyaya Grameen Kaushalya Yojana (34.4%), and Pradhan Mantri Kaushal Kendra (16.7%).

3.6 Public Distribution System

Odisha has a history of food insecurity, hunger, and starvation—that persists despite high economic growth—particularly in the lean agricultural season (Ghosh, 2024). In recent decades, the PDS has played a critical role in improving food security and also contributed to poverty reduction (Sahoo & Nayak, 2023). The survey asked questions about access to the PDS, mediated by ownership of ration cards in sample households.

At the aggregate level, 88.1% of the sample households had ration cards, of which an overwhelming majority of households were in possession of a regular ration card, and about 2% of households had the Antyodaya cards meant for the extremely poor households (Fig. 5).

The upper-caste households were nearly twice as likely to be among the households that did not have a ration card. This was followed by OBC households, while ST and SC households were more likely to have a ration card. In the case of upper-caste households, there may be voluntary exclusion from accessing the PDS entitlement on account of their better-off economic status.

By location, rural households were more likely to have regular or Antyodaya compared to urban households.[2] As expected, the percentage of households without ration cards was significantly higher in the urban areas (23.6%) compared to the rural areas (9.6%).

Regional patterns can be seen in the ownership of ration cards. In the poorest and most deprived southern region, sample households were most likely to have ration cards, and the share of Antyodaya cards was the highest (see Appendix Table 38). Thus, households in the southern region relied most on the PDS entitlements in the state. On the other hand, the more advanced coastal and northern regions had a lower

[2] 88.2% of the rural households had ration cards compared to 75.6% urban households. 2.3% of rural households had the Antyodaya ration card, compared to 0.8% of urban households.

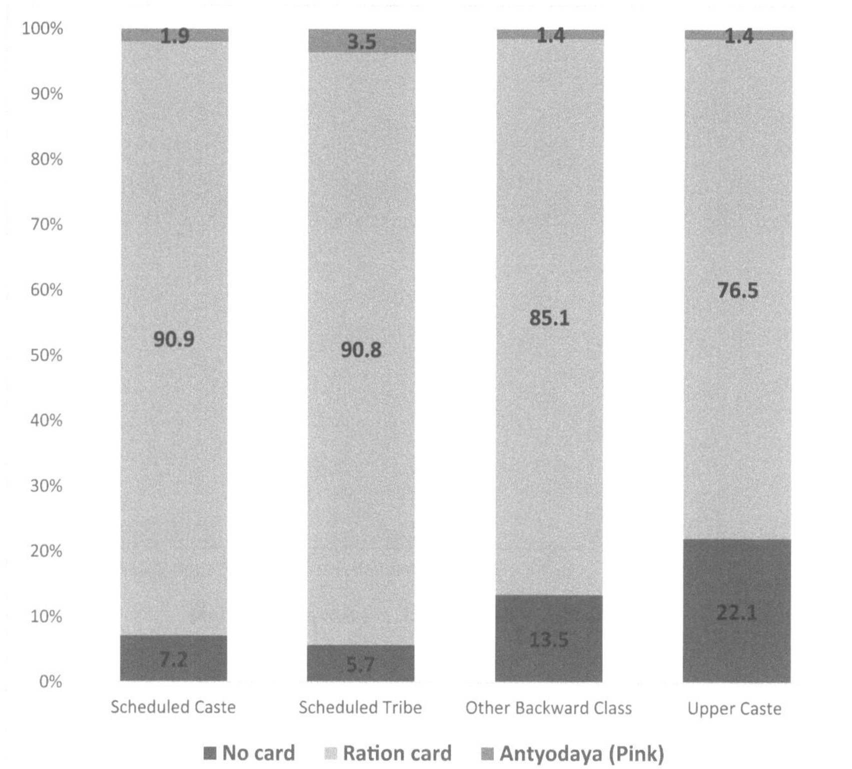

Fig. 5 Distribution of ration cards by social group (% of households). *Source* Odisha migration survey 2023, Household sample

share of households having the Antyodaya card, and a higher share of households choosing not to have ration cards (Appendix Table 39).

By district, sample households in the relatively well-off districts of Khordha (24.1%) and Cuttack (19.3%) in the coastal region, in Jharsuguda (22.9%), Angul (18.2%), and Bargarh (15.8%) districts in the northern region, and Ganjam district (18.6%) in the southern region were most likely not to have ration cards. Ganjam—the district with the highest rate of outmigration from Odisha—is located in the deprived southern region where government schemes generally seem to do well in catering to the poorest and most marginalized social groups and districts. For instance, apart from Ganjam, all other districts in the southern regions had a higher-than-average likelihood of having ration cards.

Ration card status also varies by the migration status of the household. Return migrant households are about twice as more likely to have ration cards compared to resident or current migrant households (Fig. 6). It may be noted that, on account of their definition (see Chap. 1 for details), return migrant households in our survey tend to include seasonal and short-term migrants. This stream of seasonal and short-term

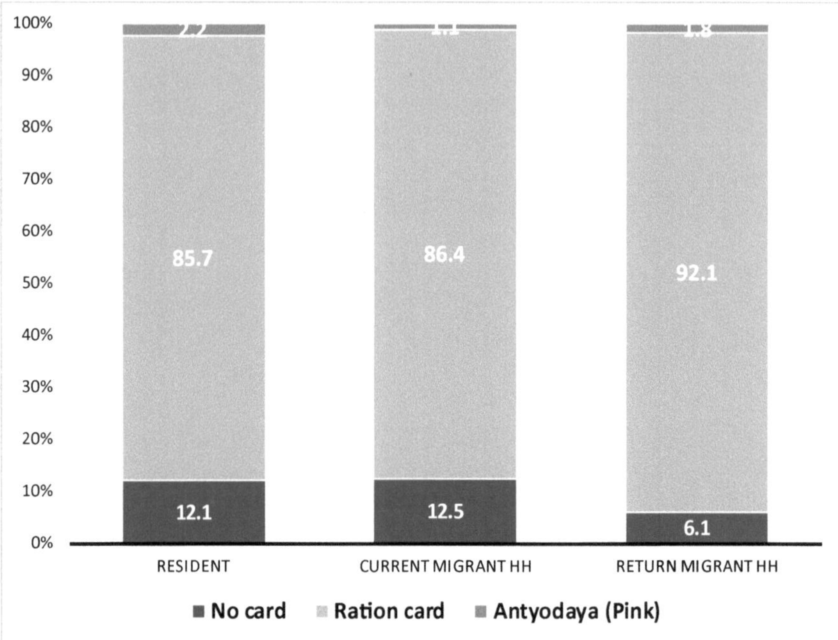

Fig. 6 Distribution of ration cards by migration status (% of households). *Source* Odisha migration survey 2023, Household sample

migrants is particularly vulnerable and deprived and thus relies the most on their PDS entitlements. Return migrant households are also more likely than average to have the Antyodaya card.

3.7 MGNREGA

The Mahatma Gandhi National Rural Employment Guarantee Act, enacted in 2005, is an important rights-based public works program to enhance the livelihood security of poor households in rural India. It is a legal entitlement that operationalizes the right to work by guaranteeing 100 days of employment to members of any rural household willing to do unskilled manual work. It is thus a demand-driven program that ensures the self-selection of households. In the context of this research, it is essential to note that one of the objectives of MGNREGA is to check seasonal distress migration from the rural areas. In Odisha, empirical studies have shown that by providing employment, the MGNREGA is able to improve household incomes and reduce distress migration (Parida, 2016), and rural workers prefer being employed locally through the MGNREGA to long-distance migration (Sahu, 2024).

3.7.1 Households with MGNREGA Job Cards

How does the MGNREGA program fare in rural Odisha? In this section, we examine survey results related to the percentage of households with the MGNREGA cards and the number of days worked in MGNREGA in 2022, disaggregated by social group, district, and region. At the aggregate level, survey results show that 46.9% of the sample households in rural Odisha had an MGNREGA job card. We find that MGNREGA is positively selected for the more deprived ST and SC households, while there is negative selection for the relatively better-off upper-caste and OBC households (Table 17). The higher likelihood of Adivasi households and lower likelihood of upper-caste households demonstrate that the demand-driven self-selection, as envisaged by the program, is in place.

By region, the variation in MGNREGA card ownership is relatively low; sample households in the northern region (50.7%) are more likely to have this card compared to the southern region (46.4%) and the coastal region (44.5%). However, disaggregated by district, we find wide variation. Districts where job card ownership was among the highest included Kandhamal (74.6%), Malkangiri (71.1%), Dhenkanal (68.7%), Nuapada (67.1%), and Gajapati (65.0%), while Ganjam (20.9%), Khordha (24.4%), Boudh (24.6%), and Bargarh (25.9%) reported the lowest incidence of MGNREGA job card ownership.

One of the aims of MGNREGA, as noted earlier, is to check distress migration from the rural areas. It is pertinent to note here that the households with migrants—both return migrants and current migrants—are more likely to have job cards than resident households (Table 18). This shows that households with migrants are interested in MGNREGA work, and we will see in the next section the number of days worked by migrant and non-migrant households in MGNREGA.

Table 17 Households with MGNREGA card and average number of days worked in MGNREGA in 2022 by social group (% of rural households)

Social group	Rural households with MGNREGA card	Average number of days worked	
		Mean	Median
Scheduled caste	48.8	33.1	20
Scheduled tribe	58.0	41.0	25
Other backward class	43.4	36.3	10
Upper caste	35.8	30.8	8
Total	46.9	36.6	16

Source Odisha migration survey 2023, Household sample

Table 18 Households with MGNREGA card and average number of days worked in MGNREGA in 2022 by households with and without migrants (% of rural households)

	Resident households	Households with current migrants	Households with return migrants
Households with MGNREGA job cards	38.1	45.6	61.3
Average number of days worked in MGNREGA in the last 1 year			
Mean	37.4	34.7	35.3
Median	20	14	16

Source Odisha migration survey 2023, Household sample

3.7.2 Number of Days Worked in MGNREGA

The average number of days worked in MGNREGA in 2022 was quite low (Table 18). Survey results show that among the rural households that had the MGNREGA card, about 39% had not worked at all in MGNREGA in the previous year. 5.5% of the households had worked 10 days or less; 31.8% had worked between 11 and 50 days; and 22.8% had worked more than 50 days in MGNREGA in 2022.

Just as with MGNREGA card ownership, clear patterns by social groups can be seen in the number of days worked in MGNREGA in 2022. ST households worked the maximum number of days, while upper-caste households worked the least. By district, the maximum number of days worked under MGNREGA was predominantly in the poorer districts of southern Odisha—Boudh and Kandhamal—while the least number of days were worked in the relatively better-off districts of Puri, Dhenkanal, Jajpur, and Khordha in coastal and southern Odisha.

4 Assets

4.1 Agricultural Assets

Tractor ownership—reported by less than 1% of the survey households—is very low in Odisha. Resident households are more likely to own tractors than migrant households, as are upper-caste and OBC households, compared to SC and ST households. Tractor ownership is more common in the northern region, and by district, Jharsuguda and Malkangiri households report the highest tractor ownership. Interestingly, tractor ownership is higher in urban areas compared to rural areas. This suggests urban–rural linkages and the involvement of urban households in agricultural production. The use of tractors is also likely for urban transportation, from agricultural operations in rural areas.

Ownership of agricultural machinery such as pumpsets, threshers, and tillers is quite low (3.2% households). In line with the results of tractor ownership discussed

Table 18a Agricultural assets, non-agricultural assets, and vehicles (% of households)

Agricultural assets		Non-agricultural assets	Vehicles		
Tractors	Other agricultural assets: pumpsets, threshers, tillers		Mechanized four-wheelers	Mechanized two-wheelers	Bicycles or cycle rickshaws
0.9	3.2	1.1	3.1	49.7	76.2

Source Odisha migration survey 2023, Household sample

above, the northern region is more mechanized, as are resident households. The OBCs, followed by the upper castes, report the highest ownership of agricultural machinery. Unlike tractor ownership, the sample households in the rural areas are more likely to own other agricultural machinery compared to the urban areas (Table 18a).

4.2 Non-agricultural Assets

The ownership of non-agricultural machinery such as flour mills and oil presses is quite low in survey households. In line with the pattern of ownership of agricultural machinery, the northern region, upper-caste, and OBC households are more likely to own non-agricultural machinery. It is interesting to note that in comparison with urban households, rural households are more likely to report ownership of non-agricultural assets. This suggests that there is some diversification in the rural economy through non-agricultural activities in Odisha. In addition, migrant households are more likely to own non-agricultural assets, indicating that migration may play a role in the adoption of non-agricultural activities in rural areas.

4.3 Vehicle and Mobile Phone Ownership

3.1% of the survey households report owning a four-wheeler vehicle. Resident households are more likely to own four-wheelers, and as expected, this incidence is higher in households in the urban areas and in upper-caste households. By district, Jharsuguda and Malkangiri report the highest four-wheeler vehicle ownership. In contrast, two- and three-wheeler vehicle ownership is widespread among survey households. Nearly half the survey households had a two-wheeler or a three-wheeler, its incidence being the highest in the advanced coastal region, followed by the northern and southern regions. Current migrant households, upper-caste and OBC households, and urban households are more likely to have these. By district, Khordha, Subarnapur, and Jharsuguda report the highest ownership of two- and three-wheeler vehicles. Going down the transport asset ladder, we now come to bicycles and cycle rickshaws. The ownership of these is widespread—with three-fourths of the survey households owning bicycles or cycle rickshaws—but there were substantial variations. Here too, migrant households were more likely to have these, as were upper-caste and OBC households. While the difference in ownership by rural and urban areas was negligible, region mattered; in the backward southern region of the state, bicycle and rickshaw ownership was substantially lower than average.

Three-fourths of the households reported owning a basic mobile phone, and nearly 70% households possessed a smartphone. Both types of phones were more likely to be owned by current migrant households and households in the coastal regions. However, the variations by social group and locality were sharper in the case of smartphone ownership compared to basic mobile phones.

4.4 Consumer Durables

More than half of the survey households owned color televisions. Regional patterns persisted, with households in the coastal region reporting the highest ownership, followed by the northern and southern regions. Current migrant households were significantly more likely to own TVs compared to resident households, as were urban households compared to rural households. Again, there was a clear pattern by social group: ST households (29%) were least likely to own color TVs, while upper-caste households (69%) were most likely to do so. Refrigerator ownership was significantly lower than color TV ownership, and the same patterns by region, location, household migration status, and social group persisted. Upper-caste households were six times more likely to own refrigerators than ST households.

The penetration of computers, laptops, and internet connections was quite low (Table 18b). Here, too, there was a clear pattern by locality, social group, and household migration status. Urban households, upper castes, and current migrant households were more likely to have computers, laptops, and internet connections compared to rural households, SC and ST households, and resident households, respectively. Household ownership of consumer durables—air conditioners, washing machines, and microwave ovens—is quite low (Table 18b) and follows a similar pattern mentioned above by region, locality, social group, and household migration status. Radio ownership patterns are somewhat different, with resident households reporting the highest ownership, and by social group, OBC households reported the same, followed by the SC and ST households.

Last, we discuss the household ownership of beds. Lack of a bed—or to sleep on the floor—indicates material hardship at a very fundamental level. While more than 70% of the survey households own beds, households in the southern region (61%), in rural localities (70%), and SC (70%) and ST (52%) groups are less likely to own beds. However, material deprivation is compounded when location, social group, and

Table 18b Ownership of mobile phones, consumer durables, and others (% of households)

Mobile phones		Consumer durables						Others		
Basic mobile phone	Smart phone	Color TV	Refrigerator	Air-conditioner	Washing machine	Computer	Laptop	Internet	Radio	Bed
75.1	69.8	51.3	20.1	2.3	5.8	1.5	3.3	1.3	2.7	72.7

Source Odisha migration survey 2023, Household sample

region intersect; in ST households in rural areas in the southern region, household bed ownership is as low as 46%.

4.5 *COVID-19 Pandemic and Income Levels*

To gauge the impact of COVID-19 on household income, the survey asked what the current household income level was compared to the pre-COVID period. At the time of data collection in the first half of 2023—about 3 years since the pandemic—nearly 70% of the sample households reported that their household income level hadn't changed since the pandemic, about 20% reported a decline in the level of their household income, and 12% reported an increase (Table 19).

Disaggregated by social group, the upper-caste households were most likely to report an increase in household income and least likely to report a decline (Appendix Table 40). On the other hand, ST households were least likely to report an increase in income and most likely to report a decline. SC and OBC households were somewhere in the middle, with the latter being marginally worse. This shows that—caste matters, and—the relatively better-off upper-caste households were less adversely impacted

Table 19 Change in household (HH) income compared to the pre-COVID period by social group and residential status (% of households)

Social group		Change in household income since COVID-19			
	Residential status	Increased	Decreased	Same as before	Total
Scheduled caste	Resident	11.3	13.4	75.2	100
	Current migrant HH	15.6	29.6	54.8	100
	Return migrant HH	10.4	38.8	50.8	100
Scheduled tribe	Resident	5.8	16.6	77.6	100
	Current migrant HH	12.0	34.2	53.8	100
	Return migrant HH	2.4	43.1	54.5	100
Other backward class	Resident	10.8	18.6	70.6	100
	Current migrant HH	16.7	27.6	55.6	100
	Return migrant HH	7.0	38.5	54.5	100
Upper caste	Resident	16.1	15.4	68.5	100
	Current migrant HH	27.3	15.9	56.9	100
	Return migrant HH	16.5	26.2	57.3	100
Total	Resident	10.4	16.7	72.9	100
	Current migrant HH	17.8	26.8	55.4	100
	Return migrant HH	7.7	38.2	54.0	100
	Total	11.6	19.5	68.9	100

Source Odisha migration survey 2023, Household sample

by COVID-19 and could bounce back more quickly than other social groups—particularly the STs, who reported the worst income outcomes among all social groups.

Residential status matters too. Overall, resident households are associated with more stable (and stagnant) incomes, but also a lesser likelihood of increasing or declining household income post-pandemic. Migrant households, on the other hand, are more likely to report more volatility—*both* an increase and a decline in household income. But the type of migration matters; current migration is associated with better income outcomes, while return migration is associated with worse outcomes.

Disaggregated by *social group and residential status* of households, the variations in the change in household income since COVID–19 are even more striking (Table 19). The worst-off have been the ST or Adivasi return migrants, with 43% of households reporting that their income is still below pre-pandemic levels (and only 2% of households report an increase in income). Diametrically opposite to the Adivasi return migrant households are the upper-caste current migrant households that are more than 11 times more likely than the former to report an increase in income and 40% less likely to report a decrease in income.

By region, there was not much variation in the decrease in household income. 20.1% of households in the coastal region reported a decrease, followed by 19.6% in the southern region, and 18.7% in the northern region. However, in terms of reporting an increase in household income, the likelihood of households in the coastal region (15.5%) was far higher than that of the northern (9.3%) and southern regions (7.9%). Thus, it may be reasonable to infer here that the more advanced coastal region has bounced back much better than the other regions.

On the whole, however, the assessment is not quite positive. Even in the coastal districts, nearly two-thirds of the districts reported stagnant incomes since the pandemic. Overall, in 17 of the 30 districts, a greater percentage of households reported income decline compared to an increase in income. Of the households that reported a decline in household income, what was the magnitude of the decline? And what were the reasons for the decline in income? Survey results reveal that the magnitude of decline was quite large. Among sample households where income declined, 33% reported a 0–20% decline; 55% reported a 20–50% decline, and 13% reported a decline of more than 50%. The two main reasons reported for the decline in income were loss of employment and salary cuts by the employer. Again, migration status mattered. Resident households were more likely to experience lower levels of income decline compared to current migrant households (see Appendix Table 41).

5 Land

5.1 Landownership

Land is a marker of socioeconomic status and outcomes. Landownership is closely intertwined with caste, class, and wealth. This section discusses the OMS results related to the ownership of cultivable land, migration, and agriculture.

Table 20 demonstrates the extent of landlessness in Odisha. Nearly 45% of the survey households did not own cultivable land. Even when they own cultivable land, the size of landholding is quite small, as can be seen in the fact that nearly 30% of the households have one acre or less. Those who have between 1–5 acres are not a huge number either; it is only 24% approximately. Landlords, i.e., those owning five acres or more, are less than 2% of the survey households. Thus, we find that landownership is very skewed, and the majority of households are either landless or have small and marginal landholdings.

If this distribution is seen from the lens of caste, the figures present interesting findings (Table 21). SC households have less land compared to ST households in Odisha. As discussed in Chap. 8, among STs, attachment to land is high, and in turn, their rate of migration is relatively lower than SCs in Odisha. There are nearly negligible landholdings among SCs when it comes to land of one acre or less, but in every other category, STs have more land than SCs, and, in some cases, OBC households. For instance, about 30% of SC households have between one and five acres of land, compared to 25.5% of OBC households and 20.5% of upper-caste households.

Among households that own land, the average area of land owned per household is 1.56 acres. STs have more landownership in Odisha among all groups, as can be seen in Table 22. One reason for this may be that STs tend to be concentrated in the Scheduled Areas, which are less densely populated (Gaurav & Mishra, 2016). When we disaggregate landownership by social group and region, we find distinct landownership patterns by region (Table 23).

The above pattern of higher-than-average land size among ST households is found in both the southern and the northern regions, which are also regions where the tribal population is concentrated. In the more developed coastal region, landownership

Table 20 Distribution of survey households by cultivable landownership categories (% of households)

Cultivable landownership	Percentage of households
Landless	44.8
0–1 acres	29.9
1–5 acres	23.8
5+ acres	1.6
Total	100.0

Source Odisha migration survey 2023, Household sample

Table 21 Distribution of survey households by social group and cultivable landownership categories (% of households)

Cultivable landownership	SC	ST	OBC	Upper caste	Total
Landless	54.7	39.8	42.6	46.8	44.8
0–1 acres	29.1	28.9	30.2	31.1	29.9
1–5 acres	15.2	29.5	25.5	20.5	23.8
5+ acres	1.1	1.7	1.6	1.7	1.6
Total (N=15,000)	100.0	100.0	100.0	100.0	100.0

Source Odisha migration survey 2023, Household sample

Table 22 Average landownership size by social group (in acres)

Social group	Average landownership size (in acres)
Scheduled caste	1.24
Scheduled tribe	1.74
Other backward class	1.61
Upper caste	1.43
All households	1.56

Source Odisha migration survey 2023, Household sample

Table 23 Average landownership size by region and social group (in acres)

Regions	Social group	Mean area of land owned
Coastal	Scheduled caste	0.94
	Scheduled tribe	1.25
	Other backward class	1.23
	Upper caste	1.28
Southern	Scheduled caste	1.69
	Scheduled tribe	2.38
	OBC	2.08
	Upper caste	2.10
Northern	Scheduled caste	1.46
	Scheduled tribe	1.58
	Other backward class	1.95
	Upper caste	1.90

Source Odisha migration survey 2023, Household sample

follows a clear caste hierarchy, with the average size of landownership being the highest for the upper castes, followed by the OBCs, STs, and SCs. In the northern region, too, the OBCs and upper castes own larger tracts of land compared to SC and ST households (Table 23).

Table 24 Distribution of survey households by migration status and landownership categories (% of households)

Landownership	Non-migrant	Current migrant	Return migrant	Total
Landless	48.2	34.6	26.3	44.8
0–1 acre	27.2	37.6	45.2	29.9
1–5 acres	23.1	26.1	27.7	23.8
5+ acres	1.6	1.8	0.8	1.6
Total	100.0	100.0	100.0	100.0

Source Odisha migration survey 2023, Household sample

Table 25 Average landownership size by household migration status (in acres)

Migration status	Average landownership size (in acres)
Resident	1.62
Current migrant	1.42
Return migrant	1.35
All households	1.56

Source Odisha migration survey 2023, Household sample

Landownership seems to improve upon migration, as is shown by Table 24. While the landless constitute 48% of the non-migrant households, the number falls to 35% in households with a current migrant. In households where a migrant has returned (after a brief or long stay away), the proportion of landless falls even further, to 26%. Clearly, having a—current or return—migrant in a household is associated with landownership or land acquisition. When it comes to large landholdings, however, the difference between a household with no migrants and one with current or return migrant/s is negligible (Table 25).

Table 25, however, cautions us against assuming such direct links between migration and landownership (or acquisition). The data suggests that those who have more land may not have the push to migrate as much as those who do not have much land.

Does landownership have a spatial dimension? It would appear so, from Table 26. As is well known, coastal areas are well-developed compared to the southern part of Odisha. Landlessness is 50% in the southern and northern districts compared to 37% in the coastal areas. Land inequality is highest in the southern part of Odisha; it is in the southern districts that one sees a higher percentage of households with five or more acres of land.

As can be seen from Table 27 and discussed earlier in Table 23, the average land size is also higher in the southern region due to the same reason (more households with 5+ acres of land).

If we look closely within the regions, southern districts such as Kandhamal, Kalahandi, and Rayagada have average land holding of above two acres (Table 28), even though southern districts see more deprivation. This may be due to the increased presence of ST households in these regions.

Table 26 Distribution of survey households by regions and landownership categories (% of households)

Landownership	Coastal	Northern	Southern	Total
Landless	36.7	50.3	51.0	44.8
0–1 acre	40.4	24.5	19.6	29.9
1–5 acres	21.5	24.0	27.2	23.8
5+ acres	1.4	1.3	2.2	1.6
Total	100.0	100.0	100.0	100.0

Source Odisha migration survey 2023, Household sample

Table 27 Average landownership size by region (in acres)

Region	Average landownership size (in acres)
Coastal	1.19
Southern	2.04
Northern	1.74
All households (in acres)	1.56

Source Odisha migration survey 2023, Household sample

What about gender and landownership? The OMS data shows that female-headed households own less land compared to male-headed households (Table 29). This is in line with empirical evidence in the OMS and elsewhere that female-headed households tend to be more deprived than male-headed households and have relatively worse socioeconomic outcomes (World Bank, 2011).

5.2 *Source of Irrigation*

Agriculture in Odisha is predominantly rainfed, and the OMS data shows that nearly two thirds of the households that owned land reported that their land had no irrigation source and depended on rainfall for irrigation (Table 30). Among households that practiced agriculture on their own land, canal irrigation was the most preferred option.

It is interesting to note that the primary source of irrigation varied by the type of land. In the case of rented in land and sharecropped land, the share of land under canal irrigation was significantly higher. In fact, nearly half of the land under sharecropped land was under canal irrigation. This suggests that tenancy cultivation arrangements may result in higher productivity and output as they are more likely to be under a reliable and assured source of irrigation.

Table 28 Average landownership size by district (in acres)

District	Average landownership size (in acres)
Bargarh	2.28
Jharsuguda	1.88
Sambalpur	1.78
Debagarh	1.98
Sundargarh	1.79
Kendujhar	1.39
Mayurbhanj	1.27
Baleshwar	0.91
Bhadrak	0.99
Kendrapara	2.18
Jagatsinghpur	0.85
Cuttack	0.85
Jajpur	1.37
Dhenkanal	1.49
Angul	1.31
Nayagarh	1.85
Khordha	1.46
Puri	1.03
Ganjam	1.57
Gajapati	1.68
Kandhamal	2.51
Boudh	1.57
Subarnapur	1.86
Balangir	1.71
Nuapada	1.84
Kalahandi	2.50
Rayagada	2.44
Nabarangpur	1.81
Koraput	2.07
Malkangiri	3.13
Total	1.56

Source Odisha migration survey 2023, Household sample

5.3 Crops

Rice is, unsurprisingly, the most widely cultivated crop in Odisha. Monocropping is the common practice, with little diversification (Table 31). Pulses are more likely to be grown in the coastal region, while millets and vegetables are more commonly

Table 29 Average landownership size by sex of household head (in acres)

Household headship	Average landownership size (in acres)
Female-headed households	1.36
Male-headed households	1.59
All households (in acres)	1.56

Source Odisha migration survey 2023, Household sample

Table 30 Source of irrigation by own land, rented in land, and sharecropped land (%)

Irrigation source	Own land	Rented in land	Sharecropped land
Rainfed/no irrigation	65.5	49.8	28.9
Electric tubewell	5.0	12.3	11.3
Diesel tubewell	0.6	0.5	1.6
Canal	22.3	34.5	45.9
Pond/river/stream	1.9	2.1	3.2
Lift irrigation	4.2	0.8	8.8
Others	0.5	0.0	0.4
Total	100.0	100.0	100.0

Source Odisha migration survey 2023, Household sample

grown in the southern region compared to the northern and coastal regions of the state (see Table 32 below).

Table 31 Crops grown by cultivating sample households (% of households)

Crop	% of households
Rice	97.2
Pulses/Legumes	2.3
Vegetables	6.1
Millet	2.5
Others (specify)	1.3

Source Odisha migration survey 2023, Household sample

Table 32 Crops grown by cultivating sample households by region (% of households)

Crop	Coastal	Southern	Northern
Rice	96.5	95.7	99.8
Pulses/Legumes	3.9	1.6	0.1
Vegetables	5.1	12.1	2.0
Millet	0.0	9.7	0.0
Others (specify)	0.2	4.4	0.2

Source Odisha migration survey 2023, Household sample

Table 33 Crops grown by cultivating sample households by social group (% of households)

Crop	SC	ST	OBC	Upper caste
Rice	96.8	97.6	97.1	97.1
Pulses/Legumes	3.7	1.0	1.8	4.8
Vegetables	6.7	6.3	6.1	4.9
Millet	3.7	5.7	0.6	0.0
Others (specify)	1.0	2.5	0.8	0.5

Source Odisha migration survey 2023, Household sample

Table 33 presents survey data related to cropping patterns by social group. Rice cultivation is nearly universal among all social groups. There is not much variation in vegetable cultivation by social group. Millet cultivation is most likely to be undertaken by ST households, followed by SC households. On the other hand, pulses are most likely to be grown by upper-caste households, followed by SC, OBC, and ST households.

5.4 Change in Cropping Pattern

The OMS asked questions about changes in household cropping patterns in the past 5 years. It can be seen in Table 34 that at the aggregate level, while the cropping pattern did not change much, nearly 8% of the households reported a decrease in cultivated area, while 4% reported an increase. By crops, the overall pattern was dominated by rice; the area under pulses and millets changed much less than the average, and the area under vegetable cultivation seems to have both declined and increased disproportionately compared to the average change.

What were the reasons for the change in the cropping pattern? The most important reasons for the decrease in the cultivated area were the lack of labor availability or the reduced supply of labor at the household and village level; about half of the households attributed the decline in the cultivated area to this reason. Apart from

Table 34 Change in cropping pattern in the last 5 years (% of households)

Change in cultivation pattern	Crops					
	Rice	Pulses	Vegetables	Millets	Others	Total
Increased	3.9	0.0	9.6	2.4	1.6	4.1
Decreased	7.5	3.8	16.6	1.6	8.1	7.8
Remained the same	88.6	96.2	73.8	96.0	90.3	88.1
Total	100.0	100.0	100.0	100.0	100.0	100.0

Source Odisha migration survey 2023, Household sample

Table 35 Reasons for decline in cultivated area in the last 5 years (% of households)

Change in cultivation pattern	Crops					
	Rice	Pulses	Vegetables	Millets	Others	Total
Labor-intensive, less labor available in the household	35.3	50.0	76.0	0.0	0.0	40.0
Less labor available for hiring in the village	10.5	25.0	8.0	0.0	0.0	10.1
Incurs high cost of labor	9.6	0.0	0.0	0.0	20.0	8.4
Incurs high cost of material inputs	3.6	0.0	2.0	0.0	0.0	3.3
Owns a smaller area now after selling portion/s of land	3.6	0.0	0.0	50.0	0.0	3.3
Owns a smaller area now after renting out portion/s of land	3.0	0.0	0.0	0.0	0.0	2.5
Low market demand/market price	7.2	0.0	4.0	50.0	0.0	6.8
Not enough knowledge about its cultivation	14.1	0.0	0.0	0.0	20.0	12.2
Others	13.2	25.0	10.0	0.0	60.0	13.4
Total	100.0	100.0	100.0	100.0	100.0	100.0

Source Odisha migration survey 2023, Household sample

this, high costs of labor and material inputs and reduced access to land also emerged as some of the other reasons for the decline in cultivated area.

Why did the area under cultivation for some crops increase? OMS results show that households gaining knowledge about the cultivation of new crops and a high market demand and prices for such crops were the primary reasons for the increase in cultivated area. Less labor intensity also emerged as a reason for the increase in the cultivated area of some crops (Table 36).

Table 36 Reasons for increase in cultivated area in the last 5 years (% of households)

Change in cultivation pattern	Crops					
	Rice	Pulses	Vegetables	Millets	Others	Total
Less labor-intensive	9.7	0.0	20.7	0.0	0.0	11.0
Incurs less cost of labor	2.3	0.0	3.5	0.0	0.0	2.4
Incurs less cost of material inputs	2.8	0.0	0.0	0.0	0.0	2.4
Owns larger area now after buying more land	5.1	0.0	0.0	0.0	0.0	4.3
Owns larger area now after renting in more land	5.1	0.0	0.0	0.0	0.0	4.3
High market demand/market price	34.1	0.0	27.6	33.3	0.0	33.0
Knowledge on its cultivation	40.3	0.0	44.8	66.7	0.0	41.2
To diversify production	0.6	0.0	3.5	0.0	100.0	1.4
Total	100.0	0.0	100.0	100.0	100.0	100.0

Source Odisha migration survey 2023, Household sample

6 Conclusion

This chapter presented key characteristics of survey households focusing on housing, amenities, access to government programs, asset ownership, impact of COVID-19, landownership, and cropping patterns. The chapter found significant variations by social group, region, locality (rural/urban), and migration status. While home ownership was near-universal in Odisha, the quality of housing was a serious concern, as nearly one in two households lived in *kutcha* or *poor* dwellings. Electricity was the most common source of lighting (91%), but relatively less used by rural (90%) and ST households (86%). A majority—71% of households—used wood for cooking; cleaner cooking fuels such as LPG seemed unaffordable and were least accessed by SC and ST households and return migrant households that tended to have seasonal and short-term migrants. For drinking water, 55% of the households used community sources of water such as a community tap, tank, handpump, or well. Again, there was a clear caste pattern—upper-caste and urban households in the relatively better-off coastal region were more likely to rely on private sources of water, while SCs, STs, rural households, and households in the poorer regions of the north and the deprived southern region were more likely to rely on community and public sources of water. What about household-level toilet facilities? Pit latrines of various kinds were most commonly used (42.3%). This was followed by flush to piped sewer/septic tank systems (18.8%), composting toilets (6.6%), and flush or pour flush type of toilets (2.7%). Nearly 30% of the households had no sanitation facilities and practiced open defecation.

Ownership of documents for government schemes and programs varied considerably. Nearly all households had election/voter ID cards (98.7%) and Aadhaar (99.9%). This was followed by the ration card (88.1%) and the popular health scheme—Biju Swasthya Kalyan Yojana—card (87.6%). Nearly 60% of the households had members registered on the e-Shram portal, while the membership in SHG Mission Shakti (44.8%) was relatively lower. At the aggregate level, 88.1% of the sample households had ration cards, of which an overwhelming majority of households were in possession of a regular ration card, and about 2% of households had the *Antyodaya* cards meant for the extremely poor households. In the poorest and most deprived southern region, households were most likely to have ration cards, and the share of *Antyodaya* cards was the highest in this region, thus showing that households in this region relied most on their PDS entitlements. On the other hand, both the more advanced coastal region and the northern region had a lower share of households with *Antyodaya* cards and a higher share of households choosing not to have ration cards.

In the rural areas, 46.9% of households had an MGNREGA job card. MGNREGA was positively selected for the more deprived ST and SC households, while there was negative selection for the relatively better-off upper caste and OBC households. The higher likelihood of Adivasi households and lower likelihood of upper-caste households demonstrated that the demand-driven self-selection mechanism, as envisaged by the program, was in place. The average number of days worked in MGNREGA was quite low; about 39% of households with the card had not worked at all in MGNREGA in the previous year, 5.5% of the households had worked 10 days or less, 31.8% of households had worked between 11 and 50 days, and 22.8% households had worked more than 50 days in MGNREGA in the previous year.

The ownership of agricultural and non-agricultural machinery, such as tractors (0.9%), pumpsets/threshers/tillers or flour mills/oil presses, etc. (1.1%), was quite low. On the other hand, the ownership of vehicles and consumer durables varies substantially; 3.1% of the households had mechanized four-wheeler(s), 49.7% own two-wheeler(s), and 76.2% of households owned bicycles or cycle rickshaws. Mobile phone ownership was widespread (basic mobile phone—75.1%, smartphone—69.8%), and a majority of households owned a color TV (51.3%), while refrigerators (20.1%), washing machines (5.8%), computers (laptop —3.3% and desktop—1.5%), and air conditioners (2.3%) were less commonly owned. Upper-caste households, and households in the urban and coastal regions were better-off in terms of asset ownership compared to the SC and ST households and households in the rural and southern regions.

To gauge the impact of COVID-19 on household income, the survey asked what the current household income level was compared to the pre-COVID period. At the time of data collection in the first half of 2023, about 3 years since the pandemic, nearly 70% of the sample households reported that their household income level hadn't changed since the pandemic. About 20% reported a decline in the level of their household income, and about 12% reported an increase. It is noteworthy that the relatively better-off upper-caste households were less adversely impacted by COVID-19 and could bounce back more quickly than other social groups, particularly the STs, who reported the worst income outcomes among all social groups. Residential status mattered too. Overall, resident households were associated with more stable (and stagnant) incomes, but also a lower likelihood of household income volatility, post-pandemic. Migrant households, on the other hand, were more likely to experience income volatility. But the type of migration mattered; current migration was associated with better income outcomes, while return migration was associated with worse outcomes.

Landownership was highly unequal. Landlessness was widely prevalent; 44.8% households did not own any cultivable land. Three in 10 households owned less than one acre of land, and nearly one quarter owned 1–5 acres of land. The percentage of households with more than five acres of land was less than 2%. SC households were most likely to be landless and had the lowest average landholding. While landlessness was higher among resident households, these households also tended to have larger landholdings, suggesting that ownership of large land size may deter migration. At the same time, a majority of cultivated land was rainfed, with monocultures of rice. Survey households reported a decline in cultivated area in the last 5 years, predominantly due to less labor available *both* within the household as well as in the village. Agriculture and migration are closely intertwined; the agriculture-migration nexus is discussed in Chap. 9.

Appendix

Table 37 Housing quality by migration status (% of households)

Social group	Type of housing					
	Luxurious	Very good	Good	Poor	Kutcha	Total
Resident	2.2	12.4	34.7	28.6	22.3	100.0
Current migrant	5.2	19.7	33.3	23.9	17.8	100.0
Return migrant	1.9	8.7	35	32.8	21.6	100.0
Total	2.7	13.5	34.4	27.9	21.5	100.0

Source Odisha migration survey 2023, Household sample

Table 38 Distribution of regions by ration card (% of households)

‘	No card	Ration card	Antyodaya (Pink)	Total
Coastal	12.2	86.8	1.0	100.0
Southern	10.4	86.4	3.2	100.0
Northern	12.8	84.9	2.4	100.0
Total	11.9	86.1	2	100.0

Source Odisha migration survey 2023, Household sample

Table 39 Distribution of ration cards by region (% of households)

	No card	Ration card	Antyodaya (Pink)	Total
Coastal	44.2	43.5	21.8	43.2
Southern	23.2	26.6	42.1	26.5
Northern	32.6	29.9	36.1	30.4
Total	100.0	100.0	100.0	100.0

Source Odisha migration survey 2023, Household sample

Table 40 Change in household income compared to the pre-COVID period, by social group (% of households)

	Increased	Decreased	Same as before	Total
SC	12.0	17.6	70.4	100.0
ST	6.4	20	73.6	100.0
OBC	11.7	21.3	67.0	100.0
Upper caste	18.6	15.8	65.5	100.0
Total	11.6	19.5	68.9	100.0

Source Odisha migration survey 2023, Household sample

Table 41 Magnitude of decline in income by household (HH) migration status (% of households)

	0–20%	20–50%	More than 50%	Total
Resident HH	34.3	55.6	10.1	100.0
HH with current migrants	27.2	51.2	21.5	100.0
Total	32.6	54.6	12.8	100.0

Source Odisha migration survey 2023, Household sample

References

Atmashakti Trust. (2024). A study on the status of safe drinking water in tribal areas of Odisha. *Atmashakti trust, Shramajeebee mancha and mahila shramajeebee mancha.*

Datta, D. (2004). Microcredit in rural Bangladesh: Is it reaching the poorest? *Journal of Microfinance, 6*(1), 55–81.

Gaurav, S., & Mishra, S. (2016). Land ownership and tenancy in Odisha. In P. B. Nayak, S. C. Panda, & P. K. Pattanaik (Eds.), *The economy of Odisha* (pp. 54–86). Oxford University Press.

Ghosh, R. (2024). Hunger, food insecurity deepen in an Adivasi Odisha village, as govt schemes for work, nutrition fail. *Article 14. https://tribe.article-14.com/post/hunger-food-insecurity-deepen-in-an-adivasi-odisha-village-as-govt-schemes-for-work-nutrition-fail--67687592d2159*

Government of Odisha. (2020). *Odisha rural sanitation policy.* Panchayati Raj and Drinking Water Department, Government of Odisha.

Government of Odisha (2021). *Annual Activity Report 2020-2021.* Energy Department, Government of Odisha.

Government of Odisha. (2024). *Odisha urban sanitation policy.* Department of Housing and Urban Development, Government of Odisha.

Kaur, P. (2016). Efficiency of microfinance institutions in India: Are they reaching the poorest of the poor? *Vision, 20*(1), 54–65.

Parida, J. K. (2016). MGNREGS, distress migration and livelihood conditions: A study in Odisha. *Journal of Social and Economic Development, 18*, 17–39.

Sahoo, P., & Nayak, R. K. (2023). Impact of public distribution system on poverty in Odisha. *Economic and Political Weekly, 58*(1) *https://www.epw.in/sites/default/files/engage_pdf/2023/01/06/2524-1672985463.pdf*

Sahu, G. (2024). *Response of mahatma Gandhi National Rural Employment Guarantee Scheme in vulnerability reduction in the context of Covid-19: A study in migration hotspot districts of Odisha*. Institute for Social and Economic Change.

World Bank. (2011). *World development report 2012: Gender equality and development*. World Bank.

Chapter 3
The Migration Story—I

S. Irudaya Rajan, Amrita Datta, and Sunitha S.

Abstract Based on results from the Odisha Migration Survey (OMS), this chapter estimates migration from Odisha and presents its key characteristics. It estimates 2.98 million current migrants and 0.77 million return migrants from Odisha. The chapter finds that 17.1% of households had at least one current migrant, and 4.5% of households had at least one return migrant. Migration was masculinized, and out-migration to other states within India was the dominant form of migration from Odisha. Ganjam and Baleshwar were the largest migrant-sending districts to other states, and the predominant migration corridors were Ganjam–Gujarat, Baleshwar–Tamil Nadu, Bhadrak–Karnataka, and Balangir–Andhra Pradesh/Telangana. The chapter finds that migration patterns varied significantly by region and social group. Rural–urban and urban-urban migration was predominant from the relatively prosperous central or coastal region, while the more precarious rural-rural migration stream was the highest among Scheduled Caste (Dalit) and Scheduled Tribe (Adivasi) community households compared to the Other Backward Classes (OBCs) and upper caste groups. The chapter suggests that the *type of migration* mattered; while well-off households with more educated members benefited more from migration, poor, and marginalized households with scarce resources used migration as a livelihood strategy for their survival.

Keywords Migration estimates · Migration patterns · Odisha Migration Survey

---

S. I. Rajan (✉) · Sunitha S.
The International Institute of Migration and Development, Thiruvananthapuram, India
e-mail: rajan@iimad.org

A. Datta
Indian Institute of Technology, Hyderabad, India
e-mail: amritadatta@la.iith.ac.in

A. Datta and S. I. Rajan (eds.), *Migration, Livelihoods and Gender*, International Perspectives on Migration, https://doi.org/10.1007/978-981-95-5465-2_3

1 Introduction

This chapter is involved in the estimation of migration. It first presents district-wise estimates of current and return migrants from Odisha, followed by the characteristics of migrant households. The chapter then discusses migration streams, destinations, work, and occupations, before and after migration, sources of information on migration, reasons for migration, and reasons for return. In doing so, we examine the impact of migration in Odisha and offer a comprehensive exploration of its multifaceted aspects, including the inter-state migration routes. This analysis delves into the diverse economic endeavors undertaken by migrants. Additionally, the chapter aims to gain deeper insights into the variations in migration patterns across different regions, social groups, and wealth quartiles. This inquiry entails an examination of factors such as the drivers behind migration, the preferred destinations, and the socio-economic dynamics prevalent within each region, social group, and wealth quartile.

2 Migration Pattern

The Odisha Migration Survey (OMS) 2023 asked about the migration status of the members of the sample households. Three broad categories can be identified through this study: (i) non-migrants (individual household members who had not migrated), (ii) current migrants (individual household members who were away on migration at the time of the survey), and (iii) return migrants (individual household members who had migrated in the past). Within the current migrant category, further classifications are made based on the purpose of migration: current labor migrants temporarily at home for festivals, current labor migrants temporarily at home for other reasons, current migrants at the destination, migrants for education, and migrants for reasons other than work or education. Return migrants are classified based on the duration of their stay at the destination: return migrant who stayed at the destination for up to 3 months, for 4–6 months, 6–9 months, 9–12 months, for more than 12 months, and migrant who returned home due to the unavailability of work is also considered a return migrant (Table 1). The migration status question thus covers the duration of residence and the place of last residence.

As noted in Chap. 1, official data sources such as the census and NSSO—albeit dated—report a consistent upward trend in out-migration rates from Odisha. This phenomenon can be attributed to a range of factors, including agricultural challenges, economic prospects, societal influences, and social networks that drive migration. Compared to all-India figures, Odisha is overrepresented in short-term and seasonal migration streams, and migration is predominantly a coping mechanism during the lean agricultural season (Mishra, 2020; NSSO, 2010). In recent years, the agriculture sector in the state has been characterized by low employment growth, while employment growth in the manufacturing sector has been negative. Simultaneously,

Table 1 Migration status of individual household members, OMS 2023

Migration status	Number	Percent
Resident	53,823	92.6
Current migrant labor temporarily at home for festival	283	0.5
Current migrant labor temporarily at home for other reasons	289	0.5
Current labor migrant and present at work destination	2,504	4.3
Return labor migrant (last episode duration up to 3 months)	193	0.3
Return labor migrant (last episode duration 4–6 months)	126	0.2
Return labor migrant (last episode duration 7–9 months)	33	0.1
Return labor migrant (last episode duration 10–12 months)	45	0.1
Return labor migrant (last episode duration more than 12 months)	488	0.8
Spouse of current migrant	78	0.1
Child of current migrant	89	0.2
Migrated for studies	159	0.3
Migration other than employment and education	26	0.0
Total	**58,136**	**100.0**
Non-migrant	53,893	92.7
Current migrant	3,358	5.8
Return migrant	885	1.5
Total	**58,136**	**100.0**

Source Odisha Migration Survey 2023, household sample

agricultural output has been adversely impacted by climate change (Mishra et al., 2016; Panda & Padhi, 2021). It is in this broad context of rural distress that migration from the state is understood to have been on the rise, and in 2018, the Government of Odisha identified 11 of the state's 30 districts as migration-prone.[1]

3 Migration Estimation

For the estimation of migration, the study broadly focused on two main migration types: current migration and return migration. In each category, there were subcategories based on destination, which included: (i) migration within Odisha, i.e., inter-district migration within the state; (ii) migration from Odisha to other states within India, i.e., inter-state migration; and (iii) international migration, i.e., migration from Odisha to foreign countries. Notably, inter-state migration, i.e., migration outside Odisha within India, emerged as the dominant pattern of movement, followed by

[1] The 11 districts include Balangir, Bargarh, Kalahandi, Nuapada, Saharanpur, Ganjam, Gajapati, Rayagada, Koraput, Nabarangpur, and Khordha. A majority of these districts are located in the deprived, tribal-dominated region of southern Odisha.

inter-district migration within Odisha, and international migration, the last category being very limited.

3.1 Methods of Estimating Current and Return Migrants

There are three estimates at different levels for current and return migrants from Odisha, namely: state-level estimates, district-level estimates, and locality-level estimates. These estimates were calculated by using the ratio method of estimation by households and population. The process of estimation was done to calculate the overall number of current migrants, regardless of whether they had moved within the state, outside the state but within India, or outside India altogether. This same approach was used for estimating the total number of return migrants.

3.2 Ratio Methods at Different Levels

The ratio method is a useful approach for estimating the number of migrants at various levels, including the state level, district level, and regional level. One of the simplest applications of this method is to calculate the number of migrants at the state level. Here, the ratio method is applied at the district level based on the respective number of households and population present, where estimates are calculated for each district. Then, the aggregate of these district-level estimates is calculated to obtain a state-level estimate. It is important to note that as the area unit increases, the estimate of state-level migration tends to become smaller. Conversely, when using smaller locality units, such as at the sub-district level, the estimate of migration tends to be a larger figure compared to the state-level estimate.

Here, estimations at both the household and population levels were performed. Since OMS is a household-level survey, it provides more accuracy when estimating household-based migration.

Estimation Based on Household and Population

$$\begin{aligned}\text{Current migrants in a district of Odisha} = {} & (\text{No. of current migrants in a district})/\\ & \text{Sample households for OMS2023}\\ & * \text{total no. of households in Odisha Estimated to2023})\end{aligned}$$

$$\text{Current migrants in Odisha} = \text{Sum of current migrants in all the districts}$$

A similar method can be applied to estimate the return migrants.

The estimation of current and return migrants in Odisha based on population can be employed by substituting "sample households" with "sample population" and replacing "total number of households in Odisha" with "total population of Odisha." This approach is used for the specific purpose of comparing and selecting a more accurate estimation.

The OMS estimates 2.92 million current migrants and 0.78 million return migrants in Odisha (Table 2). The districts of Ganjam, Cuttack, and Balasore have the highest number of estimated current migrants. Migrants from Ganjam and Balasore largely reside in other states in India, while most of the migrants from Cuttack moved within Odisha itself. Districts with the next least number of migrants are Jharsuguda, Gajapati, and Nabarangpur (Table 3). Return migration in Odisha is highest in Balangir district, with a large proportion of migrants returning from other states. Cuttack and Nuapada are the next districts with the highest number of return migrants (Table 4).

An examination of regional patterns revealed that the central or coastal division holds the predominant share of migration movements outside Odisha, within India, with the southern division coming next, and the northern region being the last in line (Table 5). While a majority of the migrants in the coastal and southern divisions are migrants outside Odisha, the majority of migration in the northern division occurs within Odisha. The southern and northern divisions have comparatively fewer migrants compared to the coastal/central regions. Among the return migrants, the coastal region has the highest number of returnees, followed by the northern and southern regions, respectively. In the northern division, a majority of individuals returned from other states within India, as compared to other regional divisions. There is a higher proportion of return migrants from within India in the northern division compared to the coastal and southern divisions.

4 Top 10 Migration Districts

According to data from the Government of Odisha, certain districts, namely, Balangir, Bargarh, Kalahandi, Nuapada, Saharanpur, Ganjam, Gajapati, Rayagada, Koraput, Nabarangpur, and Khordha, were identified as migration-prone districts. However, the OMS 2023, conducted in the post-pandemic period, has produced contrasting results, revealing a different set of top 10 districts in terms of estimates of *both* current and return migrants. It is noteworthy that only three districts (Ganjam, Nuapada, and Balangir) from the government's list align with the OMS, in terms of the share of households with migrants, and it is only two districts (Ganjam and Balangir) when we take migrant estimates into account.

Ganjam district is the source of the highest concentration of current migrants, with a total of 2,84,342 individuals residing in various states within India (Table 6). Internal migration within the state of Odisha reveals a significant population moving within the Cuttack district. This phenomenon is primarily attributed to the bustling urban center of Cuttack, often referred to as the "Millennium City," which experiences a notable demand for labor, particularly in sectors such as construction, domestic services, and transportation. Furthermore, its strategic proximity to the state capital,

Table 2 District-level estimates of current and return migration in Odisha, 2023; based on households (HH) and population (Pop)

Districts	Estimation based on household				Estimation based on population			
	Sample HH	HH 2023 (projected)	Estimated current migrants	Estimated return migrants	Sample pop	Pop (projected)	Estimated current migrants	Estimated return migrants
Bargarh	570	4,95,638	25,217	0	2,007	16,61,122	24,002	0
Jharsuguda	240	1,85,449	0	0	732	6,75,977	0	0
Sambalpur	360	3,26,468	28,113	1,814	1,335	11,83,496	27,482	1,774
Debagarh	240	1,05,333	23,700	3,072	632	3,65,785	31,254	4,051
Sundargarh	750	6,08,972	43,846	7,308	2,881	24,59,003	46,090	7,682
Kendujhar	600	5,28,704	1,10,147	5,287	2,238	21,38,478	1,19,441	5,734
Mayurbhanj	870	7,69,613	1,28,269	46,000	3,077	29,27,842	1,37,971	49,480
Balasore[2]	840	7,67,906	2,80,651	38,395	3,260	27,33,432	2,57,412	35,216
Bhadrak	480	4,23,273	2,53,082	7,936	2,289	1,743,170	2,18,563	6,854
Kendrapara	510	3,97,757	91,250	58,494	1,911	16,25,930	99,547	63,812
Jagatsinghpur	420	3,22,106	22,241	1,534	1,492	12,40,077	24,103	1,662
Cuttack	870	7,63,069	3,05,228	1,05,251	3,864	30,10,156	2,71,101	93,483
Jajpur	600	5,39,906	2,04,264	2,700	2,718	21,04,325	1,75,747	2,322
Dhenkanal	450	3,75,975	1,83,810	43,446	1,924	13,63,702	1,55,933	36,857
Angul	450	4,15,252	98,738	4,614	1,883	14,55,295	82,696	3,865
Nayagarh	360	3,16,950	1,17,976	7,924	1,361	10,95,572	1,07,867	7,245
Khordha	780	6,99,248	92,337	20,619	3,190	28,00,562	90,426	20,192
Puri	570	5,04,264	79,621	9,731	1,911	19,68,036	92,686	11,328
Ganjam	1,050	9,24,332	3,73,254	64,263	4,048	40,28,217	4,21,928	72,643
Gajapati	240	1,52,832	8,278	0	982	6,57,509	8,704	0

(continued)

[2] [illegible]

Table 2 (continued)

Districts	Estimation based on household				Estimation based on population			
	Sample HH	HH 2023 (projected)	Estimated current migrants	Estimated return migrants	Sample pop	Pop (projected)	Estimated current migrants	Estimated return migrants
Kandhamal	270	2,10,543	24,953	6,238	1,046	8,49,807	25,998	6,500
Boudh	240	1,45,990	12,166	3,041	901	5,38,947	11,963	2,990
Subarnapur	240	2,16,233	28,831	12,614	848	7,03,675	26,554	11,617
Balangir	600	6,13,257	1,86,021	1,84,999	2,395	21,20,559	1,61,145	1,60,259
Nuapada	240	1,98,999	61,358	72,137	1,083	7,21,962	49,331	57,997
Kalahandi	600	5,27,714	55,410	23,747	2,099	19,24,775	57,771	24,759
Rayagada	360	2,78,181	26,273	2,318	1,527	11,62,113	25,875	2,283
Nabarangpur	420	3,41,843	11,395	11,395	1,457	15,04,784	14,459	14,459
Koraput	540	4,14,224	27,615	16,109	2,093	16,63,221	28,608	16,688
Malkangiri	240	1,81,293	20,395	18,885	952	7,75,516	21,995	20,365
Odisha	**15,000**	**1,27,51,324**	**29,24,437**	**7,79,870**	**58,136**	**4,92,03,045**	**28,16,652**	**7,42,117**

Source Estimated from Odisha Migration Survey 2023, household sample

Table 3 District-level estimates of current migration by destination type, ratio method, OMS 2023

Districts	Estimation based on household				Estimation based on population			
	Within Odisha	Outside Odisha, within India	Outside India	Total	Within Odisha	Outside Odisha, within India	Outside India	Total
Bargarh	5,217	19,999	0	25,217	4,966	19,036	0	24,002
Jharsuguda	0	0	0	0	0	0	0	0
Sambalpur	12,696	15,417	0	28,113	12,411	15,071	0	27,482
Debagarh	22,822	878	0	23,700	30,096	1,158	0	31,254
Sundargarh	24,359	19,487	0	43,846	25,606	20,485	0	46,090
Kendujhar	80,187	29,960	0	1,10,147	86,953	32,488	0	1,19,441
Mayurbhanj	76,961	51,308	0	1,28,269	82,783	55,188	0	1,37,971
Balasore	52,108	2,26,715	1,828	2,80,651	47,793	2,07,942	1,677	2,57,412
Bhadrak	31,745	2,20,455	882	2,53,082	27,416	1,90,386	762	2,18,563
Kendrapara	63,173	25,737	2,340	91,250	68,917	28,077	2,552	99,547
Jagatsinghpur	7,669	13,805	767	22,241	8,312	14,961	831	24,103
Cuttack	2,04,362	95,603	5,263	3,05,228	1,81,513	84,914	4,674	2,71,101
Jajpur	84,585	1,17,879	1,800	2,04,264	72,777	1,01,423	1,548	1,75,748
Dhenkanal	1,08,615	75,195	0	1,83,810	92,142	63,791	0	1,55,933
Angul	67,363	30,452	923	98,738	56,419	25,504	773	82,696
Nayagarh	83,640	32,575	1,761	1,17,976	76,473	29,784	1,610	1,07,867
Khordha	26,894	52,892	12,551	92,337	26,338	51,797	12,291	90,426
Puri	15,039	62,812	1,769	79,621	17,507	73,119	2,060	92,686
Ganjam	73,947	2,84,342	14,965	3,73,254	83,589	3,21,421	16,917	4,21,928
Gajapati	3,821	4,458	0	8,278	4,017	4,687	0	8,704

(continued)

Table 3 (continued)

Districts	Estimation based on household				Estimation based on population			
	Within Odisha	Outside Odisha, within India	Outside India	Total	Within Odisha	Outside Odisha, within India	Outside India	Total
Kandhamal	12,477	12,477	0	24,953	12,999	12,999	0	25,998
Boudh	2,433	9,733	0	12,166	2,393	9,571	0	11,963
Subarnapur	13,515	15,317	0	28,831	12,447	14,107	0	26,554
Balangir	35,773	1,50,248	0	1,86,021	30,989	1,30,155	0	1,61,145
Nuapada	5,804	55,554	0	61,358	4,666	44,664	0	49,331
Kalahandi	26,386	29,024	0	55,410	27,510	30,261	0	57,771
Rayagada	3,864	22,409	0	26,273	3,805	22,070	0	25,875
Nabarangpur	4,070	7,325	0	11,395	5,164	9,295	0	14,459
Koraput	10,739	14,575	2,301	27,615	11,125	15,099	2,384	28,608
Malkangiri	9,820	10,575	0	20,395	10,590	11,405	0	21,995
Odisha	**11,70,084**	**17,07,204**	**47,149**	**29,24,437**	**11,27,716**	**16,40,857**	**48,079**	**28,16,652**

Source Estimated from Odisha Migration Survey 2023, household sample

Table 4 District-level estimates of return migration by destination type, ratio method, OMS 2023

Districts	Estimation based on household				Estimation based on population			
	Within Odisha	Outside Odisha, within India	Outside India	Total	Within Odisha	Outside Odisha, within India	Outside India	Total
Bargarh	0	0	0	0	0	0	0	0
Jharsuguda	0	0	0	0	0	0	0	0
Sambalpur	907	907	0	1,814	887	887	0	1,774
Debagarh	3,072	0	0	3,072	4,051	0	0	4,051
Sundargarh	812	6,496	0	7,308	854	6,828	0	7,682
Kendujhar	881	4,406	0	5,287	956	4,778	0	5,734
Mayurbhanj	17,692	28,308	0	46,000	19,030	30,449	0	49,480
Balasore	5,485	32,910	0	38,395	5,031	30,185	0	35,216
Bhadrak	1,764	6,173	0	7,936	1,523	5,331	0	6,854
Kendrapara	25,737	31,197	1,560	58,494	28,077	34,033	1,702	63,812
Jagatsinghpur	0	1,534	0	1,534	0	1,662	0	1,662
Cuttack	44,732	59,642	877	1,05,251	39,730	52,974	779	93,483
Jajpur	900	1,800	0	2,700	774	1,548	0	2,322
Dhenkanal	13,368	30,078	0	43,446	11,341	25,516	0	36,857
Angul	2,768	1,846	0	4,614	2,319	1,546	0	3,865
Nayagarh	3,522	4,402	0	7,924	3,220	4,025	0	7,245
Khordha	896	17,033	2,689	20,619	878	16,680	2,634	20,192
Puri	0	9,731	0	9,731	0	11,328	0	11,328
Ganjam	7,043	53,699	3,521	64,263	7,961	60,702	3,980	72,643
Gajapati	0	0	0	0	0	0	0	0
Kandhamal	1,560	4,679	0	6,238	1,625	4,875	0	6,500
Boudh	1,217	1,825	0	3,041	1,196	1,794	0	2,990
Subarnapur	3,604	9,010	0	12,614	3,319	8,298	0	11,617
Balangir	17,376	1,66,601	1,022	1,84,999	15,052	1,44,322	885	1,60,259
Nuapada	8,292	63,846	0	72,137	6,666	51,331	0	57,997
Kalahandi	5,277	18,470	0	23,747	5,502	19,257	0	24,759
Rayagada	0	2,318	0	2,318	0	2,283	0	2,283
Nabarangpur	3,256	8,139	0	11,395	4,131	10,328	0	14,459
Koraput	3,835	12,273	0	16,109	3,973	12,715	0	16,688
Malkangiri	9,820	9,065	0	18,885	10,590	9,775	0	20,365
Odisha	**1,83,816**	**5,86,388**	**9,669**	**7,79,870**	**1,78,686**	**5,53,450**	**9,980**	**7,42,117**

Source Estimated from Odisha Migration Survey 2023, household sample

Table 5 Estimated current and return migrants by destination type and administrative division[3]

Divisions	Number				Percent			
Current migration estimation based on household								
	Within Odisha	Outside Odisha, within India	Outside India	Total	Within Odisha	Outside Odisha, within India	Outside India	Total
Central/coastal division	6,68,138	11,75,435	42,164	18,85,737	35.4	62.3	2.2	100.0
Southern division	87,123	1,25,892	2,301	2,15,316	40.5	58.5	1.1	100.0
Northern division	4,14,822	4,05,877	2,684	8,23,383	50.4	49.3	0.3	100.0
Total	11,70,084	17,07,204	47,149	29,24,437	40.0	58.4	1.6	100.0
Return migration estimation based on household								
Central/coastal division	99,924	2,43,797	8,648	3,52,369	28.4	69.2	2.5	100.0
Southern division	28,568	65,779	0	94,347	30.3	69.7	0.0	100.0
Northern division	55,322	2,76,811	1,022	3,33,154	16.6	83.1	0.3	100.0
Total	1,83,814	5,86,386	9,670	7,79,870	23.6	75.2	1.2	100.0

Source Estimated from Odisha Migration Survey 2023, household sample

Bhubaneswar, makes it an attractive destination for individuals seeking business opportunities and employment. Dhenkanal emerges as the second-largest district in Odisha in terms of migrant population within Odisha, renowned for its coal and mining industrial zones.

A considerable influx of return migration was observed from within Odisha, primarily to the districts of Cuttack, Kendrapara, Mayurbhanj, and Balangir, all situated in the northeastern region of the state (Table 7). When it comes to return migration from other states in India, Balangir district had the highest numbers, closely followed by Nuapada, Cuttack, and Ganjam. Notably, many districts with substantial return migration from other states were either bordering neighboring states or located in close proximity to the state's border districts. Additionally, the districts of Ganjam, Khordha, Kendrapara, Balangir, and Cuttack stood out for receiving the

[3] **Central/Coastal Division**: Cuttack, Jagatsinghpur, Kendrapara, Jajpur, Balasore, Bhadrak, Puri, Khordha, Nayagarh, and Mayurbhanj; **Southern Division**: Ganjam, Gajapati, Koraput, Nabarangpur, Rayagada, Malkangiri, Kalahandi, Nuapada, Kandhamal, and Boudh districts; **Northern Division**: Sambalpur, Deogarh, Jharsuguda, Bargarh, Balangir, Subarnapur/Sonepur, Sundargarh, Dhenkanal, Angul, and Keonjhar.

Table 6 Top 10 districts by destination type of current migration

Districts	Within Odisha	Districts	Outside Odisha, within India	Districts	Outside India
Cuttack	2,04,362	Ganjam	2,84,342	Ganjam	14,965
Dhenkanal	1,08,615	Balasore	2,26,715	Khordha	12,551
Jajpur	84,585	Bhadrak	2,20,455	Cuttack	5,263
Nayagarh	83,640	Balangir	1,50,248	Kendrapara	2,340
Kendujhar	80,187	Jajpur	1,17,879	Koraput	2,301
Mayurbhanj	76,961	Cuttack	95,603	Balasore	1,828
Ganjam	73,947	Dhenkanal	75,195	Jajpur	1,800
Angul	67,363	Puri	62,812	Puri	1,769
Kendrapara	63,173	Nuapada	55,554	Nayagarh	1,761
Balasore	52,108	Khordha	52,892	Angul	923

Source Estimated from Odisha Migration Survey 2023, household sample

highest influx of return migration from other countries. It's worth mentioning that these five districts share common borders with each other.

Table 7 Top districts by destination type of return migration

Districts	Within Odisha	Districts	Outside Odisha, within India	Districts	Outside India
Cuttack	44,732	Balangir	1,66,601	Ganjam	3,521
Kendrapara	25,737	Nuapada	63,846	Khordha	2,689
Mayurbhanj	17,692	Cuttack	59,642	Kendrapara	1,560
Balangir	17,376	Ganjam	53,699	Balangir	1,022
Dhenkanal	13,368	Balasore	32,910	Cuttack	877
Malkangiri	9,820	Kendrapara	31,197		
Nuapada	8,292	Dhenkanal	30,078		
Ganjam	7,043	Mayurbhanj	28,308		
Balasore	5,485	Kalahandi	18,470		
Kalahandi	5,277	Khordha	17,033		

Source Estimated from Odisha Migration Survey 2023, household sample

5 Types of Migration in the Households of Odisha

The determination of household migration status was established by prioritizing the recording of the presence of *current* migrants within the household, with return migrants being considered subsequently. When a household comprised both types of migration, the categorization was determined by adhering to these priorities.

Table 8 indicates that nearly 8 in 10 households were non-migrant households, and 17.5% of the households reported having migrants currently. Almost 5% were return migrant households. Hence, the majority of the households come under the non-migrant (or resident) category.

When examining households with migrants, it is observed that approximately 13% of these households have only one current migrant, with nearly 4% of these households hosting two or more current migrants (Table 9). On the other hand, 4.6% of households include at least one return migrant. There are instances where a single household accommodates both current and return migrants.

5.1 *Age at First Migration*

The average age at first migration for current migrants stands at 23 years, with females typically migrating at a younger age of 20 years and males at a slightly older age of 24 years. In contrast, return migrants exhibit a slightly higher average age at first migration, which stands at 25 years. This suggests that the average age of migration

Table 8 Migration status of the households, OMS 2023

HH migration status	Percent
Non-migrant HH	77.9
Current migrant HH	17.5
Return migrant HH	4.6
Total	**100.0**

Source Odisha Migration Survey 2023, household sample

Table 9 Households with number of current and return migrants

	Percent		Percent
HH with no current migrants	83.2	HH with no return migrants	93.5
HH with one migrant	13.1	HH with one return migrant	4.6
HH with two or more migrants	3.7	HH with two or more return migrants	1.9
Total	**100.0**	**Total**	**100.0**

Source Odisha Migration Survey 2023, household sample

has declined over time. Among return migrants, females tend to migrate at an average age of 21 years, while males typically migrate at 25 years of age.

5.2 *Change in Place of Residence*

The OMS data shows that migration from rural to urban areas is the predominant migration stream. From Odisha, which is an economically weaker state, people tend to migrate to places with better opportunities. This rural–urban migration is also accompanied by an occupational shift away from agriculture, as discussed later.

There are clear patterns in the type of migration by social group, wealth quartile, and region. Rural–urban migration is highest among the upper castes and lowest among the ST community (Table 10). As per Table 11, the rural–urban migration is predominant in the relatively advanced coastal/central division, accounting for 80% of all migration from this region, and is least predominant in the northern division, where only 56.9% of migration follows the rural–urban pattern.

As figures from Table 12 show, the majority of the rural-rural migrants belong to the lowest wealth quartile, and the majority of the urban-urban migrants belong to the highest wealth quartile. The northern division has the highest occurrence of rural-rural migration, and the central/coastal division has the highest incidence of urban-urban migration, highlighting the relative difference in economic prosperity between the two administrative divisions. It is noteworthy that migrants in the lowest

Table 10 Change in place of residence by social group of current migrants (%)

Social group	Rural-rural	Rural–urban	Urban–rural	Urban-urban	Total
SC	26.0	69.6	0.2	4.2	100.0
ST	26.8	69.3	0.4	3.5	100.0
OBC	17.4	75.0	0.5	7.0	100.0
Upper caste	14.0	75.5	0.4	10.0	100.0
Total	**19.8**	**73.2**	**0.4**	**6.6**	**100.0**

Source Odisha Migration Survey 2023, household sample

Table 11 Change in place of residence by region of current migrants (%)

Division	Rural-rural	Rural–urban	Urban–rural	Urban-urban	Total
Coastal/central	12.4	79.6	0.5	7.5	100.0
Southern	17.0	75.6	0.1	7.3	100.0
Northern	38.7	56.9	0.7	3.8	100.0
Total	**19.8**	**73.2**	**0.4**	**6.6**	**100.0**

Source Odisha Migration Survey 2023, household sample

wealth quintile are overrepresented in the precarious rural-rural migration stream (Table 12).

The most important migration stream from Odisha is to Tamil Nadu (18.8% of all inter-state migrants), followed by Karnataka (15.9%), Gujarat (14.8%), and Andhra Pradesh (14.3%) as seen in Fig. 1. An analysis of inter-state migration shows that the southern states are the most preferred migration destination. This phenomenon can be due to higher wages and socio-economic development among the southern states, making them a preferred destination for employment and migration. Among the top 10 destinations for inter-state migration, six of the preferred destinations are in the southern states, and the remaining are Gujarat, Maharashtra, Delhi, and West Bengal.

The OMS data reveals important migration corridors from districts in Odisha to other states. As Tamil Nadu is the top-most migration destination of migrants from Odisha, a major migration corridor is from Balasore (22.2%). Ganjam district stands out as part of the most significant corridor, accounting for 38% of the total current

Table 12 Change in place of residence by wealth quartile of current migrants (%)

Quartile	Rural-rural	Rural–urban	Urban–rural	Urban-urban	Total
First quartile (lowest)	33.2	65.0	0.2	1.6	100.0
Second quartile	18.8	75.1	0.3	5.8	100.0
Third quartile	14.2	80.6	0.3	4.9	100.0
Fourth quartile	16.7	70.2	0.8	12.3	100.0
Total	**19.8**	**73.2**	**0.4**	**6.6**	**100.0**

Source Odisha Migration Survey 2023, household sample

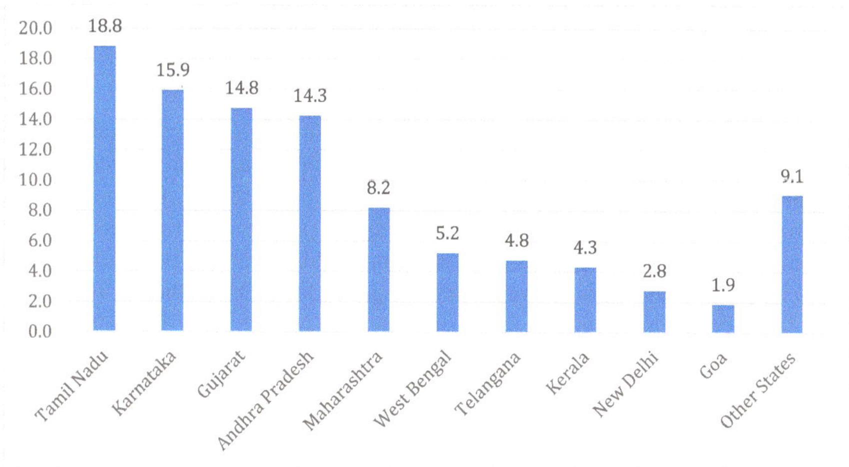

Fig. 1 Percentage of out-migrants by destination states. *Source* Odisha Migration Survey 2023, household sample

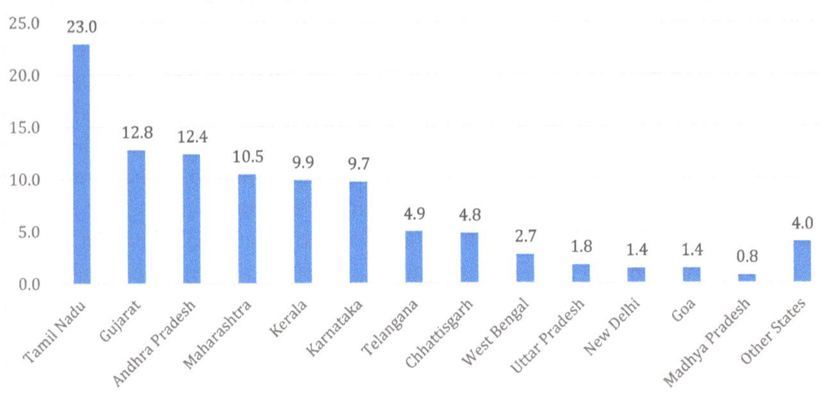

Fig. 2 Percentage of return migrants by their last destination state. *Source* Odisha Migration Survey 2023, household sample

migrants heading toward Gujarat. In contrast, the migration corridor from Bhadrak to Karnataka constitutes approximately 32.3% of the total migration from the state. The most important destination for the migrants from Balangir is Andhra Pradesh (37.4%).

The data on return migration shows Tamil Nadu as the last destination for the maximum number of return migrants in Odisha (23.0%), followed by Gujarat (12.8%), Andhra Pradesh (12.4%), Maharashtra (10.5%), Kerala (9.9%), and Karnataka (9.7%) (Fig. 2). Among the current migrants, 4.3% originate from Kerala, whereas 9.9% of the return migrants are from Kerala. The reverse is true for Karnataka; 15.9% of the current migrants are from Karnataka, while 9.7% of migrants returned from Karnataka. Notably, within Balangir district, there is a substantial number of return migrants, with the majority having returned from Tamil Nadu (29.1%), followed by Andhra Pradesh (16.6%), Chhattisgarh (12.1%), and Maharashtra (11.1%).

The Gulf migration corridor constituted the majority of the international migrants from Odisha. The United Arab Emirates was the top destination for international migrants (42.8%) (Fig. 3). Bahrain and Iraq (7.3% each), Saudi Arabia and Qatar (7.1% each), and Kuwait (6.9%) are the subsequent preferred destinations for international migrants. In Saudi Arabia, Riyadh and Jeddah are important destinations, while in Qatar, Odia migrants predominantly go to Doha. Out of the top 10 destinations for international migrants, seven of them were Middle Eastern countries, with the USA and South Africa being the exceptions (Fig. 3).

The OMS collected data on the activity status of current and return migrants *before* and *after* migration. It emerges from the data that, for current migrants, regular wage (salaried) in the private sector category has seen the highest increase post-migration (from 5.5% before migration to 48.9% after migration), indicating that migrant workers are predominantly employed in the private sector. The proportion of migrants who identified as students before migration (25.0%) decreased to

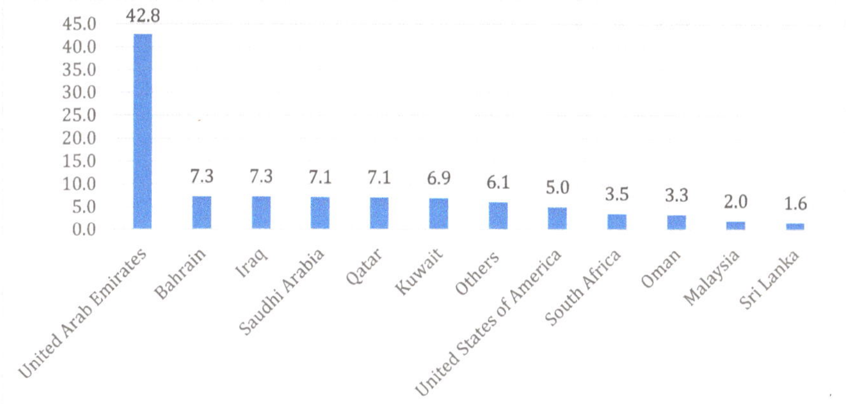

Fig. 3 Percentage of current migrants by destination countries. *Source* Odisha Migration Survey 2023, household sample

9.7% after migration, suggesting that a significant proportion of migrants moved for employment after their period of education ended, highlighting the dire employment scenario in the state. This is corroborated by the indicator on unemployment; the proportion of unemployed decreased from 24.2% to 0.1% after migration (Table 13). Similar trends are observed in the case of return migrants as well, as seen in Table 14.

As seen in Table 15, the majority of female migrants within the working population are employed in the fields of health and education (22.9%), followed by trade and repair (22.3%) and engagement in agriculture and allied activities (18.7%). Conversely, the primary occupation for the majority of the migrant men is in the construction sector (19.3%), followed by trade and repair (17.8%), manufacturing or mining industries (17.9%), and agriculture and allied occupations (11.2%) (Table 15).

For men, the majority of the migrants are engaged in three occupations before migration: construction work, agriculture, and manufacturing. The agricultural sector shows the largest decline after migration, suggesting that a large proportion of migrants have left agricultural activities in Odisha and have migrated elsewhere for jobs in other sectors, such as manufacturing and construction. When comparing male–female occupational activities, it could be observed that a large proportion of females who migrated were engaged in skilled jobs, but in the case of males, it's to the contrary (Table 16).

Table 15 shows that current migrants work in three broad occupational categories: (i) construction, (ii) manufacturing and mining, and (iii) trade and repair. Agricultural activities and hotel-hospitality occupations are the next most important. When considering return migrants and their current occupational group, nearly 40% were engaged in agriculture, followed by construction (25%). These two occupations were the predominant and easily available occupations in their hometown. In a similar vein, Table 17 shows that most of the return migrants are engaged in agriculture and allied

Table 13 Change in activity status of current migrants before and after migration

Activity status	Before migration			After migration		
	Male	Female	Total	Male	Female	Total
Own account worker (employer)	1.0	1.0	1.0	1.1	1.3	1.1
Own account worker (self-employed)	5.8	1.1	5.1	4.5	1.9	4.1
Regular wage (salaried) in public sector	1.3	2.4	1.5	6.3	5.5	6.2
Regular wage (salaried) in private sector	6.1	2.3	5.5	54.9	15.8	48.9
Casual wage labor	26.0	11.1	23.7	18.8	9.4	17.3
Unpaid family labor	7.0	3.0	6.4	0.8	1.8	1.0
Domestic work/ household chores	0.9	30.5	5.5	0.6	23.8	4.2
Student	23.0	36.0	25.0	7.2	23.0	9.7
Retired/pensioner/too old to work	0.1	0.0	0.1	0.9	1.4	1.0
Unemployed	27.6	5.9	24.2	0.1	0.0	0.1
Unable to work due to physical or mental disability	1.3	6.7	2.1	4.8	16.1	6.6
Others	1.0	1.0	1.0	1.1	1.3	1.1
Total	**100.0**	**100.0**	**100.0**	**100.0**	**100.0**	**100.0**

Source Odisha Migration Survey 2023, household sample

occupations (37.7%), followed by construction (25.3%) and trade and repair (14.7%) categories.

Disaggregated by social group, the upper castes have the highest proportion of current migrants with respect to their total population, followed by OBCs (6.2%), SCs (5.6%), and STs (3.9%). The group with the least representation in the migrant pie is STs (94.7% of STs are non-migrants). At the aggregate level, the figures suggest that there is a higher proportion of migrants among the upper castes compared to the marginalized social groups, and it is not necessarily the poorest who migrate the most. The proportion of return migrants among SCs (1.9%) is the highest, and among upper castes, the lowest (1.2%), suggesting that the migrants from the lower castes are more likely to be return migrants than the upper castes (Table 18).

A majority of the migrants have a decent educational background, with 20.3% of the migrants having completed Class 10. Only 2.9% of migrants are illiterate. In general, female migrants at the lower end of the education spectrum are relatively worse off than their male counterparts, although when it comes to higher educational

Table 14 Change in activity status of return migrants before migration and at destination before returning to place of origin

Activity status	Before migration			At destination		
	Male	Female	Total	Male	Female	Total
Own account worker (employer)	0.9	1.2	0.9	0.2	1.2	0.3
Own account worker (self-employed)	14.9	0.0	13.4	5.2	1.0	4.8
Regular wage (salaried) in public sector	0.0	0.0	0.0	4.2	2.0	4.0
Regular wage (salaried) in private sector	4.1	1.1	3.8	36.0	11.3	33.6
Casual wage labor	45.0	40.8	44.5	51.1	70.8	53.1
Unpaid family labor	5.7	4.2	5.5	1.3	1.2	1.3
Domestic work/ household chores	1.5	29.0	4.3	0.0	5.0	0.5
Student	9.1	12.1	9.4	0.3	6.2	0.9
Retired/pensioner/too old to work	0.1	0.0	0.1	0.0	0.0	0.0
Beggar	0.1	0.0	0.1	0.0	0.0	0.0
Unemployed	17.8	8.2	16.8	0.1	0.0	0.1
Unable to work due to physical or mental disability	0.0	0.0	0.0	0.0	0.0	0.0
Others	0.0	0.0	0.0	1.4	1.3	1.4
Too young to work	0.7	3.5	0.9	0.0	0.0	0.0
Total	**100.0**	**100.0**	**100.0**	**100.0**	**100.0**	**100.0**

Source Odisha Migration Survey 2023, household sample

qualifications (degree, professional degrees, postgraduate degrees), female migrants perform significantly better than male migrants. Among return migrants, illiterates over the age of seven represent 6.7% of males and 16.2% of females (Table 19).

The source of information about job opportunities for current migrants varies significantly on the basis of their sex. More than half of the male migrants learnt about their current job through their friends, while more than 60% of female migrants learnt about their current job through their family (Table 20).

The major reason for migration, as expected, is search for employment (59.2%), and this is higher for males than for females (Table 21). While only 7.9% of migrants reported "accumulating savings" as a reason for migration, accompanying family stands as the major reason for female migration (around 41%).

Family ties are a significant driver of return migration, as evident from the high percentage (26.6%) of individuals returning because they missed their families (Table 22). This emphasizes the importance of family connections in migration

Table 15 Occupation of current migrants by sex

Occupational groups	Male	Female	Total
Agriculture and allied activities	10.9	18.7	11.4
Manufacturing and mining	17.5	5.1	16.6
Construction	19.3	11.9	18.8
Law, finance, and accounting	2.5	2.0	2.4
Engineering and managerial	3.8	5.4	3.9
Transport	4.7	0.6	4.4
Hotel and hospitality	9.4	1.5	8.8
Trade and repair	17.9	22.3	18.2
Health and education	2.2	22.9	3.6
Public service	2.3	1.7	2.3
Village services	1.0	0.9	1.0
Other services	8.1	7.0	8.0
Other occupations	0.6	0.0	0.6
Total	**100.0**	**100.0**	**100.0**

Source Odisha Migration Survey 2023, household sample

decisions. COVID-19 was another major reason for return, accounting for 13.9% of all return migration. This was also evident from the year of return; we saw a large number of people return in 2020. A considerable portion of return migrants cited retirement as a reason (10.7%). This points to the circularity of migration, as individuals *eventually* return to their place of origin to retire. A total of 10.6% of return migrants desired to work in Odisha. This could be driven by a sense of community, a connection to their place of origin, or opportunities in the local job market. The data underscores the need for policies that address the economic vulnerabilities of migrants and provide support during crises such as pandemics. Understanding the factors behind the desire to work in Odisha could help in creating employment opportunities and retaining local workers, particularly the youth. Further research could explore the experiences and challenges faced by migrants during short-term migration and the implications for both the migrants and their place of origin (Tables 23 and 24).

Bhadrak (59.8), followed by Dhenkanal (48.9), Ganjam (40.4), Cuttack (40.0), Jajpur (37.8), Nayagarh (37.2), Balasore (36.5), and Nuapada (30.8), has the highest number of migrants per 100 households (Fig. 4). Nabarangpur (3.3), Bargarh (5.1), and Gajapati (5.4) have the lowest number of migrants per 100 households.

Nuapada district had the highest number of return migrants (36 return migrants per 100 households), followed by Balangir (30.2) and Kendrapara (14.7) (Fig. 5). Sambalpur, Jajpur, and Jagatsinghapur had the lowest number of return migrants, whereas three districts reported no return migrants.

The majority of current migrants are employed in factories, accounting for 38.3% of this group, with a higher representation among males (40.3%) than females

Table 16 Change in occupation of current migrants: before and after migration

Major occupation among men, before and after migration		
Male	Before	After
No occupation	49.0	0
Agriculture	24.7	10.0
Construction	11.3	14.0
Manufacturing	1.1	15.9
Cook	0.9	3.7
Salesperson	1.0	4.4
Hotel administration-related staff	0.3	3.5
Contract labor	0.4	2.1
Sewing/embroidery-related work	0.0	2.8
Site supervisor	0.3	2.5
Car/taxi driver	0.7	2.0
Doorkeepers and security staff	0.1	2.2
Engineer	0.4	1.9
Cashier, ticket clerks, clerks, accountant	0.5	1.6
Loading/unloading Worker	0.7	1.8
Heavy truck and lorry driver	0.6	1.7
Fabrication worker	0.3	2.0
Mechanic	0.3	1.5
Defense (navy, army, air force)	0.2	1.4
Electrician	0.4	1.5
Mason	1.1	1.6
Small-scale industry worker (artisan, beedi, cashew, dairy workers, food processing)	0.2	1.0
Plumber	0.3	1.1
Other occupations	5.3	19.8
Total	**100.0**	**100.0**
Female	**Before**	**After**
No occupations	59.1	0
Agriculture	16.9	14.7
Contract labor	0.0	2.1
Construction worker	5.1	10.9
Tailor/dressmaker	2.7	7.1
Nurse and nursing assistant	2.1	9.6
Teacher	1.4	7.1

(continued)

Table 16 (continued)

Major occupation among men, before and after migration		
Male	Before	After
Manufacturing worker	0.0	4.6
Fisherperson/fish-related work	0.0	4.0
Sewing/embroidery-related work	0.5	5.7
Bricklayer	1.4	3.8
Peon/office assistant/sweeper/cleaner	0.5	2.4
Computer programmer	1.0	3.5
Salesperson	0.0	2.6
Doctor	0.4	1.9
Police	0.0	1.2
Hotel administration-related staff	0.5	1.5
Cashier, ticket clerks, clerks, accountant	0.6	1.6
Household worker/maid/servant (full-time)	0.6	1.5
Laboratory/X-Ray technician	0.0	1.7
Lecturer/professor	1.1	1.5
Housekeeper/cook in households (part-time)	1.6	0.0
Service engineer (electronic equipment)	0.6	0.6
Other occupations	3.7	10.6
Total	**100.0**	**100.0**

Source Odisha Migration Survey 2023, household sample

Table 17 Current occupational group of return migrants by sex

Occupational groups	Male	Female	Total
Agriculture and allied activities	37.7	50.9	38.2
Manufacturing and mining	3.5	3.7	3.5
Construction	25.3	17.4	25.0
Law, finance and, accounting	0.4	0.0	0.4
Engineering and managerial	0.3	0.0	0.2
Transport	4.8	0.0	4.6
Hotel and hospitality	1.4	0.0	1.4
Trade and repair	14.7	7.4	14.5
Health and education	0.9	3.4	1.0
Village services	1.8	0.0	1.7
Other services	8.6	13.3	8.8
Other occupations	0.6	3.9	0.7
Total	**100.0**	**100.0**	**100.0**

Source Odisha Migration Survey 2023, household sample

Table 18 Distribution of current and return migrants by social group (% of households)

Social group	Non-migrant	Current migrant	Return migrant	Total
SC	92.5	5.6	1.9	100.0
ST	94.7	3.9	1.3	100.0
OBC	92.2	6.2	1.5	100.0
Upper caste	91.5	7.4	1.2	100.0

Source Odisha Migration Survey 2023, household sample

Table 19 Educational status of current and return migrants

Current migrants	Male	Female	Total
Illiterate	2.7	3.9	2.9
Less than or equal to primary	8.2	16.1	9.5
Classes 5–9	33.6	20.8	31.6
Class 10	21.2	15.1	20.3
Classes 11–12	13.9	15.9	14.2
Diploma and certificate course	4.5	2.8	4.3
Degree and above	15.7	25.5	17.2
Total	100.0	100.0	100.0
Return migrants	**Male**	**Female**	**Total**
Illiterate	6.7	16.2	7.6
Less than or equal to primary	16.4	28.1	17.6
Classes 5–9	44.8	33.4	43.7
Class 10	20.0	5.5	18.6
Classes 11–12	7.4	7.9	7.4
Diploma and certificate course	1.3	1.3	1.3
Degree and above	3.3	7.5	3.7
Total	**100.0**	**100.0**	**100.0**

Source Odisha Migration Survey 2023, household sample

(20.4%) (Table 25). A similar pattern is observed for those working at construction sites, where 16.3% of migrants are employed, with a higher proportion among males compared to females. In contrast, only 4.8% of migrants work in households, with a significant gender disparity—15.1% of females work in households, while only 3.6% of males do.

While both current migrants and return migrants were most likely to work in factories, as expected, the next most likely workplace for current migrants was office-based, whereas for return migrants, this was a construction site. When looking at current migrants, it becomes evident that approximately 14% of them are engaged in office-based activities, which is comparatively higher than what was observed among return migrants. Farms, which showed a similar lower prevalence in both

Table 20 Sources of job information for current migrants

Source of job information	Male	Female	Total
Family	20.2	62.7	26.6
Friends	57.9	13.9	51.3
Relatives	13.4	13.2	13.4
Middleman (brokers)	1.2	0.4	1.1
Unregistered agencies	0.3	0.2	0.3
Registered agencies	2.2	1.9	2.1
Mass media advertisement	3.8	4.4	3.9
Community	0.4	0.9	0.5
Professional network	0.1	0.0	0.1
Others (specify)	0.5	2.3	0.8
Total	**100.0**	**100.0**	**100.0**

Source Odisha Migration Survey 2023, household sample

Table 21 Reasons for current migration by sex

	Male	Female	Total
Get employment	64.8	28.7	59.2
Accumulate savings	8.2	6.5	7.9
Marriage of siblings/children	1.1	4.3	1.6
Construction/purchase of house	0.7	0.2	0.7
Repay debts	0.5	0.2	0.5
Studying	5.4	19.4	7.5
Family accompanied	19.0	40.6	22.3
Others (specify)	0.3	0.2	0.3
Total	**100.0**	**100.0**	**100.0**

Source Odisha Migration Survey 2023, household sample

cases, indicate that agriculture and related activities were the least engaged in during migration.

While considering the sex of the person who is in the position of the "head of the household," when all three forms of households (Table 26) are taken together, it is observed that males occupy this role the most (84.7%). When these three forms of households were compared, it was found that non-migrant households have a relatively larger number of female heads of households. The absence of current migrants in the household alone is not a sufficient reason for females to take the role of the household head. Several factors contribute to the higher prevalence of male household heads over female heads. These factors may include the predominant role of males as the primary earners in the household and the influence of Indian societal norms, where males are traditionally regarded as the decision-makers in various aspects of household affairs.

Table 22 Reasons for the return of return migrants

	Male	Female	Total
To retire	10.8	9.2	10.7
Missed family	27.6	17.3	26.6
To care for elderly	4.5	9.1	4.9
Accomplished goals for migration	0.7	3.5	1.0
Prefer to work in Odisha	11.0	7.2	10.6
Lost job/laid off	5.0	4.6	5.0
Illness/accident	5.9	1.0	5.4
Expiry of contract	1.1	0.0	1.0
Covid-19	12.7	24.6	13.9
Compulsory expatriation	0.3	1.3	0.4
Low wages	9.7	2.3	9.0
Poor working conditions	2.6	1.1	2.4
Social exclusion	1.9	0.0	1.7
To migrate to another destination/to migrate to same destination for different job	0.3	0.0	0.3
Short-term contract	1.2	9.4	2.0
Seasonal migrants	2.6	4.9	2.8
Short term (less than 3 months)	0.5	0.0	0.4
Short term (3 to 6 months)	1.6	4.5	1.9
Total	**100.0**	**100.0**	**100.0**

Source Odisha Migration Survey 2023, household sample

Table 23 Reasons for return by wealth quartile of return migrants

	First quartile (lowest)	Second quartile	Third quartile	Fourth quartile (highest)	Total
Normal return	26.2	31.1	27.2	15.4	100.0
Distress return	29.0	27.5	26.0	17.4	100.0
Return to re-migrate	43.0	22.0	24.0	11.1	100.0
Total	**28.5**	**29.1**	**26.5**	**15.9**	**100.0**

Source Odisha Migration Survey 2023, household sample

Table 27 shows that the current migrants and return migrants relatively have an upper hand in holding land when compared to non-migrants. Almost 48.8% of landless people are largely constituted by people who haven't migrated at all. It is found that more than 44% of return migrants hold land less than one acre, and 28% of

Table 24 Reasons for return by social group of return migrants

	SC	ST	OBC	Upper caste	Total
Normal return	20.1	22.7	46.7	10.5	100.0
Distress return	23.0	19.3	40.6	17.1	100.0
Return to re-migrate	33.5	19.8	41.3	5.5	100.0
Total	**22.1**	**21.2**	**44.0**	**12.6**	**100.0**

Source Odisha Migration Survey 2023, household sample

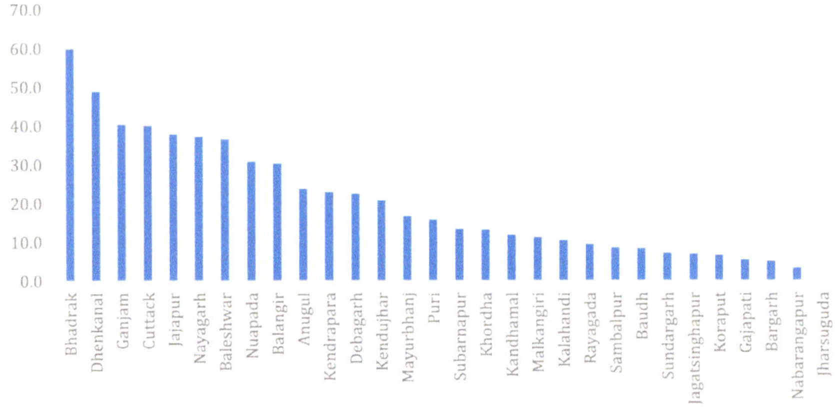

Fig. 4 Current migrants per 100 households by districts. *Source* Odisha Migration Survey 2023, household sample

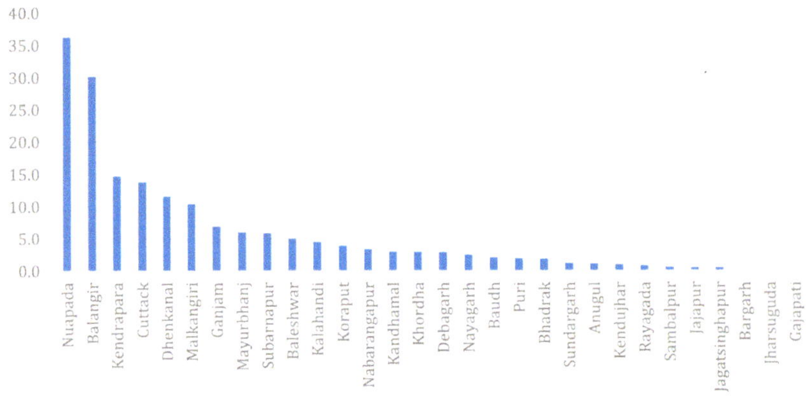

Fig. 5 Return migrants per 100 households by districts. *Source* Odisha Migration Survey 2023, household sample

Table 25 Nature of workplace of current and return migrants by sex

Current migrants			
Nature of workplace	Male	Female	Total
Office	13.6	17.2	14.0
Shop	8.4	4.7	8.1
Construction site	16.9	11.2	16.3
House	3.6	15.1	4.8
Factory	40.3	20.4	38.3
Farm	1.7	1.9	1.7
Open space	6.5	4.0	6.3
Workshop	2.1	1.8	2.1
Others	6.8	23.8	8.5
Total	**100.0**	**100.0**	**100.0**
Return migrants			
Nature of workplace	**Male**	**Female**	**Total**
Office	5.7	0.0	5.1
Shop	6.0	1.2	5.6
Construction site	34.7	24.4	33.7
House	2.0	9.9	2.8
Factory	36.8	18.3	35.1
Farm	2.4	0.0	2.2
Open space	7.2	25.5	8.9
Workshop	1.4	1.3	1.4
Others	3.8	19.3	5.3
Total	**100.0**	**100.0**	**100.0**

Source Odisha Migration Survey 2023, household sample

Table 26 Sex of the head of the household by migration status of the household

Head of the household	Non-migrant	Current migrant	Return migrant	Total
Male	83.9	86.5	90.7	84.7
Female	16.1	13.5	9.3	15.3
Total	**100.0**	**100.0**	**100.0**	**100.0**

Source Odisha Migration Survey 2023, household sample

return migrants hold land larger than one acre but less than five acres. In the case of current migrant households, landholding numbers are largely positive; around 37% hold less than one acre of land, and around 26% hold more than one acre, but less than five. Landlessness is observed mainly among non-migrant households, followed by current migrant households, and then return migrant households (Tables 28 and 29).

Table 27 Land ownership in acres by migration status of the household

Land ownership	Non-migrant	Current migrant	Return migrant	Total
Landless	48.8	35.0	26.8	45.4
0–1 acre	27.0	37.3	44.6	29.6
1–5 acres	22.6	25.8	27.7	23.4
5 + acres	1.7	1.8	0.9	1.7
Total	**100.0**	**100.0**	**100.0**	**100.0**

Source Odisha Migration Survey 2023, household sample

In the lowest wealth quartile, the proportion of current migrants (19.0%) is significantly lower when compared to non-migrants (31.1%) and return migrants (30.1%) (Table 28). The higher proportion of return migrants in the lowest quartile suggests that a significant number of migrants who returned were unable to reap the benefits of migration; although it is reassuring that the proportion of return migrants among the third quartile is higher than non-migrants (though not current migrants), indicating that some return migrants were able to improve their living conditions by migrating.

Housing conditions significantly impact quality of life, health, and overall well-being. Individuals living in poor or *kutcha* houses might face challenges related to sanitation, hygiene, and vulnerability to environmental conditions. Current migrants have significantly better houses than non-migrants and return migrants. While the percentage of kutcha houses is similar for non-migrants and return migrants at 22.3 and 21.6%, respectively, the figure is only 17.8% for current migrants (Table 29). The figures suggest that the current migrants either had better houses than non-migrants when they migrated or that the migrants were able to improve their houses after migrating. It is likely to be the former since the majority of the current migrants migrated in the last 5 years, and since the majority of them are in construction and manufacturing-rclatcd occupations.

It is also likely that having resources like land and other forms of wealth is an enabler of migration; as Table 25 on land ownership shows, the proportion of current and return migrants who own land is significantly higher than non-migrants.

Table 28 Wealth quartile by migration status of the household

Wealth status	Non-migrant	Current migrant	Return migrant	Total
Quartile 1 (lowest)	31.1	19.0	30.1	28.9
Quartile 2	24.9	27.7	31.1	25.7
Quartile 3	20.7	27.2	25.1	22.0
Quartile 4 (highest)	23.4	26.1	13.7	23.4
Total	**100.0**	**100.0**	**100.0**	**100.0**

Source Odisha Migration Survey 2023, household sample

Table 29 Current and return migrants by their house type (% of households)

Type of house	Non-migrant	Current migrant	Return migrant	Total
Luxurious	2.2	5.2	1.9	2.7
Very good	12.4	19.7	8.7	13.5
Good	34.7	33.3	35.0	34.4
Poor	28.6	23.9	32.8	27.9
Kutcha	22.3	17.8	21.6	21.5
Total	**100.0**	**100.0**	**100.0**	**100.0**

Source Odisha Migration Survey 2023, household sample

It is interesting to note that migrating for work has not improved the housing conditions of the return migrants, as the data shows more than 50% of return migrants are living in poor or kutcha houses. This could be because the majority of the return migrants in Odisha belong to the OBC, SC, and ST communities, and they have not been able to reap the benefits of migration compared to the upper castes.

6 Conclusion

This chapter provides a comprehensive analysis of migration patterns in Odisha, emphasizing distinctions between current and return migrants and categorizing migration by destination types. Through the Odisha Migration Survey 2023, various migration categories emerged, reflecting diverse migration motivations, ranging from labor and education to family and seasonal returns. The detailed classifications of migration statuses based on factors like duration of stay and reasons for migration offer insights into the distinct economic and social circumstances shaping each migration type.

The consistent upward trend in migration, as indicated by census and NSS data, underscores the complex interplay of economic and social factors driving people to move. While the COVID-19 pandemic intensified migration in the short term, it did not lead to any lasting increase in migration rates, revealing that the fundamental drivers of migration remain deeply rooted in Odisha's socio-economic landscape. This chapter underscores that migration in Odisha is a multifaceted phenomenon, shaped by diverse and dynamic factors across regions, social groups, and wealth quartiles. This understanding is essential for addressing the nuanced needs of different migrant groups and for developing targeted policies that support their varied experiences and aspirations.

References

Mishra, D., Sahu, N. C., & Sahoo, D. (2016). Impact of climate change on agricultural production of Odisha (India): A Ricardian analysis. *Regional Environmental Change, 16*, 575–584. https://doi.org/10.1007/s10113-015-0774-5

Mishra, D. K. (2020). Seasonal migration and unfree labour in globalising India: Insights from field surveys in Odisha. *Indian Journal of Labour Economics, 63*(4), 1087–1106. https://doi.org/10.1007/s41027-020-00277-8

NSSO. (2010). *Migration in India: 2007–2008* (Report No. 533). National Sample Survey Office, Ministry of Statistics & Programme Implementation, Government of India. https://www.mospi.gov.in/sites/default/files/publication_reports/533_final.pdf

Panda, S., & Padhi, B. (2021). Poverty and inequality in Odisha, India. *Journal of Public Affairs, 21*(2). https://doi.org/10.1002/pa.2220

Chapter 4
The Migration Story—II

S. Irudaya Rajan, Amrita Datta, and Sunitha S.

Abstract Extending the analysis in the previous chapter, this chapter estimates the size of remittances and discusses their patterns and impacts. It finds that among migrant households, 68.6% received remittances, and the average monthly household remittance was Rs 5,096. The estimated monthly remittances for the entire state of Odisha amounted to Rs 693.47 crore, with Ganjam district emerging as the recipient of the highest estimated remittances per month with Rs 112.76 crore, closely followed by Bhadrak (Rs 99.23 crore) and Jajpur district (Rs 78.3 crore). However, there existed significant disparities in remittance inflows across districts, as the majority of the districts (21) received remittances below 20 crores. More than 50% of the migrant households received remittances in most districts, but the actual amount received vastly varied. Remittances significantly impacted the living standards of households with migrants in Odisha. 90% of households reported using remittances for meeting expenses of everyday consumption and 73% for health and medical expenses. Among the various social groups, the Other Backward Class (OBC) community received the highest monthly average remittance (Rs 5,527), closely followed by the upper-caste (Rs 5,397), Scheduled Caste (SC) (Rs 4,815), and Scheduled Tribe (ST) (Rs 3,245) households. The STs were the worst off, with the lowest remittances, and only 47% of the ST migrant households received remittances (compared to 74.3% of OBC households, 71.9% of SC households, and 68.7% of upper-caste households). In terms of the rural-urban comparison, 68.8% of the rural migrant households received remittances compared to 52.5% of urban households.

Keywords Remittances · Migration · Odisha migration survey

S. I. Rajan · Sunitha S.
The International Institute of Migration and Development, Thiruvananthapuram, India

A. Datta (✉)
Indian Institute of Technology, Hyderabad, India
e-mail: amritadatta@la.iith.ac.in

A. Datta and S. I. Rajan (eds.), *Migration, Livelihoods and Gender*, International Perspectives on Migration, https://doi.org/10.1007/978-981-95-5465-2_4

1 Introduction

The remittances, often sent by migrants to their families residing in their places of origin, have significant socio-economic impacts that extend beyond mere financial transactions, influencing individuals, households, the economy, and society as a whole. Remittances play a vital role in sustaining the well-being of recipient families, supporting education and healthcare, and even fostering economic development at the community level. This chapter first estimates district-level household remittances and discusses their use. It then presents the percentage of migrant households receiving remittances and the size of remittances disaggregated by social group, rural and urban areas, housing quality, wealth status, landownership, administrative region, and ration card status. Last, we discuss survey findings related to advance payments and conclude.

2 Calculation of Household Remittances

The average monthly remittance per household was determined by taking the mean of remittances received across all households. However, for this calculation, only 90% of the observations were considered, and the remaining 10% were excluded by removing the lowest and highest 5% as outliers. Specifically, we included observations falling within the range of Rs 458 to Rs 14,167 in the calculation.

After the elimination of outliers, the average monthly remittance received by a household from the Odisha Migration Survey (OMS) stands at Rs 5,101, and there are a total of 1,734 households receiving remittances (Table 2). The total number of households receiving remittances, before the elimination of outliers, was 1,764. To calculate the total monthly remittance received at the state level, we multiply the average monthly remittance per household by the total number of households in Odisha that receive remittances.

Formula

$$\text{Total Remittance} = \text{Total number of remittance} - \text{receiving households} \times \text{Average remittances received by households per month}$$

2.1 Estimation

Using the formula, first, remittances were estimated at the district level and then aggregated for the entire state. For Odisha, estimated remittances amount to Rs 772.47 crore. However, it is important to note that this figure is likely to be an underestimate. This underestimation can be attributed to the fact that individuals often tend to underreport their income and remittances. In the case of the Odisha Migration Survey, we have relied on people's responses as they were provided, without any adjustments. This implies that the observed remittances may be lower than the actual amounts people receive or send (Table 1).

Before migrating, some migrants also typically receive an upfront lump sum payment. It is important to note that this lump sum payment has not been taken into account in the calculation of remittances. A total of 4.8% of households with migrants reported receiving lump sum payments, which ranged from Rs 3,600 to Rs 2,00,000. The total lump sum received by the sample households before their migration, as reported in the OMS, amounts to Rs 0.58 crore.

Remittances were widespread—more than two-thirds of the migrant households received remittances (Table 1). Among all the districts in Odisha, Ganjam district stands out as the recipient of the highest remittances, estimated at a sum of Rs 112.76 crore per month. Following closely behind are Bhadrak and Cuttack districts, ranking as the second and third highest recipients, accumulating remittances of Rs 99.23 crore and Rs 78.33 crore, respectively.

Districts falling within the range of Rs 70 crore to Rs 60 crore in remittances include Jajpur, Baleshwar, and Nayagarh. Notably, the remaining districts receive remittances below the Rs 35 crore threshold, which is significantly lower than the top recipients in the region. This data underscores the disparities in remittance inflows across Odisha's districts, with Ganjam district clearly emerging as the frontrunner in this regard.

The data highlights significant disparities in remittance inflows across the districts. While some districts, like Ganjam, Bhadrak, and Cuttack, receive substantial financial support from individuals working elsewhere, others receive much less. These remittances play a crucial role in supporting families and local economies in these districts, and the variations in these inflows underscore the economic diversity and migration patterns within the state of Odisha (Table 2).

When examining the proportion of migrant households receiving remittances in Odisha, it becomes evident that in most districts, over half of the migrant households are beneficiaries of remittances. Among all the districts in Odisha, Bhadrak (89.2%), Boudh (87.0%), Dhenkanal (85.7%), Jajpur (83.4%), Khordha (83.3%), Puri (79.7%), Cuttack (77.0%), Kalahandi (75.0%), Ganjam (74.6%), and Nayagarh (73.3%) stand out with the highest proportion of households receiving remittances. However, despite Boudh having the highest proportion of remittance-receiving households, the actual amount received as remittances is quite negligible. Similarly, Ganjam, which ranks first in terms of both the number of migrants and the total remittance volume received, appears ninth when considering the proportion of migrant households benefiting from remittances (Table 3).

Analyzing the utilization of remittances in Odisha reveals that more than 90% of households use remittances to support their daily consumption expenses. Additionally, about 73% of households use remittances to cover health and medical expenses. Furthermore, it is noteworthy that remittances are also a significant source of funding for children's education, house construction, and special occasions. Paying off debts

Table 1 Households (HH) receiving remittances (%) and remittance estimates by districts (in rupees), 2023

District	% Migrant HH receiving remittances (from sample)	HH receiving remittance (projected)	Monthly average remittance, last 12 months (in rupees)	Estimated remittances per month (in crores)
Bargarh	70.0	18,260	2,874	5.25
Sambalpur	33.3	7,255	2,311	1.68
Debagarh	32.6	6,144	3,362	2.07
Sundargarh	9.1	3,248	1,208	0.39
Kendujhar	52.8	50,227	6,293	31.61
Mayurbhanj	63.8	65,461	3,019	19.76
Baleshwar	67.5	1,46,268	4,460	65.24
Bhadrak	89.2	1,53,436	6,779	104.01
Kendrapara	51.0	41,336	5,319	21.99
Jagatsinghpur	63.0	13,038	1,755	2.29
Cuttack	77.0	1,55,245	5,513	85.58
Jajpur	83.4	1,31,377	5,362	70.44
Dhenkanal	85.7	1,10,286	5,948	65.60
Angul	42.1	29,529	4,258	12.57
Nayagarh	73.3	74,835	6,181	46.26
Khordha	83.3	62,753	6,580	41.29
Puri	79.7	52,196	5,316	27.75
Ganjam	74.6	2,01,593	5,876	118.45
Gajapati	20.0	1,274	2,792	0.36
Kandhamal	50.0	10,137	2,497	2.53
Boudh	87.0	12,166	3,349	4.07
Subarnapur	57.6	17,118	3,044	5.21
Balangir	50.9	59,282	2,205	13.07
Nuapada	53.7	29,850	2,721	8.12
Kalahandi	75.0	39,579	3,275	12.96
Rayagada	25.9	5,409	983	0.53
Nabarangpur	53.8	5,697	1,690	0.96
Koraput	34.6	6,904	3,398	2.35
Malkangiri	22.2	4,532	1,150	0.52
Total	**67.9**	**15,14,435**	**5,101**	**772.47**

Source Odisha Migration Survey 2023, Household sample

Table 2 Distribution and incidence of migrant households by remittance receipt

	Migrant HH not receiving remittances	Migrant HH receiving remittances	Total migrant HH	Percentage of HH receiving remittances
Bargarh	9	21	30	70.0
Sambalpur	16	8	24	33.3
Debagarh	29	14	43	32.6
Sundargarh	40	4	44	9.1
Kendujhar	51	57	108	52.8
Mayurbhanj	42	74	116	63.8
Baleshwar	77	160	237	67.5
Bhadrak	21	174	195	89.2
Kendrapara	51	53	104	51.0
Jagatsinghpur	10	17	27	63.0
Cuttack	53	177	230	77.0
Jajpur	29	146	175	83.4
Dhenkanal	22	132	154	85.7
Angul	44	32	76	42.1
Nayagarh	31	85	116	73.3
Khordha	14	70	84	83.3
Puri	15	59	74	79.7
Ganjam	78	229	307	74.6
Gajapati	8	2	10	20.0
Kandhamal	13	13	26	50.0
Boudh	3	20	23	87.0
Subarnapur	14	19	33	57.6
Balangir	56	58	114	50.9
Nuapada	31	36	67	53.7
Kalahandi	15	45	60	75.0
Rayagada	20	7	27	25.9
Nabarangpur	6	7	13	53.8
Koraput	17	9	26	34.6
Malkangiri	21	6	27	22.2
Total	**836**	**1,734**	**2,570**	**67.9**

Source Odisha Migration Survey 2023, Household sample

Table 3 Utilization of remittances[1] (% of households)

Items	
Everyday consumption (food/clothing/drinks/tobacco)	90.7
Health and medical expenses	73.2
Children's education	40.4
House construction or renovation	31.8
Special occasions (e.g., weddings/funerals)	29.1
Savings and fixed deposits in banks	15.3
SHG loan repayment	13.1
Religion (Pilgrimage)	12.6
Agricultural production (purchase of seeds/irrigation/water/employ workers)	12.1
Pay off other debt/loan	11.6
Purchase household/electronic goods (e.g., furniture, home utensils, computer, TV, fridge, washing machine)	9.9
Donation to temple/mosque/church/other religious or charitable organizations	9.2
Life insurance	8.1
Purchase of jewelry/gold	3.3
Purchase of agricultural equipment	2.5
Other expenses	9.1

Source Odisha Migration Survey 2023, Household sample

or loans—this encompasses both "paying off SHG loans" and "paying off other debts/loans"—represents another purpose for which remittances are utilized.

Thus, the receipt of remittances enhances the living standards and life prospects of recipient households in Odisha. It provides them with the means to meet their immediate needs, access healthcare and education, and improve their housing conditions. Additionally, remittances can alleviate financial burdens by helping families pay off debts, ultimately contributing to their economic well-being. In conclusion, remittances serve as a lifeline for many households in Odisha, addressing both short-term necessities as well as aspirations.

Table 4 shows the incidence and average remittance amount received by each social group. It can be seen that a significant proportion of households receive remittances, with the total average across all categories being 67.9%. Other Backward Classes (OBCs) have the highest percentage of remittance-receiving households, followed by Scheduled Castes (SCs) and upper castes. On the other hand, only 50% of the Scheduled Tribe (ST) households receive remittances. Hence, except for the ST households, a significant proportion of all other social groups receive remittances. This could be due to various factors, including economic, social, and regional dynamics. The table also shows that average remittances follow a pattern by social

[1] This question captures multiple responses from the same household.

Table 4 Remittance by social group (% of households)

Social group	Percentage of HH receiving remittances	Monthly average remittance, last 12 months[a] (in rupees)
SC	72.7	4,814
ST	49.9	3,261
OBC	74.0	5,536
Upper Caste	68.6	5,402
Total	**67.9**	**5,101**

[a]Only for remittance-receiving households
Source Odisha Migration Survey 2023, Household sample

Table 5 Remittance by place of residence (% of households*)

Place of residence	Percentage of HH receiving remittances	Monthly average remittance, last 12 months[a] (in rupees)
Rural	69.9	5,128
Urban	52.2	4,627
Total	**67.9**	**5,101**

[a]Only for remittance-receiving households
Source Odisha Migration Survey 2023, Household sample

group. At the top are the OBC and the upper-caste households, with the highest remittances; both groups received higher than average remittances. Conversely, households belonging to the ST and SC communities receive less than average remittances, with the STs having significantly lower remittances and faring the worst among all communities.

In Odisha, a striking 94.6% of total remittances are directed toward rural areas, whereas only 5.4% of the remittances accrue to urban households.[2] Rural households are also more likely to receive remittances compared to households in urban areas (Table 5). In addition, the magnitude of remittances is higher for rural households. That rural households receive remittances at a significantly higher rate (69.9%) than urban households (52.2%) suggests that remittances are a crucial source of financial support for rural families. In addition, rural households receive higher remittances on average (Rs 5,128) than urban households (Rs 4,627). This indicates that the reliance on remittances of rural households is somewhat greater.

The high rate of homeownership among both remittance-receiving and non-receiving households may indicate that owning a house is a common and achievable goal for many families in Odisha. This may also be due to ancestral property being passed down through generations. The data suggests that in Odisha, a high percentage of households own houses, and this trend is consistent across both

[2] As 83.3% of Odisha's population resides in rural areas and 16.7% in urban areas (Census of India 2011), the rural areas receive a disproportionately higher share of remittances.

remittance-receiving and non-receiving households. This implies that while remittances can have a significant impact on recipients' financial well-being, they may not play a decisive role in homeownership. Nearly all households that receive remittances (99.1%) own a house, while a similarly high percentage of migrant households not receiving remittances also own a house in Odisha. However, as seen in Table 3, nearly one-third of remittance-receiving households had used remittances for house construction or renovation in Odisha.

Table 6 shows the percentage of households receiving remittances and the average remittance received by these households, disaggregated by the type of housing. Remittances are not confined to any specific house type, as households across all categories receive remittances to some degree.

The "very good" house type has the highest percentage of remittance-receiving households (76%), indicating that households with better housing conditions are more likely to receive remittances. Conversely, poor and *kutcha* house types have slightly lower percentages (around 65%), suggesting that households in less favorable housing conditions also benefit from remittances. Luxurious and very good households receive substantially higher average remittances than other house types, and the average remittance declines with the fall in the standard of house type (Table 6). Hence, poor and kutcha households receive comparatively lower average remittances.

Remittances can play a role in improving the quality of housing. We saw earlier that nearly one-third of remittance-receiving households reported spending remittances on house construction and repair. As indicated by Table 6, there does not appear to be a significant relationship between owning a house and receiving remittances. However, when examining the type of houses owned, it becomes evident that a substantial proportion of relatively higher-quality house types are owned by households that receive remittances. Among migrant households that do not receive remittances, a significant proportion own houses with relatively better conditions. For example, 34.8% of these houses are rated as "Good," and 14.9% are classified as "Very Good." However, it is important to note that a considerable share of houses categorized as "Poor" (26%) also belong to households without remittance receipts. Remittances might be helping some households move up the housing quality ladder,

Table 6 Remittance by housing type

House type	Percentage of HH receiving remittances	Monthly average remittance, last 12 months[a] (in rupees)
Luxurious	66.9	6,778
Very good	76.1	6,285
Good	67.4	5,259
Poor	65.9	4,368
Kutcha	66.7	3,982
Total	**67.9**	**5,101**

[a]Only for remittance-receiving households
Source Odisha Migration Survey 2023, Household sample

while others may struggle to improve their housing conditions due to a lack of this additional income.

Table 7 illustrates the wealth status of migrant households that received remittances. Among households that do not receive remittances, the percentages are fairly evenly distributed across the four wealth status classifications. However, the numbers are notably skewed toward the households in the second wealth quartile (32.2%).

Conversely, migrant households that receive remittances tend to be more concentrated in the highest wealth quartile, indicating better economic well-being. For instance, about 32.2% of them are in the third wealth quartile, and 25.5% fall in the highest wealth quartile. Notably, the percentage of remittance-receiving households in the lowest wealth quartile is relatively lower when compared to those not receiving remittances (just 17.1%). The wealth status classifications among households receiving and not receiving remittances highlight significant disparities in economic well-being. Remittance-receiving households tend to be better off economically, while non-remittance-receiving households are more likely to fall into lower wealth status categories.

Table 7 shows how wealth status affects the remittance-receiving potential of a household. Around 80% of households from a higher (third) wealth quartile receive remittances, whereas 62% of the households from the lowest wealth quintile receive remittances. Similar to the house type, we find that average remittances received increase with improvement in wealth status, with the households in the highest quintile accounting for about Rs 6,476, while those in the lowest quintile receive around Rs 3,649 on average.

A significant percentage of migrant households were landless. When we disaggregate migrant households by households receiving remittances and households not receiving remittances, we find that the share of landless in the latter (40%) is higher than the share of landless in the former (32.3%). Despite this, almost 40% of remittance recipient households own land under one acre, and more than 26% own land between one and five acres. Furthermore, the proportion of households that own more than five acres is even less dependent on remittances. This is in line with our observation that landholding households are relatively less dependent on remittances, and land acts as an indicator of economic and social stature (Table 8).

Table 7 Remittance by wealth quartile

Wealth status	Percentage of migrant HH receiving remittances	Monthly average remittance, last 12 months[a] (in rupees)
Quartile 1 (Lowest)	62.4	3,649
Quartile 2	63.2	4,338
Quartile 3	80.3	5,504
Quartile 4 (Highest)	66.4	6,476
Total	**67.9**	**5,101**

[a]Only for remittance-receiving households

Source Odisha Migration Survey 2023, Household sample

Table 8 Remittance by land ownership

Land ownership in acres	Percentage of HH receiving remittances	Monthly average remittance, last 12 months[a] (in rupees)
Landless	62.8	5,514
0–1 Acre	74.8	4,941
1–5 Acres	68.2	4,849
5+ Acres	61.7	5,089
Total	**67.9**	**5,101**

[a]Only for remittance-receiving households
Source Odisha Migration Survey 2023, Household sample

Looking into the relation between land ownership and remittances received, we find that the highest percentage of households receiving remittances comes from those who hold less than one acre of land (74.8%). Almost 62% of the households holding more than five acres of land receive remittances, whereas for those households holding less than five acres of land, the figures are slightly higher. However, looking at the average remittances received, landless households receive more than those who hold land. This implies that remittances are a major source of financial support for a majority of migrants belonging to landless households.

Table 9 shows remittances disaggregated by administrative regions. A striking 58.8% of households from the coastal or central regions receive remittances. This is followed by the southern and northern regions. Looking at the average remittance per region, again, the coastal area accounts for about Rs 5,387, whereas the southern and northern regions get comparatively lower remittances. About 34% of the households in the northern region do not receive remittances. This could be in line with the fact that the highest number of migrants belong to the coastal and central regions of Odisha.

The survey data shows three types of households disaggregated by ration card status: households with regular ration cards, households with Antyodaya ration cards, and households with no ration cards (see Chap. 2 for details). Households that receive remittances and hold Antyodaya cards are a very small proportion of about 0.9%.

Table 9 Remittance by administrative region

Administrative region	Percentage of migrant households receiving remittances	Monthly average remittance, last 12 months[a] (in rupees)
Coastal/Central	76.4	5,387
Southern	63.8	4,791
Northern	56.2	4,582
Total	**67.9**	**5,101**

[a]Only for remittance-receiving households
Source Odisha Migration Survey 2023, Household sample

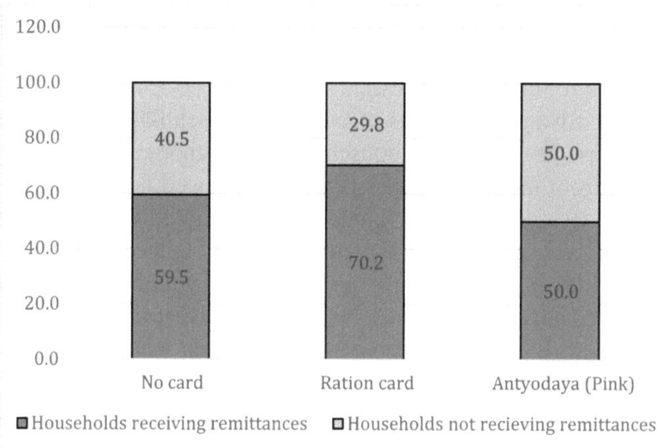

Fig. 1 Remittance by ration card status. *Source* Odisha Migration Survey 2023, Household sample

Antyodaya cardholders fall more in the category of those not receiving remittances, highlighting that economic well-being is closely related to the flow of remittances.

Figure 1 shows the remittance rate by ownership of ration cards. Amongst the ration card holder households, a significant proportion (70.2%) received remittances. Also, the majority of the households that did not have a card reported to have been receiving remittances. On the other hand, Antyodaya cardholders are least likely to receive remittances; these tend to be the poorest and most vulnerable households, where the capacity to migrate and remit is likely to be very restricted. This again shows that access to the public distribution system varies among sample households, and this, in turn, is likely to have an effect on migration patterns and influence migrant choices and the influx of remittances.

3 Advance Payments

Apart from remittances, the practice of advance payments to migrant workers or their families is prevalent in some regions of Odisha. Advance payments are typically associated with more precarious migration streams and vulnerable occupations. In the OMS data, as expected, the SC and ST households are over-represented, and the upper castes are underrepresented in the distribution of migrant households that received advances.

Figure 2 shows how the advance received by a migrant household prior to migration varies across different administrative regions. In the coastal region, almost 99% of the households reported that they did not receive any advances prior to migration. This corroborates our earlier results, which indicated that the highest remittance flow accrues to the coastal region. Similarly, we found that remittance-receiving households were significantly lower in the northern areas, and corresponding to this, we find that the maximum percentage of households that reported having received advances belonged to this area (11.8%).

Looking at the advance payments received by households across various social groups, the highest proportion of households that reported not having had any advances comes from the upper castes (98.4%), followed by OBCs (96.0%), SCs (92.3%), and STs (93.2%) (Fig. 3). In addition, OBC and SC households received relatively larger shares of advance payments compared to the other two groups.

Table 10 provides insights into the percentage of migrant households in each district that received advance payments. Notably, there is significant variation among districts. In Balangir, Bargarh, Nuapada, and Subarnapur, one-fourth of the migrant households received advances. In some districts, like Balangir and Bargarh, more than 30% of the migrant households received advances, whereas in contrast, in districts like Jharsuguda, Kendujhar, Jagatsinghapur, and several others, virtually no sample households had received advances.

Fig. 2 Advance received by migrant households by region (% migrant households). *Source* Odisha Migration Survey 2023, Household sample

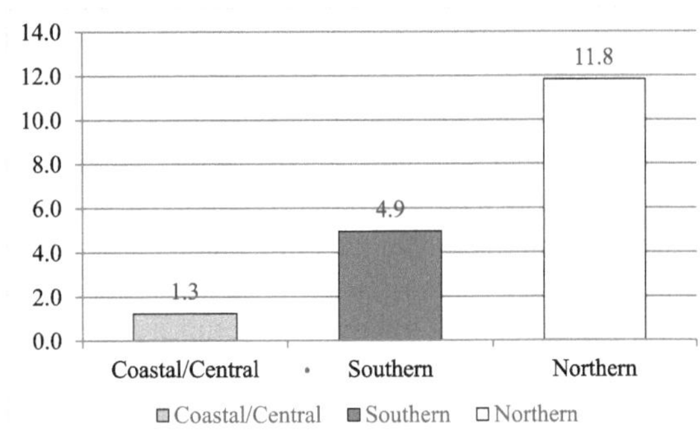

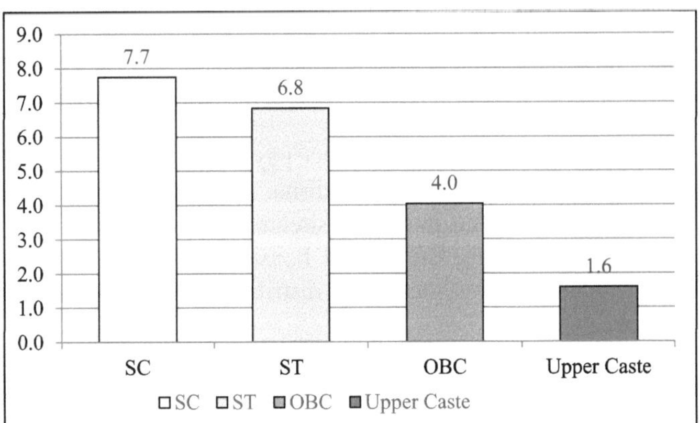

Fig. 3 Advance received by migrant households by social group (% migrant households). *Source* Odisha Migration Survey 2023, Household sample

Table 10 Advance received by migrant households by districts (% migrant households)

District	% Migrant households received advance
Balangir	38.6
Bargarh	30.0
Nuapada	29.9
Subarnapur	24.2
Boudh	17.4
Sambalpur	8.3
Debagarh	7.0
Kalahandi	5.0
Khordha	4.8
Total	4.7
Dhenkanal	4.5
Kendrapara	3.8
Sundargarh	2.3
Mayurbhanj	1.7
Cuttack	1.3
Nayagarh	0.9
Baleshwar	0.8
Ganjam	0.7
Bhadrak	0.5

Source Odisha Migration Survey 2023, Household sample

Table 11 categorizes migrant households based on their wealth quartile and their receipt of advance payments prior to migration. Approximately 11.2% of the migrant households in the lowest wealth quartile received advance payments, while only 1.5% of the households in the highest quartile received any advances. This shows that advance payments are associated with the wealth status of the household, and as expected, the incidence of such payments is the highest in households in the lowest wealth quartile.

Table 11 Advance received by migrant households by wealth quartile (% migrant households)

Wealth quartile	Advance received by migrant household prior to migration
Quartile 1 (Lowest)	11.2
Quartile 2	3.4
Quartile 3	4.5
Quartile 4 (Highest)	1.5

Source Odisha Migration Survey 2023, Household sample

4 Conclusion

The analysis of remittance inflows in Odisha highlights their critical role in shaping the socio-economic landscape of the state. Despite the estimation of remittances at Rs 772.47 crore being an apparent underestimation, the substantial financial flows underline the importance of migration-driven earnings for household sustenance and local economies. District-level disparities in remittance inflows are pronounced, with Ganjam district emerging as the dominant recipient, followed by Bhadrak and Cuttack. On the other hand, many districts, despite having a high proportion of households receiving remittances, report comparatively lower amounts, underscoring the uneven distribution of migration benefits within the state.

The utilization patterns of remittances provide insights into their impact on recipient households. The majority of households direct these funds toward essential needs such as daily consumption, healthcare, and education, while also leveraging them for house construction, debt repayment, and special occasions. This not only supports their immediate survival but also enhances their quality of life and long-term prospects, particularly in the health and education sectors. OBC households form the majority of remittance recipients, while upper-caste and SC households also receive a considerable share. However, ST households are disproportionately underrepresented, highlighting the need for targeted interventions to address this gap and ensure equitable benefits from migration-driven income. In conclusion, remittances serve as a lifeline for many households in Odisha, addressing both short-term necessities and long-term aspirations. They play a pivotal role in improving living standards, mitigating financial burdens, and fostering access to opportunities enabled by higher incomes.

Chapter 5
Food Security

Rohit Irudayarajan and Muhammed Thwoyyib K. P.

Abstract This chapter investigates several aspects of food security in Odisha through an analysis of empirical data from the Odisha Migration Survey (OMS) 2023. It draws on household-level food consumption patterns and dietary practices to identify the prevalence and magnitude of different dimensions of food insecurity. While over 90% of households surveyed under OMS reported that grains were a stable food source for them, food groups such as meat, seafood, and fruits were rarely included in the diets of more than two-thirds of households, indicating significant barriers to access. The limited accessibility to essential food items has implications for the nutritional status of these households, potentially leading to deficiencies in vital nutrients. This analysis also focuses on survey results related to qualitative dimensions of food access, including perceptions surrounding food consumption and security. It is evident from the data that vulnerable households experience more severe food insecurity and a lack of dietary diversity, subject to socio-economic characteristics such as caste, tribe, and wealth status. These vulnerable groups, including Scheduled Caste and Scheduled Tribe households, those residing in lower-quality housing, households in the southern region of Odisha, non-migrant households, those in the lowest wealth quartile, and landless and marginal landholders, are disproportionately affected by food and nutritional insecurity. The chapter concludes that the prevalence of food and nutritional insecurity among the vulnerable population underscores the pressing need for government intervention to address accessibility and affordability. By grounding the analysis in empirical evidence, it seeks to inform policy discussions and foster a more comprehensive understanding of the challenges posed by food insecurity in Odisha.

Keywords Food security · Migration · Odisha · Nutrition · Poverty · Dietary diversity · Access to food · Nutritional insecurity

---

R. Irudayarajan (✉)
The International Institute of Migration and Development, Thiruvananthapuram, India
e-mail: rohitrajan@iimad.in

Muhammed Thwoyyib K. P.
BML Munjal University, Gurugram, India

A. Datta and S. I. Rajan (eds.), *Migration, Livelihoods and Gender*, International Perspectives on Migration, https://doi.org/10.1007/978-981-95-5465-2_5

1 Introduction

Food security remains a cornerstone of sustainable development, yet it is an enduring challenge for many regions in the Global South. Urbanization, changing consumption patterns, and the transformation of agrifood systems are reshaping food security and nutrition landscapes across the globe (FAO et al., 2023). In regions like Odisha, India, where both rural and urban areas are experiencing significant transitions, these shifts substantially affect the availability, affordability, and accessibility of healthy diets (Raghunathan et al., 2020). Odisha presents a unique context characterized by a predominantly agrarian economy, high levels of poverty, and growing urbanization, all of which contribute to a complex interplay of factors influencing food security (Mohapatra, 2020).

As dietary preferences evolve with rising incomes and changing lifestyles, there has been a marked shift from traditional staples toward more diversified diets, including higher consumption of animal-sourced foods, fruits, and processed foods (Pingali, 2006). This transition has significant implications for nutrition and public health. While it reflects a global trend, its manifestation in Odisha is refracted through the region's socio-economic conditions and agrarian structure. Urbanization has driven a growing reliance on market-purchased foods, even in rural households, where traditional subsistence-based food production is increasingly supplemented—or replaced—by purchased food. However, these changes also underscore disparities, as access to healthy diets remains a challenge for low-income households, particularly in semi-urban and rural areas. Rising costs of healthy diets, coupled with low incomes, create significant barriers for rural and peri-urban households.

This chapter investigates food security in Odisha using data from the Odisha Migration Survey (OMS) 2023, analyzing household-level consumption patterns, dietary practices, and food insecurity across socio-economic and geographic contexts. Odisha's high levels of out-migration, agrarian dependence, and socio-economic disparities make it an important case for examining the links between migration, poverty, and nutrition. Migration—both seasonal and long term—critically influences food consumption and dietary diversity. Remittances from migrants enhance purchasing power but may also disrupt traditional agrarian livelihoods, impacting food security. In this context, we explore how migration shapes access to food, affordability of healthy diets, and nutrition outcomes. Our findings suggest that the acute nutritional vulnerabilities among marginalized groups, including women and children, highlight persistent disparities in food security and point to the need for targeted interventions to address the systemic inequalities shaping food insecurity in Odisha. The chapter is divided into two parts. The first part examines survey results on household consumption of key food categories such as grains, pulses, fruits, eggs, meat, and oils. The second part explores qualitative dimensions of food security, including households' experiences of food shortages, restricted diets, and reduced meals, with findings disaggregated by social group, migration status, wealth status, and region.

2 Household-Level Food Consumption Patterns

The survey reveals distinct dietary patterns among households, highlighting a reliance on staple foods and variability in the consumption of other food groups (Table 1). Grains dominate household diets, with over 90% of respondents consuming them daily, emphasizing their role as a primary and accessible food source. Similarly, nearly two-thirds of households consistently consume oil, fat, and butter, reflecting their integral role in cooking practices. In contrast, vegetables, greens, and roots/tubers show moderate regularity in consumption, with about a third of households consuming them daily and more than half including them often or occasionally in their meals. These patterns suggest their supplementary role alongside grains in daily meals.

Pulses and legumes exhibit moderate consumption levels, with only 13% of households reporting daily consumption and over half partaking often or occasionally. Their weekly inclusion highlights their importance as a protein source, albeit less frequently than staples. Sugar and honey are consumed daily by 39% of households, while about a quarter of households report rare or no consumption, suggesting that economic or health-related factors influence their inclusion. Protein-rich and nutrient-dense foods such as dairy, eggs, meat, and seafood are consumed less frequently. While 19% of households consistently include dairy, more than half rarely or never consume it. Eggs follow a similar pattern, with nearly half of households consuming them occasionally or frequently, but a notable proportion seldom or never including them in their diets. Meat and seafood, in particular, are consumed rarely, with over two-thirds of households reporting limited or no consumption, reflecting economic constraints. Fruits also exhibit low consumption rates, with more than two-thirds of households rarely or never including them in their diets.

Overall, the data depicts a dietary pattern centered on staples like grains and oils, with varying levels of access to other food groups. While vegetables, greens, pulses, and sugar are moderately consumed, the low intake of fruits, dairy, meat, and seafood points to nutritional vulnerabilities. These patterns reflect a mix of economic, cultural, and accessibility factors shaping household food consumption, as well as the need for improved access to diverse and nutrient-rich foods.

2.1 Primary Food Sources

The survey displays significant variations in the primary sources of food for different food groups, shedding light on household-level dependencies and strategies for meeting dietary needs (Table 2). Grains emerge as a critical staple, predominantly sourced through the public distribution system (41.5%), bringing to the fore the crucial role of government-provided rations in ensuring food security. A notable 30.1% of households rely on their own agricultural production for grains, which reflects the importance of subsistence farming. Purchases from local markets

Table 1 Category-wise food consumption in the past 30 days (% of households)

Frequency of consumption	Grains	Roots and tubers	Pulses and legumes	Vegetables and greens	Fruits	Eggs	Meat	Fish	Dairy products	Sugar and honey	Oil, fat, and butter	Total
Always	94.4	27.2	12.9	30	1.6	1	0.7	0.7	18.8	39.8	66.1	26.5
Often	1.5	30.5	27.4	31.1	8.3	12	6.4	9.7	9.8	18.7	12.8	15.2
Once in a while	0.7	25.1	26.7	27.1	21.5	35	29.8	32	16.3	17.9	8	22.1
Almost never	2.3	12.1	22.3	10.2	36.5	39	45	42	16.1	10.8	7.3	22.5
Never	1	5.1	10.6	1.6	30.7	12	17.9	15	39	12.7	5.8	13.5
Not eaten for religious or cultural reasons	0.1	0	0	0	1.4	0.1	0.2	0.1	0.1	0.1	0.1	0.2
Total	100	100	100	100	100	100	100	100	100	100	100	100

Note Always refers to every day; often to 3–6 times a week; once in a while to 1–2 times a week; and almost never to less than once a week
Source Odisha Migration Study 2023, Household sample

also account for a substantial share (27.6%). Thus, households rely on multiple sources to access food grains.

Roots and tubers are overwhelmingly purchased, with 92.9% of households depending on the market, indicating their integration into the local economy and limited access through other means. Own production contributes marginally (3.1%), consistent with the relatively low prevalence of cultivating these crops at the household level. Similarly, for pulses and legumes, 93.7% of households purchase these items, reflecting their essential role in diets, yet limited production within households. Gathering accounts for 2.1% of their total supply, particularly practiced by some rural or tribal households relying on traditional methods. Vegetables and greens, essential for nutritional balance, are also primarily purchased (92.9%), pointing to a dependence on market access for fresh produce. However, own production (5.5%) makes up a meaningful contribution, particularly in rural households where kitchen gardening is prevalent. The pattern for fruits mirrors that of vegetables, with 90% of households purchasing them and a smaller proportion (3.6%) obtaining them through gathering. Gifts from family members contribute to 4.8% of the total for this category, which is indicative of their sporadic availability through informal support networks.

Animal-based protein sources exhibit similar reliance on purchases. For eggs, 96.1% of households obtain them through markets, while own production contributes 2.1%, implying limited poultry rearing at the household level. Meat consumption is predominantly reliant on purchases (95%), with minimal shares sourced through hunting and gathering (2.2%) and gifts (1.3%). Similarly, fish is primarily purchased (94.1%), though fishing accounts for a minor yet significant contribution (4%). These patterns help depict the economic burden of accessing protein-rich foods, particularly for vulnerable households. Meanwhile, dairy products exhibit a somewhat more diversified sourcing pattern. While 83.4% of households purchase them, the contribution of own production is notable at 14.9%, explained by the small-scale dairy farming in rural areas. Conversely, sugar and honey, and oil, fat, or butter are almost universally purchased (98.3% and 98.5%, respectively). Household-level production or alternative sourcing of these items is uncommon.

Overall, purchasing emerges as the dominant strategy for acquiring food across all groups. While own production plays a vital role in grains and dairy, its contribution to other food groups remains limited. Gathering and gifts from relatives provide supplementary support, particularly for fruits, vegetables, and meat, albeit at minimal levels. The public distribution system plays a crucial role in addressing food security for economically vulnerable households by ensuring access to grains. These findings emphasize the need for policies that enhance household-level production and reduce reliance on markets, especially for nutrient-rich and protein-dense foods. The integration of local resources and improved access to affordable food through public distribution systems can bridge dietary gaps and ensure equitable nutrition (Morris et al., 2020).

Table 2 Main sources of food (% of households)

Main source of food	Grains	Roots and tubers	Pulses and legumes	Vegetables and greens	Fruits	Eggs	Meat	Fish	Dairy products	Sugar and honey	Oil, fat, and butter	Raw
Own production	30.1	2.7	3.1	5.5	0.5	2.1	1.0	0.4	14.9	0.2	0.3	6.3
Hunting, fishing, and gathering	0.2	0.8	2.1	0.5	3.6	0.4	2.2	4.0	0.4	0.5	0.3	1.4
Purchase	27.6	92.9	93.7	92.9	90	96.1	95	94.1	83.4	98.3	98.5	86.7
Exchange labor or items for food	0.1	0.1	0.2	0.1	0.1	0.1	0.1	0.5	0.3	0.1	0.1	0.3
Borrowed	0.1	0.4	0.4	0.5	0.6	0.4	0.2	0.2	0.3	0.7	0.4	0.4
Gift (food) from family relatives	0.3	0.4	0.6	0.4	4.8	0.5	1.3	0.8	0.6	0.2	0.2	1.1
Food aid (including from NGOs)	0	0	0	0.1	0.1	0.4	0	0	0	0	0	0.1
Ration/public distribution system	41.5	2.7	0	0	0	0	0	0	0	0	0	4.0
Others	0.1	0	0	0	0.3	0.2	0.2	0	0	0	0.1	0.2
Total	100	100	100	100	100	100	100	100	100	100	100	100

Source Odisha Migration Study 2023, Household sample

3 Household Food Insecurity and Access

This section examines the multifaceted nature of food insecurity through an analysis of nine key questions posed to 15,000 households as part of the OMS 2023. The questions covering several dimensions of food insecurity are as follows: In the past 30 days, (i) Did you worry that your household would not have enough food to eat due to a lack of resources? (ii) Were you or any household member not able to eat the kinds of foods you preferred because of a lack of resources? (iii) Did you or any household member have to eat a limited variety of foods due to a lack of resources? (iv) Did you or any household member have to eat some foods that you really did not want to eat because of a lack of resources to obtain other types of food? (v) Did you or any household member eat a smaller meal than you felt you needed because there was not enough food? (vi) Did you or any household member eat fewer meals in a day because there was not enough food? (vii) Was there ever no food at all in your household because there were no resources to get more? (viii) Did you or any household member go to sleep at night hungry because there was not enough food? (ix) Did you or any household member go a whole day without eating because there was not enough food?

Each question reveals unique patterns and disparities, offering insights into the challenges at-risk populations face in securing adequate and consistent access to food. For each question, the analysis presents cross-tabulations to provide a disaggregated analysis.

The survey revealed varying degrees of food insecurity across households, following variations in access to adequate food due to resource constraints. A majority of households reported a relatively high level of food security, with 75% never having to worry about insufficient food, and two-thirds never having to eat limited food varieties or meals due to a lack of resources. However, approximately one in five households reported having "rarely" faced challenges such as limited food variety, consuming less preferred foods, or eating smaller meals. Around 5–10% of households occasionally encountered these issues, while less than 5% faced them "often." It is concerning, however, that 2% of households reported severe food insecurity, with responses such as going a whole day without eating because there were not enough resources or having no food at all.

The findings also shed light on the constraints affecting food preferences and meal patterns. While 43% of households reported some degree of inability to eat preferred foods, 13.8% reported that they "rarely" ate smaller meals, and 11.6% reported that they "rarely" ate fewer meals in a day because there was not enough food. A majority of households (more than 90%) reported that they never experienced extreme forms of insecurity, such as going to bed hungry or having no food for an entire day. However, 6–7% of households reported these as "rare," and fewer than 2% reported experiencing them "sometimes" or "often." These results underscore the spectrum of food insecurity, from occasional constraints to severe hardships faced by a small minority (Table 3). The disaggregated findings that follow will delve further into each question,[1] to provide a deeper understanding of these challenges and their implications.

3.1 Not Having Enough Food Due to a Lack of Resources

Even though 75% of households reported not experiencing this form of food insecurity, one in four households still faces it to varying degrees. When disaggregated by locality, nearly a quarter of rural households experience some level of food insecurity, with over 5% falling into the "often" and "sometimes" categories, reflecting extreme insecurity. In urban areas, 23.6% of households reported food insecurity, with approximately 4% encountering extreme levels (Table 22).

A regional analysis reveals pronounced disparities in food security across different areas. Nearly one-fifth of households in the coastal and central regions experience food insecurity. The situation is significantly worse in the southern region, where one-third of households are affected. Extreme food insecurity further underscores these disparities. In coastal areas, 2.3% of households report extreme food insecurity, compared to 4% in the northern region. However, southern Odisha faces the gravest challenges, with 12% of households reporting extreme levels of food insecurity (Table 4).

Among Scheduled Caste (SC) and Scheduled Tribe (ST) households, approximately three in 10 report experiencing this form of food insecurity, with SC households showing a slightly higher prevalence than ST households. In comparison, less than a quarter of general-category households face food insecurity, while nearly one-fifth of Other Backward Class (OBC) households report the same. A closer look at the "often" and "sometimes" frequency categories reveals that around 9% of SC households and 9.3% of ST households experience extreme food insecurity. This figure drops significantly for OBC households (2.8%) and upper-caste households (2.1%) (Table 23).

Migration status further highlights disparities in food insecurity. Among non-migrant households, 6.1% experience extreme food insecurity, falling into the "sometimes" or "often" frequency categories. In comparison, 3.7% of return migrant households and just 2.7% of current migrant households report extreme food insecurity (Table 25). An analysis of food insecurity by wealth quartile offers a clearer picture of stark inequalities. Nearly 40% of the poorest households—those in the lowest wealth quartile—face food insecurity, followed by 30% of households in the second quartile. In contrast, only 16.7% of households in the third quartile report food insecurity, and this figure drops to 10% for the wealthiest households (Table 5).

[1] In the sub-sections that follow, the term *food insecurity* refers specifically to the dimension of insecurity addressed by the corresponding question.

Table 3 Dimensions of food insecurity experienced in the past 30 days (% of households)

	Worried about not having enough food due to a lack of resources	Unable to eat preferred food due to a lack of resources	Ate a limited variety of food due to a lack of resources	Compelled to eat certain foods due to a lack of resources to obtain other kinds of food	Ate smaller meals because there was not enough food	Ate fewer meals because there was not enough food	No food due to a lack of resources	Slept hungry at night	Went for a whole day without eating	Total
Never	74.9	57.4	64	67.6	81.4	85.4	90.9	92.2	93.0	79.3
Rarely	19.8	30.5	22.1	22.2	13.8	11.6	7.1	6.1	5.6	15.4
Sometimes	4.1	7.9	9.8	8.6	4.0	2.6	1.7	1.5	1.1	4.6
Often	1.2	4.2	4.1	1.6	0.8	0.4	0.3	0.3	0.2	0.7
Total	100	100	100	100	100	100	100	100	100	100

Note Rarely refers to 1–2 times; sometimes refers to 3–10 times; often refers to >10 times
Source Odisha Migration Study 2023, Household sample

Table 4 Households not having enough food due to a lack of resources, by region (% of households)

	Coastal/central	Southern	Northern	Total
Never	78.4	66.4	77.3	74.9
Rarely	19.3	21.7	18.8	19.8
Sometimes	1.7	8.9	3.4	4.1
Often	0.6	3.1	0.6	1.2
Total	100	100	100	100

Note Rarely refers to 1–2 times; sometimes refers to 3–10 times; often refers to >10 times
Source Odisha Migration Study 2023, Household sample

Table 5 Households not having enough food due to a lack of resources, by wealth quartile (% of households)

	Wealth quartile				
	First (lowest)	Second	Third	Fourth (highest)	Total
Never	61.1	69.5	83.3	89.7	74.9
Rarely	27.7	26.7	13.2	8.7	19.8
Sometimes	7.8	3.0	3.4	1.5	4.1
Often	3.4	0.8	0.1	0.2	1.2
Total	100	100	100	100	100

Note Rarely refers to 1–2 times; sometimes refers to 3–10 times; often refers to >10 times
Source Odisha Migration Study 2023, Household sample

3.2 *Not Able to Eat Preferred Food Due to a Lack of Resources*

About 42.5% of rural households reported experiencing this dimension of food insecurity to varying degrees (Table 3). While the overall prevalence of food insecurity in urban areas remained significant, it was comparatively lower than in rural areas, with approximately one in 10 urban households affected (Table 6). Disaggregation by social group further reveals that households experience food insecurity to different extents, with the ST households reporting the highest incidence, followed by SC, upper-caste, and OBC households, respectively (Table 28). Housing type also plays a crucial role: among households with "luxurious" homes, only 15.6% report food insecurity; whereas, more than half of those in "poor" and "kutcha" housing are food insecure (Table 29).

When disaggregated by migration status, it emerges that return migrant households face the highest food insecurity, with over half reporting it and 9% experiencing extreme food insecurity (Table 30). Similarly, households with marginal landholdings report the highest food insecurity, with almost half affected. Landless households and those with small landholdings follow, while households with middle- or large-sized landholdings report significantly lower levels of food insecurity (Table 32). These

Table 6 Households not able to eat the kinds of foods you preferred because of a lack of resources, by type of locality (% of households)

	Locality		Total
	Rural	Urban	
Never	55.8	66.5	57.4
Rarely	31.5	25.2	30.5
Sometimes	8.3	6.2	7.9
Often	4.4	3.2	4.2
Total	1000	1000	100

Note Rarely refers to 1–2 times; sometimes refers to 3–10 times; often refers to >10 times
Source Odisha Migration Study 2023, Household sample

findings reinforce the need for targeted interventions addressing both regional and socio-economic disparities in food security.

3.3 *Eating a Limited Variety of Food Due to a Lack of Resources*

Nearly one-third of survey households reported that they ate a limited variety of food due to a lack of resources (Table 3). Region-wise, this form of food insecurity is more pronounced in the northern and southern areas. In the coastal region, nearly three in 10 households report food insecurity, while this number increases to four in 10 in both the southern and northern regions. The northern region, in particular, exhibits slightly higher levels of food insecurity than the southern region, a pattern consistent with previous findings. Notably, while less than 6% of households in the coastal/central region experience extreme food insecurity, this figure rises to just over 20% in the southern region and nearly 20% in the northern region (Table 7). The regional variation highlights the need for targeted interventions in areas with the highest prevalence of extreme food insecurity.

Table 7 Households have to eat a limited variety of foods due to a lack of resources, by region (% of households)

	Coastal/central	Southern	Northern	Total
Never	70.6	59.1	58.9	64
Rarely	23.7	20.1	21.4	22.1
Sometimes	3.8	16.0	13.0	9.8
Often	1.9	4.8	6.6	4.1
Total	100	100	100	100

Note Rarely refers to 1–2 times; sometimes refers to 3–10 times; often refers to >10 times
Source Odisha Migration Study 2023, Household sample

Table 8 Households have to eat a limited variety of foods due to a lack of resources, by social group (% of households)

	SC	ST	OBC	Upper castes	Total
Never	56.1	58.0	69.2	67.8	64
Rarely	24.9	22.9	20.8	21.2	22.1
Sometimes	13.7	13.1	8.0	5.5	9.8
Often	5.4	6.0	2.0	5.5	4.1
Total	100	100	100	100	100

Note Rarely refers to 1–2 times; sometimes refers to 3–10 times; often refers to >10 times
Source Odisha Migration Study 2023, Household sample

To gain a deeper understanding of the social dimension of this form of food insecurity, disaggregating the data by social groups is essential. Nearly one-third of upper-caste households reported experiencing this form of food insecurity, with SC and ST households facing significantly higher proportions. About three in 10 OBC households reported food insecurity, a figure slightly lower than that of upper-caste households, and markedly lower than that of SC and ST households (Table 8).

Housing type further illuminates these disparities: fewer than 15% of households in the "luxurious" housing category experience food insecurity, while nearly half of those residing in "poor" and "kutcha" housing report facing food insecurity (Table 34). Disaggregating by migration status shows a similar trend, with return migrant households experiencing slightly lower levels of food insecurity compared to migrant and non-migrant households, though the overall prevalence remains high across all categories (Table 35). Wealth quartile analysis reveals a consistent pattern, where nearly half of the poorest households and three in five households in the second quartile report food insecurity, in contrast to fewer than 20% of the wealthiest households. Landless households follow closely behind, with one-third reporting food insecurity, while those with small landholdings fare somewhat better. Households with middle- or large-sized landholdings experience significantly lower levels of food insecurity, with fewer than a quarter affected (Table 37).

3.4 Have to Eat Some Foods Due to a Lack of Resources to Eat Other Kinds of Food

Nearly one-third of survey households were compelled to eat certain foods due to a lack of resources to obtain other kinds of food (Table 3). Disaggregated by locality, one in three rural households experiences this kind of food insecurity, whereas approximately one in four urban households faces the same challenge. Notably, 11% of rural households report extreme food insecurity, indicating that they *sometimes* or *often* had to eat foods they did not want in the past 30 days. In contrast, this proportion for urban households is significantly lower, at 6.3% (Table 9).

Table 9 Households had to eat some foods due to a lack of resources to obtain other types of food, by locality (% of households)

	Rural	Urban	Total
Never	66.5	73.6	67.6
Rarely	22.7	20.1	22.2
Sometimes	9.3	4.7	8.6
Often	1.6	1.6	1.6
Total	100	100	100

Note Rarely refers to 1–2 times; sometimes refers to 3–10 times; often refers to >10 times
Source Odisha Migration Study 2023, Household sample

Disaggregating the data by social group shows a pattern similar to previous dimensions of food insecurity. As one moves up the social hierarchy, the prevalence of food insecurity decreases. Among upper castes, 27% households report experiencing this kind of food insecurity, while the corresponding number for OBC households is 29%. The figures are significantly higher for ST (42%) and SC households (35%). The data clearly shows that food insecurity, particularly *extreme* food insecurity, becomes more pronounced as one moves down the social ladder (Table 39).

Examining food insecurity by housing type reveals a stark contrast in the experiences of households residing in different types of housing. While fewer than 10% of households living in "luxurious" housing report food insecurity, the incidence increases significantly for those in "good," "poor," and "kutcha" housing. In particular, a quarter of households in "good" housing report food insecurity, and the percentages rise substantially for households in "poor" and "kutcha" housing, with 39.5% and 44.3%, respectively (Table 10).

The prevalence of food insecurity differs significantly between migrant and non-migrant households, even as nearly one-third of all households experience varying degrees of food insecurity. However, non-migrant households report a notably higher incidence of extreme food insecurity at 11.2%. In comparison, 6.8% of current migrant households experience extreme food insecurity, with return migrant households reporting lower levels of food insecurity overall (Table 40). Similarly, when

Table 10 Households had to eat some foods due to a lack of resources to obtain other types of food, by type of housing (% of households)

	Luxurious	Very good	Good	Poor	Kutcha	Total
Never	92.8	79.9	74.1	60.5	55.7	67.6
Rarely	6.7	18.0	17.3	26.3	29.5	22.2
Sometimes	0.3	1.6	7.9	11.2	11.7	8.6
Often	0.3	0.5	0.8	2.0	3.1	1.6
Total	100	100	100	100	100	100

Note Rarely refers to 1–2 times; sometimes refers to 3–10 times; often refers to >10 times
Source Odisha Migration Study 2023, Household sample

examining food insecurity based on land ownership, households with marginal landholdings report a higher incidence of food insecurity, with one-third of marginal landholding and landless households facing this issue. A significant proportion of landless households experience extreme food insecurity. In contrast, households with middle- or large-sized landholdings exhibit much lower rates of food insecurity, with only one in five households owning five or more acres experiencing this issue (Table 42).

3.5 Ate Smaller Meals Because There Was Not Enough Food

Nearly 20% of the survey households ate smaller meals because there was not enough food. When understanding the disaggregation of food-insecure households by locality, it is evident that rural and urban areas display nearly identical levels of food insecurity, with urban households reporting slightly higher instances of this issue (Table 43). In terms of this specific dimension of food insecurity, fewer than 15% of households in the coastal region reported facing it. In contrast, more than one in five households in the southern and northern regions experienced this form of food insecurity. Notably, a slightly higher proportion of households in the northern region reported *extreme* food insecurity compared to those in the southern region. However, fewer than 1% of households in the coastal region experienced extreme food insecurity (Table 11).

Disaggregating the data by social group reveals nuances of this form of food insecurity. While 15.7% of upper-caste households reported experiencing food insecurity, the proportion of OBC households was slightly lower at 15.4%. In contrast, more than 25% of SC households and 20% of ST households reported facing this form of food insecurity. Although OBC households report a lower overall incidence of food insecurity than upper-caste households, the proportion of those experiencing severe food insecurity was higher for OBC households at 3.5%, compared to 1.8% for upper-caste households (Table 12).

Table 11 Households had to eat smaller meals because there was not enough food, by region (% of households)

	Coastal/central	Southern	Northern	Total
Never	85.4	78.4	78.4	81.4
Rarely	13.8	14.6	12.9	13.8
Sometimes	0.6	6.7	6.4	4.0
Often	0.2	0.3	2.3	0.8
Total	100	100	100	100

Note Rarely refers to 1–2 times; sometimes refers to 3–10 times; often refers to >10 times
Source Odisha Migration Study 2023, Household sample

Table 12 Households had to eat smaller meals because there was not enough food, by social group (% of households)

	SC	ST	OBC	Upper castes	Total
Never	74.3	79.1	84.6	84.3	81.4
Rarely	18.0	13.8	12.0	13.9	13.8
Sometimes	6.4	6.1	2.8	1.4	4.0
Often	1.3	1.0	0.7	0.4	0.8
Total	100	100	100	100	100

Note Rarely refers to 1–2 times; sometimes refers to 3–10 times; often refers to >10 times
Source Odisha Migration Study 2023, Household sample

Regarding land ownership, about one-fifth of landless households and those with marginal landholdings reported food insecurity, with the latter showing a slightly higher incidence. In contrast, 16% of households with one to five acres of land, and nearly 10% of households with more than five acres, reported food insecurity. Looking at the relationship between landholding size and food insecurity, it is evident that larger landholdings correspond to lower levels of food insecurity (Table 47).

3.6 Ate Fewer Meals Because There Was Not Enough Food

The 14.4% of households reporting food insecurity—specifically through eating fewer meals than needed due to insufficient resources—reveals discernible patterns when disaggregated by locality and region. In terms of locality, rural and urban households exhibit nearly identical levels of food insecurity, with 14.5% of rural households and 15% of urban households facing this issue to varying degrees. This suggests that food insecurity is a prevalent concern across both rural and urban areas, though localized factors may contribute to slight differences in severity (Table 13).

When examining food insecurity by region, a distinct pattern emerges. Coastal and central regions report fewer instances of food insecurity compared to the southern

Table 13 Households had to eat fewer meals in a day, by locality (% of households)

	Rural	Urban	Total
Never	85.5	85.0	85.4
Rarely	11.5	12.1	11.6
Sometimes	2.6	2.6	2.6
Often	0.4	0.3	0.4
Total	100	100	100

Note Rarely refers to 1–2 times; sometimes refers to 3–10 times; often refers to >10 times
Source Odisha Migration Study 2023, Household sample

Table 14 Households had to eat fewer meals in a day, by region (% of households)

	Coastal/central	Southern	Northern	Total
Never	88.4	80.4	85.5	85.4
Rarely	10.8	13.2	11.2	11.6
Sometimes	0.5	6.0	2.7	2.6
Often	0.2	0.4	0.6	0.4
Total	100	100	100	100

Note Rarely refers to 1–2 times; sometimes refers to 3–10 times; often refers to >10 times
Source Odisha Migration Study 2023, Household sample

and northern regions. In particular, approximately one in five households in the southern region experiences food insecurity, which is significantly higher than in the coastal areas. The northern region also shows a high prevalence of food insecurity, reinforcing the trend of greater food insecurity in southern and northern regions relative to the coastal/central regions. This regional disparity highlights the uneven distribution of food insecurity across the state, with southern and northern areas facing more severe challenges (Table 14).

Regarding migration status, 15% of non-migrant households and 12% of migrant households experience food insecurity. However, return migrant households exhibit a lower incidence, with less than 10% reporting food insecurity (Table 50). A breakdown by wealth quartile shows a clear disparity, with more than 20% of the poorest households facing food insecurity, compared to just 5% of the wealthiest households (Table 51). Finally, land ownership is a crucial factor in food insecurity. Households with marginal landholdings report the highest levels of food insecurity, followed by landless households and those with small landholdings. In contrast, fewer than 10% of households with middle- or large-sized landholdings experience food insecurity. It is also noteworthy that landless households make up a significant portion of those experiencing *extreme* food insecurity (Table 52).

3.7 No Food at All Due to a Lack of Resources

Nine percent of the survey households reported that their households had no food at all due to a lack of resources (Table 3). Disaggregating the food-insecure households based on locality, it is apparent that this percentage for urban households was slightly lower compared to rural households. Among all households, 2.2% of rural households and 1.3% of urban households experience severe food insecurity (Table 53). Looking deeper into the composition of food-insecure households by social group shows that around 15% of the SC households and almost one in 10 ST households experience this specific form of food insecurity. On the other hand, 8% of OBC households and a significantly smaller proportion of upper-caste households (less than 5%) encounter the same (Table 15). Examining the food-insecure households by the type of house occupied offers a more detailed insight into the composition. Among households with 'luxurious' houses, negligibly, less than 1% reported food insecurity. However, the prevalence of food insecurity of this form is significantly higher among households residing in 'poor' (13.5%) and 'kutcha' (16.4%) houses (Table 16).

By migration status, the data reveals notable differences in food insecurity levels. Nearly 10% of non-migrant households report experiencing food insecurity, while about 6% of current migrant households face the same issue. Return migrant households fall in between, with a slightly higher incidence than migrant households but slightly lower than non-migrant households (Table 55). An analysis of food insecurity based on land ownership reveals a consistent pattern. Around 10% of landless households report food insecurity, while this proportion decreases to approximately 5% among larger landholders. And predictably, extreme food insecurity is the highest for landless households (Table 57).

Table 15 Households had no food at all due to a lack of resources, by social group (% of households)

	SC	ST	OBC	Upper castes	Total
Never	85.4	89.6	92.1	95.8	90.9
Rarely	10.1	7.6	6.8	3.3	7.1
Sometimes	4.1	2.2	0.9	0.5	1.7
Often	0.3	0.5	0.2	0.4	0.3
Total	100	100	100	100	100

Note Rarely refers to 1–2 times; sometimes refers to 3–10 times; often refers to >10 times
Source Odisha Migration Study 2023, Household sample

Table 16 Households had no food at all due to a lack of resources, by type of housing (% of households)

	Luxurious	Very good	Good	Poor	Kutcha	Total
Never	99.5	96.7	96.1	86.5	83.6	90.9
Rarely		2.6	3.0	10.6	12.5	7.1
Sometimes	0.5	0.4	0.7	2.7	3.2	1.8
Often		0.3	0.2	0.2	0.6	0.3
Total	100	100	100	100	100	100

Note Rarely refers to 1–2 times; sometimes refers to 3–10 times; often refers to >10 times
Source Odisha Migration Study 2023, Household sample

3.8 *Had to Go to Sleep Hungry at Night Due to a Lack of Food*

Although the overall incidence of this form of food insecurity is 7.8% (Table 3), by locality, rural households face a slightly higher rate of food insecurity, with 8% of rural households affected, compared to more than 7% of urban households (Table 58). Regional disparities in food insecurity are also apparent. In the coastal region, fewer than 3% of households report food insecurity. However, this figure rises significantly in the southern region, where approximately 13% of households experience food insecurity. In the northern region, about one in 10 households reports facing food insecurity (Table 17).

While fewer than 5% of upper-caste households reported experiencing this form of food insecurity, the incidence rises significantly for SC and ST households. Specifically, 12% of SC households and nearly 9% of ST households reported experiencing food insecurity of this type. OBC households also displayed a considerable incidence, with approximately 7% reporting food insecurity. Furthermore, it is clear that SC households, followed by ST households, are disproportionately affected by severe food insecurity of this form (Table 18).

Table 17 Households had to go to sleep at night hungry because there was not enough food, by region (% of households)

	Coastal/central	Southern	Northern	Total
Never	97.2	86.9	89.6	92.2
Rarely	2.3	9.7	8.3	6.1
Sometimes	0.4	2.9	1.9	1.5
Often	0.1	0.5	0.3	0.3
Total	100	100	100	100

Note Rarely refers to 1–2 times; sometimes refers to 3–10 times; often refers to >10 times
Source Odisha Migration Study 2023, Household sample

Table 18 Households had to go to sleep at night hungry because there was not enough food, by social group (% of households)

	SC	ST	OBC	Upper castes	Total
Never	87.9	91.7	92.9	95.7	92.2
Rarely	8.5	5.8	6.1	3.7	6.1
Sometimes	3.2	2.2	0.8	0.3	1.5
Often	0.4	0.3	0.1	0.4	0.3
Total	100	100	100	100	100

Note Rarely refers to 1–2 times; sometimes refers to 3–10 times; often refers to >10 times
Source Odisha Migration Study 2023, Household sample

Table 19 Households had to go to sleep at night hungry because there was not enough food, by wealth quartile (% of households)

	Poorest	Poor	Rich	Richest	Total
Never	87.2	94.7	91.6	96.0	92.2
Rarely	9.6	4.1	7.4	2.6	6.1
Sometimes	2.7	1.1	0.8	1.2	1.5
Often	0.5	0.1	0.3	0.1	0.3
Total	100	100	100	100	100

Note Rarely refers to 1–2 times; sometimes refers to 3–10 times; often refers to >10 times
Source Odisha Migration Study 2023, Household sample

Disaggregating the data by housing type brings significant inequalities into focus. While less than 1% of households residing in "luxurious" houses report experiencing food insecurity, the incidence is much higher among those living in "poor" and "kutcha" houses, with rates of nearly 12.2% and 14%, respectively (Table 59). Additionally, analyzing food insecurity by wealth quartile reveals sharp contrasts: about 13% of the poorest households experience food insecurity, compared to only 4% of the richest households (Table 19).

3.9 *Had to Go a Whole Day Without Eating*

About 7% of households reported experiencing this specific form of food insecurity (Table 3), with deeper analysis revealing distinct patterns among these vulnerable groups. Rural households are slightly more affected, with 7.3% encountering food insecurity, compared to 5.4% of urban households. Severe food insecurity further highlights this disparity, affecting 1.5% of rural households, compared to less than 1% of urban households (Table 62). Disaggregation by migration status provides additional insights. Approximately 8% of non-migrant households face food insecurity, compared to less than 5% of current migrant and return migrant households (Table 20). Finally, an analysis by wealth quartile highlights significant disparities, with 11% of the poorest households reporting food insecurity, a figure that drops to less than 4% among the wealthiest households (Table 66).

Examining food-insecure households based on land ownership uncovers recurring patterns. Approximately 8.3% of landless households experience food insecurity, compared to only 5% of households with large landholdings. Households with small and marginal landholdings exhibit comparable levels of food insecurity, falling between the higher rates observed among landless households and the lower rates reported by households with large landholdings (Table 21).

Table 20 Households (HH) had to go the whole day without eating due to a lack of food, by migration status (% of households)

	Non-migrant HH	Current migrant HH	Return migrant HH	Total
Never	92.1	95.9	96.9	93
Rarely	6.3	3.4	2.6	5.6
Sometimes	1.3	0.5	0.4	1.1
Often	0.2	0.2		0.2
Total	100	100	100	

Note Rarely refers to 1–2 times; sometimes refers to 3–10 times; often refers to >10 times
Source Odisha Migration Study 2023, Household sample

Table 21 Households had to go the whole day without eating due to a lack of food, by land ownership (% of households)

	Landless	0–1 acre	1–5 acres	5+ acres	Total
Never	91.7	94.0	94.1	94.9	93.0
Rarely	6.6	5.0	4.6	4.8	5.6
Sometimes	1.4	0.8	1.1	0.4	1.1
Often	0.3	0.2	0.1	0.0	0.2
Total	100	100	100	100	100

Note Rarely refers to 1–2 times; sometimes refers to 3–10 times; often refers to >10 times
Source Odisha Migration Study 2023, Household sample

4 Conclusion

The findings from our analysis in this chapter reveal the intricacies of food insecurity in Odisha, shaped by socioeconomic inequalities, migration patterns, and regional disparities. While grains form the dietary staple for most households, they cannot compensate for the lack of diversity in nutrition, with access to protein- and vitamin-rich foods remaining limited for many. Vulnerable groups, such as SC and ST households, non-migrant families, and those in the lower wealth quartiles, face the brunt of food insecurity, often influenced by structural inequalities and economic constraints. The heavy reliance on market-purchased food exposes low-income households to the risks of price volatility, further intensifying their vulnerability.

Addressing these persistent challenges requires a well-rounded approach combining effective public policies and local empowerment strategies. Strengthening the public distribution system to include nutrient-rich and fortified foods can play a crucial role in bridging nutritional gaps, particularly for marginalized communities. Additionally, supporting small-scale farmers and promoting sustainable agricultural practices can enhance local food production and reduce dependency on markets. Such initiatives, along with targeted programs to address the specific needs of vulnerable populations, are essential for reducing disparities and ensuring long-term food security. Looking to the future, food security in Odisha must align with broader sustainable development goals by incorporating technological advancements, climate-resilient agricultural practices, and community-driven initiatives. Government efforts should focus on addressing regional imbalances, particularly in the southern and northern regions, where food insecurity is most severe. Policies must also consider the role of migration, ensuring that remittances and mobility contribute positively to household nutrition. By fostering inclusive growth and resilience, Odisha can not only address current food security challenges but also lay the groundwork for sustainable and equitable development.

Appendix

See Tables 22, 23, 24, 25, 26, 27, 28, 29, 30, 31, 32, 33, 34, 35, 36, 37, 38, 39, 40, 41, 42, 43, 44, 45, 46, 47, 48, 49, 50, 51, 52, 53, 54, 55, 56, 57, 58, 59, 60, 61, 62, 63, 64, 65, and 66.

Table 22 Households not having enough food due to a lack of resources, by locality (% of households)

	Rural	Urban	Total
Never	74.6	76.4	74.9
Rarely	19.8	19.6	19.8
Sometimes	4.3	3.3	4.1
Often	1.4	0.7	1.2
Total	100	100	100

Note Rarely refers to 1–2 times; sometimes refers to 3–10 times; often refers to >10 times
Source Odisha Migration Survey 2023, Household sample

Table 23 Households not having enough food due to a lack of resources, by social group (% of households)

	SC	ST	OBC	Upper castes	Total
Never	69.6	66.9	81.0	76.1	74.9
Rarely	21.6	23.8	16.1	21.8	19.8
Sometimes	6.8	7.0	2.3	1.7	4.1
Often	2.1	2.3	0.6	0.4	1.2
Total	100	100	100	100	100

Note Rarely refers to 1–2 times; sometimes refers to 3–10 times; often refers to >10 times
Source Odisha Migration Survey 2023, Household sample

Table 24 Households not having enough food due to a lack of resources, by type of housing (% of households)

	Luxurious	Very good	Good	Poor	Kutcha	Total
Never	97.0	89.6	77.6	71.3	63.2	74.9
Rarely	1.7	8.4	19.4	21.8	27.2	19.8
Sometimes	1.3	1.5	2.6	5.8	6.4	4.1
Often	0.0	0.5	0.5	1.1	3.3	1.2
Total	100	100	100	100	100	100

Note Rarely refers to 1–2 times; sometimes refers to 3–10 times; often refers to >10 times
Source Odisha Migration Survey 2023, Household sample

Table 25 Households (HH) not having enough food due to a lack of resources, by migration status (% of households)

	Non-migrant HH	Current migrant HH	Return migrant HH	Total
Never	74.2	77.2	77.7	74.9
Rarely	19.8	20.1	18.6	19.8
Sometimes	4.6	2.3	3.2	4.1
Often	1.5	0.4	0.5	1.2
Total	100	100	100	100

Note Rarely refers to 1–2 times; sometimes refers to 3–10 times; often refers to >10 times
Source Odisha Migration Survey 2023, Household sample

Table 26 Households not having enough food due to a lack of resources, by land ownership (% of households)

	Landless	0–1 acre	1–5 acres	5+ acres	Total
Never	73.6	72.6	79.4	86.3	74.9
Rarely	20.2	21.9	17.0	8.6	19.8
Sometimes	5.1	4.0	2.5	2.3	4.1
Often	1.1	1.5	1.1	2.8	1.2
Total	100	100	100	100	100

Note Rarely refers to 1–2 times; sometimes refers to 3–10 times; often refers to >10 times
Source Odisha Migration Survey 2023, Household sample

Table 27 Households not able to eat preferred food due to a lack of resources, by region (% of households)

	Coastal/central	Southern	Northern	Total
Never	64.3	53.6	50.9	57.4
Rarely	29.5	29.6	32.7	30.5
Sometimes	4.0	11.6	10.3	7.9
Often	2.1	5.2	6.1	4.2
Total	100	100	100	100

Note Rarely refers to 1–2 times; sometimes refers to 3–10 times; often refers to >10 times
Source Odisha Migration Survey 2023, Household sample

Table 28 Households not able to eat preferred food due to a lack of resources, by social groups (% of households)

	SC	ST	OBC	Upper castes	Total
Never	69.6	66.9	81.0	76.1	57.4
Rarely	21.6	23.8	16.1	21.8	30.5
Sometimes	6.8	7.0	2.3	1.7	7.9
Often	2.1	2.3	0.6	0.4	4.2
Total	100	100	100	100	100

Note Rarely refers to 1–2 times; sometimes refers to 3–10 times; often refers to >10 times
Source Odisha Migration Survey 2023, Household sample

Table 29 Households not able to eat preferred food due to a lack of resources, by type of housing (% of households)

	Luxurious	Very good	Good	Poor	Kutcha	Total
Never	84.4	72.9	63.9	46.9	47.7	57.4
Rarely	11.0	19.7	26.8	37.7	36.3	30.5
Sometimes	1.8	3.9	7.2	10.6	8.8	7.9
Often	2.8	3.5	2.1	4.8	7.2	4.2
Total	100	100	100	100	100	100

Note Rarely refers to 1–2 times; sometimes refers to 3–10 times; often refers to >10 times
Source Odisha Migration Survey 2023, Household sample

Table 30 Households not able to eat preferred food due to a lack of resources, by migration status (% of households)

	Non-migrant HH	Current migrant HH	Return migrant HH	Total
Never	58.2	57.3	45.5	57.4
Rarely	29.3	31.8	45.7	30.5
Sometimes	8.2	6.5	7.6	7.9
Often	4.3	4.3	1.2	4.2
Total	100	100	100	100

Note Rarely refers to 1–2 times; sometimes refers to 3–10 times; often refers to >10 times
Source Odisha Migration Survey 2023, Household sample

Table 31 Households not able to eat preferred food due to a lack of resources, by wealth quartile (% of households)

	First (lowest)	Second	Third	Fourth (highest)	Total
Never	45.7	51.2	56.3	79.8	57.4
Rarely	35.1	37.6	32.3	15.3	30.5
Sometimes	11.0	7.8	7.8	4.3	7.9
Often	8.1	3.3	3.6	0.6	4.2
Total	100	100	100	100	100

Note Rarely refers to 1–2 times; sometimes refers to 3–10 times; often refers to >10 times
Source Odisha Migration Survey 2023, Household sample

Table 32 Households not able to eat preferred food due to a lack of resources, by land ownership (% of households)

	Landless	0–1 acre	1–5 acres	5+ acres	Total
Never	58.4	50.4	63.2	75.9	57.4
Rarely	29.1	34.7	28.9	17.8	30.5
Sometimes	8.9	8.8	5.3	2.3	7.9
Often	3.7	6.0	2.6	4.0	4.2
Total	100	100	100	100	100

Note Rarely refers to 1–2 times; sometimes refers to 3–10 times; often refers to >10 times
Source Odisha Migration Survey 2023, Household sample

Table 33 Households have to eat a limited variety of foods due to a lack of resources, by locality (% of households)

	Rural	Urban	Total
Never	62.8	69.8	64.0
Rarely	22.4	20.4	22.1
Sometimes	10.6	5.9	9.8
Often	4.2	3.8	4.1
Total	100	100	100

Note Rarely refers to 1–2 times; sometimes refers to 3–10 times; often refers to >10 times
Source Odisha Migration Survey 2023, Household sample

Table 34 Households have to eat a limited variety of foods due to a lack of resources, by type of housing (% of households)

	Luxurious	Very good	Good	Poor	Kutcha	Total
Never	86.2	75.0	72.7	54.9	52.2	64.0
Rarely	8.7	17.8	15.0	27.6	30.5	22.1
Sometimes	1.8	4.0	10.1	12.6	10.5	9.8
Often	3.4	3.2	2.2	5.0	6.8	4.1
Total	100	100	100	100	100	100,100

Note Rarely refers to 1–2 times; sometimes refers to 3–10 times; often refers to >10 times
Source Odisha Migration Survey 2023, Household sample

Table 35 Households have to eat a limited variety of foods due to a lack of resources, by migration status (% of households)

	Non-migrant HH	Current migrant HH	Return migrant HH	Total
Never	63.7	64.3	67.2	64.0
Rarely	22.2	22.0	20.4	22.1
Sometimes	9.9	9.3	11.1	9.8
Often	4.2	4.4	1.3	4.1
Total	100	100	100	100

Note Rarely refers to 1–2 times; sometimes refers to 3–10 times; often refers to >10 times
Source Odisha Migration Survey 2023, Household sample

Table 36 Households have to eat a limited variety of foods due to a lack of resources, by wealth quartile (% of households)

	First (lowest)	Second	Third	Fourth (highest)	Total
Never	52.7	60.0	64.6	81.7	64.0
Rarely	26.3	26.7	21.8	11.9	22.1
Sometimes	13.2	9.8	10.0	5.6	9.8
Often	7.7	3.6	3.6	0.8	4.1
Total	100	100	100	100	100

Note Rarely refers to 1–2 times; sometimes refers to 3–10 times; often refers to >10 times
Source Odisha Migration Survey 2023, Household sample

Table 37 Households have to eat a limited variety of foods due to a lack of resources, by land ownership (% of households)

	Landless	0–1 acre	1–5 acres	5+ acres	Total
Never	65.9	57.9	67.1	76.6	64.0
Rarely	20.4	25.6	21.3	13.8	22.1
Sometimes	9.6	10.7	9.4	8.0	9.8
Often	4.1	5.8	2.2	1.5	4.1
Total	100	100	100	100	100

Note Rarely refers to 1–2 times; sometimes refers to 3–10 times; often refers to >10 times
Source Odisha Migration Survey 2023, Household sample

Table 38 Households had to eat some foods due to a lack of resources to obtain other types of food, by region (% of households)

	Coastal/central	Southern	Northern	Total
Never	71.9	64.1	64.7	67.6
Rarely	26.5	16.7	21.1	22.2
Sometimes	1.4	17.9	10.7	8.6
Often	0.3	1.4	3.5	1.6
Total	100	100	100	100

Note Rarely refers to 1–2 times; sometimes refers to 3–10 times; often refers to >10 times
Source Odisha Migration Survey 2023, Household sample

Table 39 Households had to eat some foods due to a lack of resources to obtain other types of food, by social group (% of households)

	SC	ST	OBC	Upper castes	Total
Never	57.7	64.6	71.3	73.4	67.6
Rarely	29.2	17.3	22.0	22.4	22.2
Sometimes	10.8	15.4	5.9	3.1	8.6
Often	2.3	2.7	0.8	1.1	1.6
Total	100	100	100	100	100

Note Rarely refers to 1–2 times; sometimes refers to 3–10 times; often refers to >10 times
Source Odisha Migration Survey 2023, Household sample

Table 40 Households had to eat some foods due to a lack of resources to obtain other types of food, by migration status (% of households)

	Non-migrant HH	Current migrant HH	Return migrant HH	Total
Never	67.2	67.8	74.7	67.6
Rarely	21.7	25.5	19.5	22.2
Sometimes	9.5	5.5	5.2	8.6
Often	1.7	1.3	0.6	1.6
Total	100	100	100	100

Note Rarely refers to 1–2 times; sometimes refers to 3–10 times; often refers to >10 times
Source Odisha Migration Survey 2023, Household sample

Table 41 Households had to eat some foods due to a lack of resources to obtain other types of food, by wealth quartile (% of households)

	First (lowest)	Second	Third	Fourth (highest)	Total
Never	59.4	62.9	65.6	84.9	67.6
Rarely	23.6	27.5	26.4	10.8	22.2
Sometimes	13.5	8.2	7.4	4.0	8.6
Often	3.5	1.4	0.6	0.3	1.6
Total	100	100	100	100	100

Note Rarely refers to 1–2 times; sometimes refers to 3–10 times; often refers to >10 times
Source Odisha Migration Survey 2023, Household sample

Table 42 Households had to eat some foods due to a lack of resources to obtain other types of food, by land ownership (% of households)

	Landless	0–1 acre	1–5 acres	5+ acres	Total
Never	66.4	64.6	73.0	80.0	67.6
Rarely	20.9	26.9	19.7	10.2	22.2
Sometimes	10.7	6.8	6.7	8.8	8.6
Often	2.0	1.7	0.6	1.1	1.6
Total	100	100	100	100	100

Note Rarely refers to 1–2 times; sometimes refers to 3–10 times; often refers to >10 times
Source Odisha Migration Survey 2023, Household sample

Table 43 Households had to eat smaller meals because there was not enough food, by locality (% of households)

	Rural	Urban	Total
Never	81.5	81.1	81.4
Rarely	13.8	13.5	13.8
Sometimes	4.0	3.9	4.0
Often	0.7	1.5	0.8
Total	100	100	100

Note Rarely refers to 1–2 times; sometimes refers to 3–10 times; often refers to >10 times
Source Odisha Migration Survey 2023, Household sample

Table 44 Households had to eat smaller meals because there was not enough food, by housing (% of households)

	Luxurious	Very good	Good	Poor	Kutcha	Total
Never	98.5	94.6	87.4	75.5	69.1	81.4
Rarely	1.5	5.0	9.7	16.0	24.5	13.8
Sometimes		0.3	2.6	6.9	5.2	4.0
Often		0.1	0.4	1.6	1.2	0.8
Total	100	100	100	100	100	100

Note Rarely refers to 1–2 times; sometimes refers to 3–10 times; often refers to >10 times
Source Odisha Migration Survey 2023, Household sample

Table 45 Households had to eat smaller meals because there was not enough food, by migration status (% of households)

	Non-migrant HH	Current migrant HH	Return migrant HH	Total
Never	80.6	83.6	87.5	81.4
Rarely	14.1	13.2	10.9	13.8
Sometimes	4.5	2.5	1.5	4.0
Often	0.9	0.7		0.8
Total	100	100	100	100

Note Rarely refers to 1–2 times; sometimes refers to 3–10 times; often refers to >10 times
Source Odisha Migration Survey 2023, Household sample

Table 46 Households had to eat smaller meals because there was not enough food, by wealth quartile (% of households)

	Poorest	Poor	Rich	Richest	Total
Never	72.8	77.9	84.6	92.8	81.4
Rarely	19.5	18.3	10.9	4.4	13.8
Sometimes	6.1	3.1	4.0	2.4	4.0
Often	1.6	0.7	0.5	0.4	0.8
Total	100	100	100	100	100

Note Rarely refers to 1–2 times; sometimes refers to 3–10 times; often refers to >10 times
Source Odisha Migration Survey 2023, Household sample

Table 47 Households had to eat smaller meals because there was not enough food, by land ownership (% of households)

	Landless	0–1 acre	1–5 acres	5+ acres	Total
Never	81.0	79.5	84.0	90.1	81.4
Rarely	12.4	17.2	12.6	6.7	13.8
Sometimes	5.2	2.8	3.2	2.8	4.0
Often	1.5	0.4	0.2	0.4	0.8
Total	100	100	100	100	100

Note Rarely refers to 1–2 times; sometimes refers to 3–10 times; often refers to >10 times
Source Odisha Migration Survey 2023, Household sample

Table 48 Households had to eat fewer meals in a day, by social group (% of households)

	SC	ST	OBC	Upper castes	Total
Never	80.1	84.2	88.0	86.1	85.4
Rarely	14.9	10.8	10.4	12.5	11.6
Sometimes	4.4	4.5	1.4	1.2	2.6
Often	0.6	0.5	0.2	0.3	0.4
Total	100	100	100	100	100

Note Rarely refers to 1–2 times; sometimes refers to 3–10 times; often refers to >10 times
Source Odisha Migration Survey 2023, Household sample

Table 49 Households had to eat fewer meals in a day, by housing (% of households)

	Luxurious	Very good	Good	Poor	Kutcha	Total
Never	98.5	96.1	92.2	80.2	72.9	85.4
Rarely	0.5	3.3	6.7	14.7	22.0	11.6
Sometimes	0.5	0.4	0.9	4.7	4.3	2.6
Often	0.5	0.2	0.1	0.4	0.8	0.4
Total	100	100	100	100	100	100

Note Rarely refers to 1–2 times; sometimes refers to 3–10 times; often refers to >10 times
Source Odisha Migration Survey 2023, Household sample

Table 50 Households had to eat fewer meals in a day, by migration status (% of households)

	Non-migrant HH	Current migrant HH	Return migrant HH	Total
Never	84.6	87.9	90.2	85.4
Rarely	12.0	10.5	8.3	11.6
Sometimes	3.0	1.3	1.2	2.6
Often	0.4	0.2	0.3	0.4
Total	100	100	100	100

Note Rarely refers to 1–2 times; sometimes refers to 3–10 times; often refers to >10 times
Source Odisha Migration Survey 2023, Household sample

Table 51 Households had to eat fewer meals in a day, by wealth quartile (% of households)

	Poorest	Poor	Rich	Richest	Total
Never	78.2	82.7	88.0	94.9	85.4
Rarely	16.6	15.5	9.2	3.4	11.6
Sometimes	4.6	1.6	2.6	1.3	2.6
Often	0.7	0.2	0.2	0.3	0.4
Total	100	100	100	100	100

Note Rarely refers to 1–2 times; sometimes refers to 3–10 times; often refers to >10 times
Source Odisha Migration Survey 2023, Household sample

Table 52 Households had to eat fewer meals in a day, by land ownership (% of households)

	Landless	0–1 acre	1–5 acres	5+ acres	Total
Never	85.6	83.9	86.7	91.3	85.4
Rarely	10.2	14.4	11.2	6.8	11.6
Sometimes	3.7	1.5	2.0	1.9	2.6
Often	0.6	0.2	0.1		0.4
Total	100	100	100	100	100

Note Rarely refers to 1–2 times; sometimes refers to 3–10 times; often refers to >10 times
Source Odisha Migration Survey 2023, Household sample

Table 53 Households had no food at all due to a lack of resources, by locality (% of households)

	Rural	Urban	Total
Never	90.8	91.4	90.9
Rarely	7.0	7.4	7.1
Sometimes	1.9	1.0	1.7
Often	0.3	0.3	0.3
Total	100	100	100

Note Rarely refers to 1–2 times; sometimes refers to 3–10 times; often refers to >10 times
Source Odisha Migration Survey 2023, Household sample

Table 54 Households had no food at all due to a lack of resources, by regions (% of households)

	Coastal/central	Southern	Northern	Total
Never	96.8	86.1	86.6	90.9
Rarely	2.7	9.9	10.8	7.1
Sometimes	0.3	3.6	2.1	1.7
Often	0.2	0.4	0.5	0.3
Total	100	100	100	100

Note Rarely refers to 1–2 times; sometimes refers to 3–10 times; often refers to >10 times
Source Odisha Migration Survey 2023, Household sample

Table 55 Households had no food at all due to a lack of resources, by migration status (% of households)

	Non-migrant HH	Current migrant HH	Return migrant HH	Total
Never	90.1	94.2	91.8	90.9
Rarely	7.7	4.6	6.0	7.1
Sometimes	1.9	1.0	1.8	1.7
Often	0.3	0.2	0.5	0.3
Total	100	100	100	100

Note Rarely refers to 1–2 times; sometimes refers to 3–10 times; often refers to >10 times
Source Odisha Migration Survey 2023, Household sample

Table 56 Households had no food at all due to a lack of resources, by wealth quartile (% of households)

	Poorest	Poor	Rich	Richest	Total
Never	84.7	93.4	90.9	95.8	90.9
Rarely	11.4	5.2	8.2	2.6	7.1
Sometimes	3.4	1.1	0.8	1.3	1.7
Often	0.6	0.2	0.2	0.3	0.3
Total	100	100	100	100	100

Note Rarely refers to 1–2 times; sometimes refers to 3–10 times; often refers to >10 times
Source Odisha Migration Survey 2023, Household sample

Table 57 Households had no food at all due to a lack of resources, by land ownership (% of households)

	Landless	0–1 acre	1–5 acres	5+ acres	Total
Never	89.2	92.3	92.1	94.8	90.9
Rarely	7.9	6.6	6.2	4.8	7.1
Sometimes	2.4	1.0	1.5	0.4	1.7
Often	0.5	0.2	0.2		0.3
Total	100	100	100	100	100

Note Rarely refers to 1–2 times; sometimes refers to 3–10 times; often refers to >10 times
Source Odisha Migration Survey 2023, Household sample

Table 58 Households had to go to sleep at night hungry because there was not enough food, by locality (% of households)

	Rural	Urban	Total
Never	92.0	92.9	92.2
Rarely	6.1	5.9	6.1
Sometimes	1.6	0.9	1.5
Often	0.2	0.4	0.3
Total	100	100	100

Note Rarely refers to 1–2 times; sometimes refers to 3–10 times; often refers to >10 times
Source Odisha Migration Survey 2023, Household sample

Table 59 Households had to go to sleep at night hungry because there was not enough food, by housing (% of households)

	Luxurious	Very good	Good	Poor	Kutcha	Total
Never	99.3	96.9	96.8	87.9	86.3	92.2
Rarely	0.5	2.8	2.4	9.2	10.8	6.1
Sometimes		0.2	0.7	2.6	2.4	1.5
Often	0.3	0.2	0.1	0.3	0.5	0.3
Total	100	100	100	100	100	100

Note Rarely refers to 1–2 times; sometimes refers to 3–10 times; often refers to >10 times
Source Odisha Migration Survey 2023, Household sample

Table 60 Households had to go to sleep at night hungry because there was not enough food, by migration status (% of households)

	Non-migrant HH	Current migrant HH	Return migrant HH	Total
Never	91.2	95.6	95.3	92.2
Rarely	6.9	3.2	3.7	6.1
Sometimes	1.6	1.1	0.7	1.5
Often	0.3	0.2	0.3	0.3
Total	100	100	100	100

Note Rarely refers to 1–2 times; sometimes refers to 3–10 times; often refers to >10 times
Source Odisha Migration Survey 2023, Household sample

Table 61 Households had to go to sleep at night hungry because there was not enough food, by land ownership (% of households)

	Landless	0–1 acre	1–5 acres	5+ acres	Total
Never	90.5	93.4	93.6	94.9	92.2
Rarely	7.1	5.5	5.1	3.1	6.1
Sometimes	2.0	0.9	1.2	1.6	1.5
Often	0.4	0.2	0.1	0.4	0.3
Total	100	100	100	100	100

Note Rarely refers to 1–2 times; sometimes refers to 3–10 times; often refers to >10 times
Source Odisha Migration Survey 2023, Household sample

Table 62 Households had to go the whole day without eating due to a lack of food, by locality (% of households)

	Rural	Urban	Total
Never	92.7	94.6	93.0
Rarely	5.8	4.8	5.6
Sometimes	1.3	0.4	1.1
Often	0.2	0.3	0.2
Total	100	100	100

Note Rarely refers to 1–2 times; sometimes refers to 3–10 times; often refers to >10 times
Source Odisha Migration Survey 2023, Household sample

Table 63 Households had to go the whole day without eating due to a lack of food, by region (% of households)

	Coastal/central	Southern	Northern	Total
Never	98.3	87.6	90.2	93.0
Rarely	1.3	9.3	8.7	5.6
Sometimes	0.2	2.7	1.0	1.1
Often	0.2	0.4	0.2	0.2
Total	100	100	100	100

Note Rarely refers to 1–2 times; sometimes refers to 3–10 times; often refers to >10 times
Source Odisha Migration Survey 2023, Household sample

Table 64 Households had to go the whole day without eating due to a lack of food, by housing (% of households)

	Luxurious	Very good	Good	Poor	Kutcha	Total
Never	99.5	96.9	97.6	88.7	88.0	93.0
Rarely	0.3	2.6	1.9	9.0	9.8	5.6
Sometimes		0.3	0.4	2.2	1.7	1.1
Often	0.3	0.3	0.1	0.1	0.5	0.2
Total	100	100	100	100	100	100

Note Rarely refers to 1–2 times; sometimes refers to 3–10 times; often refers to >10 times
Source Odisha Migration Survey 2023, Household sample

Table 65 Households had to go the whole day without eating due to a lack of food, by social group (% of households)

	SC	ST	OBC	Upper castes	Total
Never	88.9	93.3	93.3	96.4	93.0
Rarely	7.9	4.9	6.1	3.0	5.6
Sometime	2.9	1.5	0.5	0.3	1.1
Often	0.3	0.3	0.1	0.3	0.2
Total	100	100	100	100	100

Note Rarely refers to 1–2 times; sometimes refers to 3–10 times; often refers to >10 times
Source Odisha Migration Survey 2023, Household sample

Table 66 Households had to go the whole day without eating due to a lack of food, by wealth quartile (% of households)

	Poorest	Poor	Rich	Richest	Total
Never	88.8	95.4	92.2	96.3	93.0
Rarely	8.6	3.8	7.1	2.7	5.6
Sometimes	2.1	0.8	0.5	0.9	1.1
Often	0.4	0.1	0.2	0.2	0.2
Total	100	100	100	100	100

Note Rarely refers to 1–2 times; sometimes refers to 3–10 times; often refers to >10 times
Source Odisha Migration Survey 2023, Household sample

References

FAO, IFAD, UNICEF, WFP, & WHO. (2023). *The state of food security and nutrition in the world 2023: Urbanization, agrifood systems transformation and healthy diets across the rural–urban continuum*. FAO, IFAD, UNICEF, WFP, WHO. https://doi.org/10.4060/cc3017en

Mohapatra, B. K. (2020). Poverty and food insecurity disparities and their causes in the eastern Indian state of Odisha. *The International Journal of Community and Social Development, 2*(4), 426–448. https://doi.org/10.1177/2516602620980595

Morris, S. S., Garg, A., & Black, R. E. (2020). Nutrient gaps and affordability of complementary foods in Eastern and Southern Africa and South Asia. *Nutrition Reviews, 79*(Suppl. 1), 1–3. https://doi.org/10.1093/nutrit/nuaa149

Pingali, P. (2006). Westernization of Asian diets and the transformation of food systems: Implications for research and policy. *Food Policy, 32*(3), 281–298. https://doi.org/10.1016/j.foodpol.2006.08.001

Raghunathan, K., Headey, D., & Herforth, A. (2020). Affordability of nutritious diets in rural India. *Food Policy, 99*, 101982. https://doi.org/10.1016/j.foodpol.2020.101982

Chapter 6
Education

Subhadarshee Nayak and Rohit Irudayarajan

Abstract Based on the Odisha Migration Survey, 2023, this chapter presents an overview of the educational attainments of the general and youth population in Odisha. It finds that the highest percentage of people (13.4%) have completed secondary education (Class 10), 12.6% of the population was illiterate, and illiteracy was higher among women (16.5%) compared to men (8.9%). Overall, males had higher educational attainments than females, and furthermore, gender disparity was more pronounced at higher levels of education, such as graduate and professional education. There was a continuation of the rural-urban divide in educational attainments. The coastal region had better educational attainments in Odisha compared to the northern and southern regions, and educational outcomes varied for different caste groups, as overall educational attainments were better for upper castes, followed by Other Backward Classes, Scheduled Castes, and Scheduled Tribes. The chapter thus shows the different ways in which inequality in educational attainments exists in Odisha, highlighting disparities across different categories, including gender, region, and caste. This chapter is an important contribution to a discussion about the state's development trajectory, as it provides an update on the 2011 Census results and discusses the most up-to-date status of educational attainments in Odisha.

Keywords Odisha migration survey · Educational attainments · Professional education · Odisha · Employment

1 Introduction

Education has long been recognized as a cornerstone of human-capital development and social equity. Since Independence, Odisha has made significant strides in expanding basic literacy. Between 1991 and 2011, the state's literacy rate rose from

S. Nayak (✉)
Manager, Education, Collectives for Integrated Livelihood Initiatives, Jamshedpur, India

R. Irudayarajan
International Institute of Migration and Development, Thiruvananthapuram, India

A. Datta and S. I. Rajan (eds.), *Migration, Livelihoods and Gender*, International Perspectives on Migration, https://doi.org/10.1007/978-981-95-5465-2_6

52% to 73.5% (Government of India, 2011), and further to an estimated 77.3% by 2018, with male literacy at 84% and female literacy at 70% (National Sample Survey Office [NSSO], 2018).

Different studies and reports suggest near-universal enrollment with primary-level gross enrollment ratios (GERs) exceeding 95% and dropout rates falling from over 40% in 2000 to below 5% by 2005 (Agrawal, 2014). Yet, these aggregate achievements mask persistent challenges. Retention beyond primary grades remains uneven: secondary GER hovers around 84%, but progression to higher secondary (Classes 10–12) drops sharply to 20–25% (Ministry of Education, 2020). Existing research suggests that socio-economic disadvantages, such as household poverty, limited parental educational attainment, and customary early marriage practices, significantly contribute to school dropout rates (Garg et al., 2024; Venkatesanet al., 2024; Kumar et al., 2023). Spatial disparities compound these issues. Dash and Swain (2025) suggest that school-related issues, including poor infrastructure contribute significantly to dropout rates, especially among children from disadvantaged groups. These barriers are likely to be more pronounced in tribal-dominated and rural areas. Nayak et al., (2016) argue that the high incidence of school dropouts in Odisha is a significant concern, especially in the state's backward districts.

Gender and social group inequities further characterize Odisha's educational landscape. Female literacy, though improved from 4.0% in 1951 to 64.0% in 2011, still lags male literacy (82.0%) by nearly 18 percentage points (Government of India, 2011). While gender gaps in enrollment narrow at primary levels, they widen at higher secondary and tertiary stages (Mishra, 2022). Scheduled Tribes (STs) and Scheduled Castes (SCs) face compounded disadvantages: in 2011, literacy among STs was only 52.2%, over 20 points below the state average, and literacy among SCs was 70.4% (Government of India, 2011). Caste-based hierarchies in educational outcomes are well documented (Kamat, 2011; Nambissan, 1996), reflecting structural barriers such as poverty, discrimination, and limited schooling access in marginalized habitations (Thorat, 2009).

Parallel to general schooling, Odisha has sought to expand higher and professional education. Since the establishment of the Indian Institute of Technology Bhubaneswar in 2008, the state has seen rapid institutional growth. Nevertheless, its tertiary GER remains at 21–22%, below the national figure of 27% (Ministry of Education, Government of India, 2022). Rural and interior students continue to encounter financial and logistical hurdles, and enrollments are disproportionately concentrated in urban coastal centers (Tilak, 2011). Recognizing that academic pathways do not suit all learners, the state has also invested in vocational and skill training. By 2023, the Odisha Skill Development Authority reported over 1,50,000 training seats across Industrial Training Institutes (ITIs) and polytechnics (Odisha Skill Development Authority [OSDA], 2023). Although enrollment in vocational streams remain modest (approximately 3–4% of the workforce), these programs are viewed as vital for enhancing employability, especially among youth who do not pursue higher secondary or tertiary education (World Bank, 2021).

Drawing on the household survey data collected across 15,000 households in all 30 districts of Odisha in 2023, this chapter systematically explores patterns of educational attainment. Section 2 examines the overall educational profile of the population, disaggregated by sex, urban-rural locality, migration status, and caste. Section 3 focuses on the educational status of the 15–19 age group with a similar disaggregation. Section 4 concludes with reflections on policy implications. By situating the 2023 survey data within the broader literature on Odisha's education, the chapter aims to identify enduring challenges and potential pathways for more inclusive educational development.

1.1 Data and Methodology

This chapter uses the household data collected in the Odisha Migration Survey (OMS) to discuss different aspects of education in Odisha. The data collected in 2023 provides an up-to-date status of educational attainments in Odisha. The survey asked respondents about the educational attainments of each member of the household, along with the socio-economic and socio-cultural profiles of the household. For each person from the household, the completed education was recorded on the day of the survey; for example, if a person was pursuing an undergraduate course at the time, the completed education recorded was Class 12. The OMS considered those who had ever attended school and those who were literate without going to school to be literate.

As discussed earlier (see Chap. 1 for details), the survey followed a stratified random sampling method to ensure comprehensive coverage across all 30 districts of Odisha, enhancing the reliability of findings. A total of 15,000 households were included in the study, carefully selected to represent diverse regions, including urban and rural areas, as well as various socio-economic groups. This sampling approach minimizes bias and provides a more accurate reflection of the state's educational landscape. By encompassing such a broad and representative sample, the survey results offer valuable insights into educational achievements in Odisha.

The tables in this chapter show educational attainments for different levels and categories. These categories represent either a level of education and/or the type of education. The figures in the tables show the percentage of persons who have completed the level or type of education. For example, "Industrial Training Institutes (ITIs), certificate courses" or "diploma" categories represent the percentage of persons who have completed vocational or industry-specific skill education and not above. The data provides a clear and detailed picture of educational attainments in Odisha, breaking down different aspects of attainments for various groups.

The analysis focuses on general education, encapsulating milestones such as primary (Class 8), secondary (Class 10), and higher secondary education (Class 12). These foundational stages serve as pillars upon which subsequent educational pursuits are erected, making them pivotal in assessing educational access and progression.

The analysis also examines the educational achievements in technical and professional courses at both undergraduate and postgraduate levels in Odisha. It explores performances of different socio-economic categories in specialized fields such as engineering, medicine, law, management, and other professional or technical programs.

Vocational education (ITI, certificate courses, and diplomas) is another aspect that this chapter discusses regarding educational attainments, with a focus on the proportion of individuals who pursued specialized courses to hone their skills and competencies. Education in institutes like ITIs provides training for specific trades like electrician, fitter, and plumber, which equip an individual for employment. Apart from ITIs, different schemes like Deen Dayal Upadhyaya Grameen Kaushalya Yojana are also aimed at training rural youth for employment. Odisha has its own urban employment program called Mukhyamantri Karma Tatpara Abhiyan (MUKTA). These programs train individuals and provide opportunities to gain skills so that they can be employed in different sectors, industrial settings, or be self-employed. Additionally, diploma programs offered in different polytechnics and in many private institutions impart education to train individuals in employable skills. Diploma programs offered by such institutes include education in food technology, diploma engineering in different sectors, like the automobile sector, etc. By showing how common vocational training is among different age groups, the chapter helps understand how well education matches job market needs, supporting better policies and programs.

Throughout the chapter, the tables act as visual aids, presenting complex data in a more accessible format. Each percentage point reflects more than just a statistic; it represents the aspirations, efforts, and progress of countless individuals striving for educational advancement in Odisha. Moreover, the utilization of stratified random sampling ensures that the findings are representative of the diverse tapestry of the state's population, mitigating biases, and conferring credibility to the conclusions drawn.

2 Educational Profile of the General Population

2.1 Educational Attainments by Sex

Disparities based on sex in educational attainment are a widespread phenomenon, observed across most societies. Historically, these disparities have often favored men, largely due to the influence of patriarchy, which, consequently, leads to lower educational attainments for women in many regions. This analysis specifically examines the differences in educational attainment between females and males within Odisha. By focusing on these categories, we aim to shed light on how these broader societal trends manifest in this context, and to what extent historical patriarchal norms continue to influence current educational outcomes for women in the state.

Table 1 shows that in Odisha, 12.6% of individuals were illiterate at the time of the survey. The percentage was 8.9 among men and 16.5 among women. It shows a very noticeable disparity (7.6 percentage points) in sex-wise illiteracy percentages, with illiteracy among females being nearly double that among males.

Table 1 also shows that a higher percentage (13.4%) of education completed in Odisha was Class 10 for both sexes. When disaggregated, more men (14.1%) than women (12.6%) had completed 10 years of school education. For higher secondary (Class 12) education too, men have better attainment than women, with 8.7% of men and 7.1% of women having completed education up to Class 12.

Table 1 Educational status by sex, all ages (% of individuals)

Education	Male	Female	Total
Pre-primary	6.7	9.1	7.8
Class 1	2.3	2.6	2.4
Class 2	3.5	4.2	3.9
Class 3	4.1	4.7	4.4
Class 4	4.0	3.9	3.9
Class 5	8.0	8.2	8.1
Class 6	3.8	3.7	3.8
Class 7	5.9	6.2	6.0
Class 8	5.5	4.2	4.8
Class 9	10.5	8.2	9.4
Class 10	14.1	12.6	13.4
Class 11	1.8	1.2	1.5
Class 12	8.7	7.1	7.9
ITI, certificate course	1.2	0.2	0.7
Diploma	0.8	0.2	0.5
Degree (BA, BSc, BCom, BLISc, etc.)	6.7	4.6	5.7
PG diploma (PGDCA, etc.)	0.2	0.1	0.2
Professional degree (BTech, LLB, MBBS, BDS, BSc (N), BPharm, BHMS, BAMS)	0.7	0.2	0.5
PG (MA, MSc, MCom, etc.)	0.4	0.3	0.4
Professional PG (MTech, MBA, MCA, MLISc, MSW, MCJ, BEd, MEd, LLM, MD, MS, medical PG diploma, MDS, MLT, MSc)	0.7	0.3	0.5
Others (specify)	0.1	0.1	0.1
Illiterate	8.9	16.5	12.6
Literate without school education	1.4	1.6	1.5
Total	100.0	100.0	100.0

Source Odisha migration survey 2023, Household sample

At the aggregate level, 5.7% of the sample population were graduates (BA, BSc, BCom, etc.). Disaggregated by sex, 6.7% among men and 4.6% among women were reported to be graduates. At the postgraduate level, in total, 0.4% held a postgraduate degree or higher. Among the two sexes, 0.4% of men and 0.3% of women were found to have attained this level of education in Odisha. Men fared better in attaining professional degrees as well, at 0.7%, compared to 0.2% of women who had a professional bachelor's degree.

In vocational education, too, the survey found notable sex-wise disparities. In total, 1.2% studied vocational education, whereas 2% among men and 0.4% among women did so (Table 1). The gap is clear and significant.

In summary, the comparison of educational attainments between men and women in Odisha shows that men have higher levels of education than women. This difference is especially evident at advanced levels, including degree programs and professional courses such as engineering and law. A similar trend is observed in vocational education—which imparts practical job skills like carpentry or computer training—with more men than women having completed these programs. This gap highlights the need to support women's access to higher education and vocational training to create equal opportunities.

2.2 *Educational Attainments by Locality*

The rural-urban divide in educational attainments has been well-studied. As urban populations have better access to education infrastructure and services (see Agrawal, 2014), educational attainment is often found to be better in urban places. The analysis here also compares rural and urban educational attainments. In most cases—the comparison shows—the outcomes are more favorable for urban locations in Odisha.

Table 2 shows that in Odisha, the percentage of illiteracy is higher in rural areas at 13.2% compared to 9.8% in urban areas. Overall, 12.6% reported being illiterate. The table also shows that a higher percentage, for both rural and urban areas, had completed 10 years of education. 13% in rural areas and 15.5% in urban areas had studied up to Class 10. This indicates that a lower percentage of individuals in rural areas have studied up to Class 10 than in urban areas. In higher secondary education (Class 12), a similar trend emerges, with 10% in urban areas and 7.5% in rural areas having completed 12 years of school education.

As far as graduates (BA, BSc, BCom, etc.) in rural and urban areas are concerned, the latter have a higher share (8.5%) than the former (5.1%). The share stands at 0.3% in rural areas and 0.7% in urban areas for postgraduate education, and at 0.3% and 1.4% respectively, for professional degree education at the graduate level.

Table 2 also illustrates the share of vocational education across Odisha, highlighting a gap between urban and rural areas. As anticipated, a higher percentage of individuals in urban regions had completed vocational training compared to their rural counterparts. Specifically, the study found that 1.7% of people in urban areas

Table 2 Educational status by locality, all ages (% of individuals)

Education	Rural	Urban	Total
Pre-primary	8.3	5.4	7.8
Class 1	2.6	1.8	2.4
Class 2	4.1	2.7	3.9
Class 3	4.4	3.8	4.4
Class 4	3.9	3.9	3.9
Class 5	8.3	7.3	8.1
Class 6	3.8	3.4	3.8
Class 7	6.1	6.0	6.0
Class 8	4.7	5.5	4.8
Class 9	9.7	7.8	9.4
Class 10	13.0	15.5	13.4
Class 11	1.5	1.8	1.5
Class 12	7.5	10.0	7.9
ITI, certificate course	0.7	0.9	0.7
Diploma	0.4	0.8	0.5
Degree (BA, BSc, BCom, BLISc, etc.)	5.1	8.5	5.7
PG diploma (PGDCA, etc.)	0.1	0.3	0.2
Professional degree (BTech, LLB, MBBS, BDS, BSc (N), BPharm, BHMS, BAMS)	0.3	1.4	0.5
PG (MA, MSc, MCom, etc.)	0.3	0.7	0.4
Professional PG (MTech, MBA, MCA, MLISc, MSW, MCJ, BEd, MEd, LLM, MD, MS, medical PG diploma, MDS, MLT, MSc)	0.4	1.0	0.5
MPhil, PhD, etc.	0.0	0.1	0.0
Others (specify)	0.1	0.1	0.1
Illiterate	13.2	9.8	12.6
Literate without school education	1.5	1.5	1.5
Total	100.0	100.0	100.0

Source Odisha migration survey 2023, Household sample

had successfully completed vocational education programs, while only 1.1% of individuals in rural areas had done so. This urban-rural divide underscores the varying access to and participation in vocational training opportunities. These findings point to the need for targeted efforts to expand vocational education in rural areas, bridging the gap and promoting equal opportunities for skill development and employment across the state. The analysis shows that educational attainment is better in urban locations, as expected, and the difference is more pronounced in higher and professional education.

2.3 *Educational Attainments by Migration Status*

As shown in Table 3, migrants are less likely to be illiterate than residents. It shows that at the aggregate level, the illiteracy in the state stands at 12.6%. Among residents, the percentage climbs up to 13.3% compared to 2.9% of current migrants and 9.7% of return migrants.

Table 3 also shows that for all migration status categories, higher percentages of individuals had studied up to Class 10. A total of 13.4% had completed education up to Class 10. Among residents, the share was 12.8%; whereas it stood at 20.4%

Table 3 Educational attainment by migration status, all ages (% of individuals)

Education	Non-migrant	Current migrant	Return migrant	Total
Pre-primary	8.2	2.5	4.5	7.8
Class 1	2.6	0.5	1.1	2.4
Class 2	4.0	1.6	1.6	3.9
Class 3	4.5	2.3	4.6	4.4
Class 4	4.0	2.4	4.2	3.9
Class 5	8.2	6.6	8.8	8.1
Class 6	3.8	2.6	4.5	3.8
Class 7	6.1	4.8	7.9	6.0
Class 8	4.8	4.9	8.9	4.8
Class 9	9.1	12.5	13.6	9.4
Class 10	12.8	20.4	18.6	13.4
Class 11	1.5	1.8	1.5	1.5
Class 12	7.7	12.4	5.9	7.9
ITI, certificate course	0.6	2.1	0.9	0.7
Diploma	0.4	2.2	0.5	0.5
Degree (BA, BSc, BCom, BLISc, etc.)	5.4	11.2	2.8	5.7
PG diploma (PGDCA, etc.)	0.2	0.3	0.0	0.2
Professional degree (BTech, LLB, MBBS, BDS, BSc (N), BPharm, BHMS, BAMS)	0.4	2.5	0.3	0.5
PG (MA, MSc, MCom, etc.)	0.3	1.0	0.0	0.4
Professional PG (MTech, MBA, MCA, MLISc, MSW, MCJ, BEd, MEd, LLM, MD, MS, medical PG diploma, MDS, MLT, MSc)	0.4	1.9	0.6	0.5
Others (specify)	0.1	0.1	0.0	0.1
Illiterate	13.3	2.9	7.6	12.6
Literate without school education	1.6	0.5	1.6	1.5
Total	100.0	100.0	100.0	100.0

Source Odisha migration survey 2023, Household sample

among current migrants and 18.6% among return migrants. At the same time, 7.7% of residents, 12.4% of current migrants, and 5.9% of return migrants had studied up to Class 12.

In Odisha, 5.4% of residents, 11.2% of current migrants, and 2.8% of return migrants had obtained a general bachelor's degree. Meanwhile, 0.4% in total reported having studied at the postgraduate level or above. This share was 0.3% among residents and 1% among current migrants. For professional degrees, 0.5% in total reported having completed them. The survey found that 0.8% of residents, 2.5% of current migrants, and 0.3% of return migrants had a professional bachelor's degree.

Furthermore, the survey found that 1.2% had completed vocational education. Among residents, 1% had pursued vocational education compared to 4.3% of current migrants and 1.4% of return migrants.

2.4 *Educational Attainments by Caste*

Like the rest of India, members of different social groups live in Odisha. Social science researchers (Kamat, 2011; Nambissan, 1996; Nayak et al., 2016; Thorat, 2009; Tilak, 2011) have widely discussed caste-based disparities in educational outcomes. Hence, the analysis here also focuses on caste-based outcomes.

It can be seen in Table 4 that among the different social groups, the STs had the highest percentage of illiterate population, at 18.5%. The second-highest percentage was reported among SCs at 14%, followed by 10% among Other Backward Classes (OBCs), and 7.9% among the upper castes.

Table 4 also shows that for all caste groups, the percentage of people having completed Class 10 was higher than at other levels of education. A total of 13.4% had studied up to Class 10 in Odisha; the upper castes (16.8%) had the highest percentage of persons who had studied up to Class 10, followed by OBCs (14.9%), SCs (12.3%), and STs (9.3%).

For higher secondary, the upper castes again had the highest share of individuals who had completed 12 years of education at 10.6%; among OBCs, 8.7% had studied up to Class 12, followed by SCs at 7%. Among all social groups, STs had the lowest percentage of individuals, at 5.6%, who had completed higher secondary education.

As far as the share of graduates (BA, BSc, BCom, etc.) in different caste groups is concerned, 5.7% in total were graduates. When disaggregated, the highest share of graduates was reported among the upper castes at 10.7%, compared to 6.6% among OBCs, 3.9% among SCs, and 2.1% among STs. Additionally, 0.4% reported having studied at the postgraduate level in Odisha. Disaggregated by caste groups, the share was 0.9% among the upper castes, 0.4% among OBCs, 0.2% among SCs, and 0.1% among STs. Similarly, 0.5% in total held professional degrees. Among different caste groups, the upper castes had the highest percentage of professional degree holders at 1.4%, compared to 0.5% among OBCs, 0.2% among SCs, and 0.1% among STs.

There were considerable disparities in vocational education outcomes by social group. The OMS data shows that 1.7% of the upper-caste individuals had completed

Table 4 Educational status by social group, all ages (% of individuals)

Education	SC	ST	OBC	General	Total
Pre-primary	8.9	11.9	6.4	4.2	7.8
Class 1	2.6	3.3	2.2	1.5	2.4
Class 2	4.4	4.1	4.0	2.6	3.9
Class 3	5.0	4.4	4.4	3.4	4.4
Class 4	3.7	4.2	4.2	3.2	3.9
Class 5	8.2	8.3	8.5	6.7	8.1
Class 6	3.8	4.0	3.9	3.3	3.8
Class 7	5.9	5.8	6.4	5.7	6.0
Class 8	5.2	4.8	4.8	4.7	4.8
Class 9	10.6	7.9	9.3	10.3	9.4
Class 10	12.3	9.3	14.9	16.8	13.4
Class 11	1.2	1.6	1.5	1.9	1.5
Class 12	7.0	5.6	8.7	10.6	7.9
ITI, certificate course	0.6	0.7	0.7	0.9	0.7
Diploma	0.4	0.3	0.6	0.8	0.5
Degree (BA, BSc, BCom, BLISc, etc.)	3.9	2.1	6.6	10.7	5.7
PG diploma (PGDCA, etc.)	0.1	0.1	0.2	0.3	0.2
Professional degree (BTech, LLB, MBBS, BDS, BSc (N), BPharm, BHMS, BAMS)	0.2	0.1	0.5	1.4	0.5
PG (MA, MSc, MCom, etc.)	0.2	0.1	0.4	0.9	0.4
Professional PG (MTech, MBA, MCA, MLISc, MSW, MCJ, BEd, MEd, LLM, MD, MS, medical PG diploma, MDS, MLT, MSc)	0.2	0.1	0.6	1.3	0.5
MPhil, PhD, etc.	0.0	0.0	0.0	0.1	0.0
Others (specify)	0.1	0	0.1	0.1	0.1
Illiterate	14	18.5	10	7.9	12.6
Literate without school education	1.5	2.8	1.1	0.7	1.5
Total	100.0	100.0	100.00	100.0	100.0

Source Odisha migration survey 2023, Household sample

vocational education compared to 1.3% among OBCs, and 1% each among SCs and STs.

Thus, social group- and caste-wise analysis of educational attainments for Odisha shows that members of marginalized groups, STs and SCs, are left behind in all levels of educational attainments. There is a clear and consistent social hierarchy in educational outcomes for different caste groups. Educational attainments were found to be better for the upper castes, followed by OBCs, SCs, and STs. The disparities become more pronounced as one moves from lower levels of education to higher levels of education.

3 Educational Status of the 15–29 Age Group in Odisha

3.1 Educational Attainments by Sex

Table 5 shows that in the 15–29 age group, 1.5% of men and 3.5% of women were found to be illiterate. Though overall literacy rates are much higher for this younger age cohort compared to other age groups (Table 1), the percentage of illiterate young women is higher than illiterate men in Odisha, suggesting continuation of sex disparities in educational outcomes.

Table 5 Educational status by sex, age 15–29 (% of individuals)

Education	Male	Female	Total
Pre-primary	0.8	1.5	1.1
Class 1	0.2	0.3	0.2
Class 2	0.5	0.9	0.7
Class 3	0.9	1.5	1.2
Class 4	1.4	1.3	1.3
Class 5	3.3	4.1	3.7
Class 6	1.7	2.2	1.9
Class 7	3.7	4.5	4.1
Class 8	4.9	4.3	4.6
Class 9	14.7	12.2	13.5
Class 10	24.2	26.2	25.1
Class 11	3.9	3.3	3.7
Class 12	18.7	19.2	19.0
ITI, certificate course	3.0	0.4	1.8
Diploma	2.0	0.5	1.3
Degree (BA, BSc, BCom, BLISc, etc.)	11.5	11.5	11.5
PG diploma (PGDCA, etc.)	0.4	0.3	0.4
Professional degree (BTech, LLB, MBBS, BDS, BSc (N), BPharm, BHMS, BAMS)	1.2	0.6	0.9
PG (MA, MSc, MCom, etc.)	0.5	0.6	0.5
Professional PG (MTech, MBA, MCA, MLISc, MSW, MCJ, BEd, MEd, LLM, MD, MS, medical PG diploma, MDS, MLT, MSc)	0.7	0.5	0.6
MPhil, PhD, etc.	0.1	0.0	0.0
Others (specify)	0.0	0.0	0.0
Illiterate	1.4	3.4	2.4
Literate without school education	0.3	0.7	0.5
Total	100.0	100.0	100.0

Source Odisha migration survey 2023, Household sample

Table 5 also shows that for both sexes in the 15–29 age group, a higher percentage had completed Class 10 compared to other levels. A total of 25.1% had completed 10 years of education; whereas when disaggregated, more women (26.2%) had completed 10 years of education compared to men (24.2%). In higher secondary education, females had better attainment than males again, as 19.2% of females and 18.7% of males were found to have completed education up to Class 12.

As far as the percentage of graduates (BA, BSc, BCom, etc.) is concerned, 11.5% in total held graduate degrees. Between the two sexes, there was no difference in the percentages of graduates, as both stood at 11.5% within the 15–29 age group. In postgraduate education, however, women had better educational attainments than men. On the other hand, more men had pursued professional degrees compared to women, as 1.2% of men and 0.6% of women in the 15–29 age group held professional bachelor's degrees. The survey also found noticeable sex-wise disparities in vocational education within the age group. Data shows that 5% of men and only 0.9% of women obtained vocational education (Table 5).

To sum up, a comparison of educational attainments between males and females in the 15–29 age group shows that females have better educational attainments in general education. More females had completed Class 10 and Class 12, whereas a higher percentage of males had completed professional education in the 15–29 age group in Odisha.

3.2 *Educational Attainments by Locality*

Table 6 shows that in the 15–29 age group, the percentage of illiteracy was higher in rural areas (2.6%) compared to urban areas (2%). It also shows that, within the age group, higher percentages of individuals had completed Class 10 in both rural and urban areas than at any other level. The share was 26% in rural and 20.7% in urban places for those who had completed 10 years of education. It shows that a higher percentage of individuals in rural areas had completed 10 years of education compared to urban areas. However, in higher secondary education (Class 12), this is true for individuals from urban locations, as 18.8% in rural and 19.8% in urban locations were found to have completed Class 12.

As far as percentages of graduates (BA, BSc, BCom, etc.) in rural and urban areas are concerned, urban locations had a higher share (16%) of graduates than rural (10.6%). In postgraduate education, 0.5% in rural areas and 0.7% in urban areas had education at the postgraduate level. For professional degree education in the 15–29 age group, 0.7% in rural areas and 2.2% in urban areas held professional bachelor's degrees.

Vocational education attainment is expected to be better in urban areas, as such education often provides better employment opportunities in cities. The expectation also reflects the unequal availability of vocational education in India, shaped by the urban-rural divide. In line with this, the study found disparities with 4% in urban and

Table 6 Educational status by locality, age 15–29 (% of individuals)

Education	Rural	Urban	Total
Pre-primary	1.2	0.8	1.1
Class 1	0.2	0.2	0.2
Class 2	0.7	0.6	0.7
Class 3	1.2	1.4	1.2
Class 4	1.3	1.4	1.3
Class 5	3.8	3.2	3.7
Class 6	1.9	1.9	1.9
Class 7	4.2	3.4	4.1
Class 8	4.6	4.9	4.6
Class 9	14.0	10.6	13.5
Class 10	26.0	20.7	25.1
Class 11	3.6	3.8	3.7
Class 12	18.8	19.8	19.0
ITI, certificate course	1.8	1.8	1.8
Diploma	1.1	2.2	1.3
Degree (BA, BSc, BCom, BLISc, etc.)	10.6	16.0	11.5
PG diploma (PGDCA, etc.)	0.3	0.7	0.4
Professional degree (BTech, LLB, MBBS, BDS, BSc (N), BPharm, BHMS, BAMS)	0.7	2.2	0.9
PG (MA, MSc, MCom, etc.)	0.5	0.7	0.5
Professional PG (MTech, MBA, MCA, MLISc, MSW, MCJ, BEd, MEd, LLM, MD, MS, medical PG diploma, MDS, MLT, MSc)	0.5	1.0	0.6
Illiterate	2.6	2.0	2.4
Literate without school education	0.4	0.7	0.5
Total	100.0	100.0	100.0

Source Odisha migration survey 2023, Household sample

2.9% in rural areas having completed vocational education in Odisha, in the 15–29 age group.

Thus, the analysis in this section shows that educational attainment is better in urban locations, as expected. The rural areas outperform the urban areas in the 15–29 age group only at the secondary education level (Class 10).

3.3 Educational Attainments by Migration Status

The survey collected data on the migration status of each member of the household and their educational attainment. Table 7 here shows educational attainments of the 15–29 age group for Odisha, disaggregated by migration status.

It can be seen in Table 7 that in the 15–29 age group, 2.4% were illiterate in total, while 2.8% of non-migrants were illiterate compared to 1% of current migrants and 0.8% of return migrants.

Table 7 also shows that the percentage of people having completed Class 10 across categories was higher than at other levels of education in the 15–29 age group

Table 7 Educational attainment by migration status, age 15–29 (% of individuals)

Education	Non-migrant	Current migrant	Return migrant	Total
Pre-primary	1.2	0.6	0.4	1.1
Class 1	0.2	0.1	0.5	0.2
Class 2	0.7	0.3	0.7	0.7
Class 3	1.2	0.6	2.0	1.2
Class 4	1.3	1.1	1.8	1.3
Class 5	3.6	3.5	6.7	3.7
Class 6	1.8	2.1	3.3	1.9
Class 7	4.0	3.9	7.5	4.1
Class 8	4.5	4.8	11.0	4.6
Class 9	13.5	13.1	15.6	13.5
Class 10	25.0	25.7	29.2	25.1
Class 11	3.8	2.8	2.8	3.7
Class 12	19.4	16.9	10.5	19.0
ITI, certificate course	1.6	2.9	2.1	1.8
Diploma	1.1	3.3	0.8	1.3
Degree (BA, BSc, BCom, BLISc, etc.)	11.7	11.0	2.5	11.5
PG diploma (PGDCA, etc.)	0.4	0.4	0.0	0.4
Professional degree (BTech, LLB, MBBS, BDS, BSc (N), BPharm, BHMS, BAMS)	0.7	3.0	0.4	0.9
PG (MA, MSc, MCom, etc.)	0.5	0.8	0.0	0.5
Professional PG (MTech, MBA, MCA, MLISc, MSW, MCJ, BEd, MEd, LLM, MD, MS, medical PG diploma, MDS, MLT, MSc)	0.5	1.6	0.7	0.6
Illiterate	2.8	1.0	0.8	2.4
Literate without school education	0.5	0.4	0.8	0.5
Total	100.0	100.0	100.0	100.0

Source Odisha migration survey 2023, Household sample

in Odisha. Within this age group, 25.1% in total had completed education up to Class 10. Among non-migrants, 25% had studied up to Class 10, whereas 25.7% among current migrants and 29.2% among return migrants had reached this level. On the other hand, 19.4% of non-migrants, 16.9% of current migrants, and 10.5% of return migrants had studied up to Class 12 in Odisha in the 15–29 age group.

As far as percentages of graduates (BA, BSc, BCom, etc.) are concerned in the 15–29 age group, 11.7% of non-migrants, 11% of current migrants, and 2.5% of return migrants had obtained a general bachelor's degree. At the postgraduate level (MA, MSc, MCom, etc.), a total of 0.5% held such degrees.

In the 15–29 age group, only 0.9% in total had attained professional degrees. The survey found that 0.7% among non-migrants, 3% among current migrants, and 0.4% among return migrants held professional degrees. In addition, a total of 3.1% had completed vocational education. Among non-migrants, this share was 2.7% compared to 6.2% among current migrants and 2.9% among return migrants within the age group.

3.4 Educational Attainments by Region

Odisha is one of the largest states in India, with 30 districts. Area-wise, it ranks eighth among the Indian states. Hence, comparison of educational attainments in different regions of Odisha will provide a nuanced overview of their performances and specific contexts. For this purpose, we have divided Odisha into three regions: Coastal, Southern, and Northern.

Table 8 shows that illiteracy is higher in the Southern region compared to the Coastal and Northern regions, and it is the lowest in the Coastal region. The survey found that 4% of individuals in the 15–29 age group in the Southern region reported being illiterate, compared to 2% each in the Northern and Coastal regions.

Table 8 also demonstrates that across regions, the percentages of individuals having completed Class 10 were higher than at other levels of education in the 15–29 age group. A total of 25.1% had completed 10 years of education. Disaggregated by region, 25.9% in the Northern, 25.3% in the Coastal, and 24.3% in the Southern regions had completed education up to Class 10. In higher secondary education, the Northern region had the highest share of individuals completing Class 12 at 20.2%, compared to 19.3% in the Coastal and 17.2% in the Southern region.

A total of 11.5% of individuals across regions in the 15–29 age group were graduates (BA, BSc, BCom, etc.). The highest percentage of graduates was reported in the Coastal region at 14%, followed by 9.8% in the Northern and 9.6% in the Southern region. At the postgraduate level (MA, MSc, MCom, etc.), a total of 0.5% reported having these degrees. When disaggregated, the share was 0.7% for the Coastal region, 0.6% for the Northern region, and 0.2% for the Southern region. There was variation in the incidence of professional bachelor's as well; the share was 1.3% in the Coastal region, 0.8% in the Southern, and 0.6% in the Northern region of Odisha. The survey found that within the 15–29 age group in Odisha, 3.1%

Table 8 Educational attainment by migration status, age 15–29 (% of individuals)

Education	Coastal	Southern	Northern	Total
Pre-primary	0.6	1.5	1.4	1.1
Class 1	0.1	0.4	0.2	0.2
Class 2	0.5	0.9	0.8	0.7
Class 3	0.8	1.9	1.1	1.2
Class 4	1.0	1.8	1.3	1.3
Class 5	2.5	5.7	3.2	3.7
Class 6	1.3	2.8	1.8	1.9
Class 7	3.0	5.7	3.9	4.1
Class 8	3.8	5.2	5.2	4.6
Class 9	15.0	11.5	13.2	13.5
Class 10	25.3	24.3	25.9	25.1
Class 11	3.2	3.7	4.2	3.7
Class 12	19.3	17.2	20.2	19.0
ITI, certificate course	2.2	1.0	2.0	1.8
Diploma	1.8	0.6	1.2	1.3
Degree (BA, BSc, BCom, BLISc, etc.)	14.0	9.6	9.8	11.5
PG diploma (PGDCA, etc.)	0.2	0.3	0.6	0.4
Professional degree (BTech, LLB, MBBS, BDS, BSc (N), BPharm, BHMS, BAMS)	1.3	0.8	0.6	0.9
PG (MA, MSc, MCom, etc.)	0.7	0.2	0.6	0.5
Professional PG (MTech, MBA, MCA, MLISc, MSW, MCJ, BEd, MEd, LLM, MD, MS, medical PG diploma, MDS, MLT, MSc)	0.9	0.3	0.4	0.6
Illiterate	2.0	4.0	2.0	2.4
Literate without school education	0.5	0.6	0.4	0.5
Total	100.0	100.0	100.0	100.0

Source Odisha migration survey 2023, Household sample

had completed vocational education. The disaggregated share was 4% in the Coastal region, compared to 3.2% in the Northern and 1.6% in the Southern regions.

Thus, data from the survey shows that among the three regions, the Coastal region has better educational attainments in Odisha compared to the Northern and the Southern regions in the 15–29 age group. One can clearly see that educational attainments are lower in the Southern region, particularly in higher and professional education. The region lags behind in vocational education as well.

3.5 Educational Attainments by Caste

Table 9 shows social group-wise educational attainments in the 15–29 age group. The age group represents the population that, in general, looks for employment or is already employed. It is worth noting here that according to the Right to Education Act, eight years of education is compulsory in India, and it has been more than 10 years since the Act was implemented. Prior to the Act, Sarva Shiksha Abhiyan (Universal Elementary Education) aimed to provide education for all in the 6–14 age group. Hence, individuals in the 15–29 age group are supposed to have attained at least eight years of education.

Table 9 Educational status by social group, age 15–29 (% of individuals)

Education	SC	ST	OBC	General	Other
Pre-primary	1.5	2.2	0.5	0.4	1.1
Class 1	0.1	0.4	0.2	0.1	0.2
Class 2	0.8	1.2	0.5	0.2	0.7
Class 3	1.3	2.3	0.8	0.3	1.2
Class 4	1.3	2.1	1.0	0.9	1.3
Class 5	3.8	6.7	2.4	1.7	3.7
Class 6	2.0	2.8	1.6	1.1	1.9
Class 7	4.4	6.0	3.3	2.5	4.1
Class 8	6.0	6.0	3.7	2.9	4.6
Class 9	17.2	14.4	11.9	11.4	13.5
Class 10	25.4	21.5	27.8	23.8	25.1
Class 11	3.2	4.3	3.6	3.2	3.7
Class 12	18	14.9	20.7	22.7	19
ITI, certificate course	1.5	1.7	1.8	2.3	1.8
Diploma	1.1	0.6	1.7	1.8	1.3
Degree (BA, BSc, BCom, BLISc, etc.)	8.5	5.5	14.2	18.5	11.5
PG diploma (PGDCA, etc.)	0.2	0.4	0.3	0.6	0.4
Professional degree (BTech, LLB, MBBS, BDS, BSc (N), BPharm, BHMS, BAMS)	0.5	0.3	1.0	2.3	0.9
PG (MA, MSc, MCom, etc.)	0.3	0.1	0.7	1.0	0.5
Professional PG (MTech, MBA, MCA, MLISc, MSW, MCJ, BEd, MEd, LLM, MD, MS, medical PG diploma, MDS, MLT, MSc)	0.3	0.1	0.8	1.4	0.6
Illiterate	2.1	5.5	1.2	0.8	2.4
Literate without school education	0.5	1.0	0.3	0.1	0.5
Total	100.0	100.0	100.0	100.0	100.0

Source Odisha migration survey 2023, Household sample

Table 9 shows that in the 15–29 age group, overall, 2.5% were illiterate. Among the different caste groups, the ST group had the highest percentage of illiterate individuals at 5.5%. The second-highest percentage was reported for the SC group, at 2.1%. Among OBCs and upper castes, only 1.2% and 0.8%, respectively, were found to be illiterate.

It can be seen that for all caste groups, higher percentages of education completed were in the "up to Class 10" category, within the 15–29 age group. A total of 25.1% had completed 10 years of education, whereas among different caste groups, the highest share was among the OBCs (27.8%), followed by SCs (25.4%). Among upper castes, 23.8% had completed 10 years of education, and among the STs, the share was 21.5% in this age group.

At the higher secondary level, the upper castes had the highest percentage of persons who had completed 12 years of education (22.7%). Among OBCs, 20.7% had completed Class 12, followed by SCs (18%). The STs had the lowest percentage of persons, at 14.9%, in the 15–29 age group, who had completed higher secondary education.

Within the age group, 11.5% were graduates (BA, BSc, BCom, etc.). Among different caste groups, the highest share of graduates was reported among the upper castes, at 18.5%, compared to 14.2% among OBCs, 8.5% among SCs, and 5.5% among STs. At the postgraduate degree level, a total of 0.5% held such degrees. When disaggregated, the shares were 1% for the upper castes, 0.8% for OBCs, 0.3% for SCs, and 0.1% for STs. Only 0.9% in total reported having professional degrees. The highest percentage of professional degree holders was among upper castes (2.3%), compared to 1% among OBCs, 0.5% among SCs, and 0.3% among STs.

The survey found that in the 15–29 age group in Odisha, 3.1% had completed vocational education. The caste-wise shares were 4.1% among the upper castes, followed by 3.5% among the OBCs, 2.6% among the SCs, and 2.3% among the STs.

Thus, our analysis of educational attainments shows that in the 15–29 age group population of Odisha, members of marginalized caste groups—particularly STs and SCs—are left behind. In fact, except for the attainments in secondary education (Class 10), one can find a caste-like hierarchy in educational outcomes for different caste groups, as overall educational attainments were found to be better for the upper castes, followed by OBCs, SCs, and STs.

4 Conclusion

This chapter has presented an overview of educational attainments, first for the entire population, i.e., for all ages, and then specifically for the youth population (age group of 15–29) in Odisha. The analysis of educational attainment data for all ages showed that the highest percentage of people (13.4%) had completed secondary education (Class 10) compared to any other level of education. However, 12.9% of the population was illiterate, and illiteracy was higher among women (16.5%)

compared to men (8.9%). Overall, males had higher educational attainments than females, and furthermore, gender disparity was more pronounced at higher levels of education, such as graduate and professional education. There was a continuation of the rural-urban divide in educational attainments in Odisha, as the urban locations fared better than rural ones. Further, the analysis showed caste-wise disparities; upper castes had better educational attainments than other caste groups, and a comparison of all caste groups showed a caste-like social hierarchy in educational outcomes, as the attainments of the upper castes were followed by OBCs, SCs, and STs. Additionally, as one moved from lower to higher levels of education, caste-wise differences in educational attainment became more pronounced.

For the 15–29 age group, the data showed that a higher percentage of females had completed Class 10 and Class 12 compared to males. However, a greater percentage of males had completed professional education compared to women. Further, the chapter showed that the Coastal region had better educational attainments in Odisha compared to the Northern and Southern regions. Educational attainments in the Southern region were lower, particularly in higher and professional education, as well as in vocational education. Caste-wise analysis of educational attainments showed that in the 15–29 age group, STs and SCs were left behind. In fact, except for the attainments in secondary education (Class 10), there was a caste-like hierarchy in educational outcomes for different caste groups, as overall educational attainments were better again for the upper castes, followed by OBCs, SCs, and STs.

In summary, this analysis mapped the educational status and attainments of Odisha. It showed how education levels differ across the state, underscoring inequalities that need to be addressed. It pointed out clear differences in educational achievements based on factors, including gender, location (urban versus rural), and caste. For example, urban areas often have higher education rates than rural ones, and certain caste groups may face barriers to accessing quality education. These gaps highlight the need for action to create a fairer education system. Policymakers, educators, and community leaders should collaborate to address these inequalities, ensuring everyone in Odisha has equal opportunities to learn and succeed.

References

Agrawal, T. (2014). Educational inequality in rural and urban India. *International Journal of Educational Development, 34*(1), 11–19. https://doi.org/10.1016/j.ijedudev.2013.05.002

Garg, M. K., Chowdhury, P., & Sheikh, I. (2024). Determinants of school dropouts in India: A study through survival analysis approach. *Journal of Social and Economic Development, 26*(1), 26–48.

Government of India. (2011). *Census of India 2011: Provisional population totals*. Registrar General & Census Commissioner of India. https://censusindia.gov.in/nada/index.php/catalog/42611/download/46274/Census%20of%20India%202011-Provisional%20Population%20Totals.pdf

Kamat, S. (2011). Education and social equity in elementary education. In R. Govinda (Ed.), *Who goes to school? Exploring exclusion in Indian education* (pp. 87–122). Oxford University Press.

Kumar, P., Patel, S. K., Debbarma, S., & Saggurti, N. (2023). Determinants of school dropouts among adolescents: Evidence from a longitudinal study in India. *PLoS one, 18*(3), e0282468.
Ministry of Education, Government of India. (2020). *Educational statistics at a glance 2020.*
Ministry of Education, Government of India. (2022). *All India survey on higher education 2021–22.* https://cdnbbsr.s3waas.gov.in/s392049debbe566ca5782a3045cf300a3c/uploads/2024/02/20240214825688998.pdf
Mishra, A. (2022). *Educational Status of Women in Odisha.* Available at SSRN 4054581.
Nambissan, G. B. (1996). Equity in education? Schooling of dalit children in India. *Economic and Political Weekly, 31*(16/17), 1011–1024. http://www.jstor.org/stable/4404063
National Sample Survey Office. (2018). *Key indicators of household social consumption in India: Education.* Ministry of Statistics and Programme Implementation, Government of India.
Nayak, N. C., Dhar, S., & Mahakur, P. K. (2016). Educational outcomes in Odisha. In P. B. Nayak, S. C. Panda, & P. K. Pattanaik (Eds.), *The economy of Odisha: A profile* (pp. 303–349). Oxford University Press. https://doi.org/10.1093/ACPROF:OSO/9780199464784.003.0010
Odisha Skill Development Authority. (2023). *Annual report 2022–23.* Government of Odisha.
Swain, S. D. M. (2025). Economic inequality and child education: A study of school dropouts in Odisha. *Journal on the Rights of the Child of National Law University Odisha, 6*(2), 29–48.
Thorat, S. (2009). *Dalits in India: Search for a common destiny.* Sage Publications. https://doi.org/10.4135/9788132101086
Tilak, J. B. G. (2011). *Higher education in India: In search of equality, quality, and quantity.* Orient Blackswan.
Venkatesan, R. G., Karmegam, D., & Mappillairaju, B. (2024). Exploring determinants of school dropout across regions in India: a comprehensive meta-analysis. *Journal of Computational Social Science, 7*(2), 1665–1697.
World Bank. (2021). *Skills for employability in Odisha: Challenges and opportunities.* World Bank Publications.

Chapter 7
Labor Market and Employment

Nandini Ramamurthy and Amrita Datta

Abstract Based on the Odisha Migration Survey, this chapter presents the work and employment scenario in Odisha. Using the survey data, we estimated the workforce participation rate (WPR) and found that the WPR in the state varied considerably by sex (the male WPR was 73.3% and the female WPR was 15.9%). Migrants had a higher WPR than residents, and WPRs were higher for individuals in the marginalized communities such as the Scheduled Castes and Scheduled Tribes, and those in the poorest and poor wealth quartiles. WPR by age took an inverted U curve, where it was lower among younger age cohorts, peaked at varying ages for men and women, and then declined again for older age cohorts. Agriculture emerged as the predominant occupation in Odisha, employing 40.1% of all workers; this was followed by service occupations (36.7%), construction (19%), and manufacturing and mining (3.7%). The data suggested a feminization of employment in agriculture, as 57.7% of female workers were engaged in the agricultural sector as compared to 35.9% of male workers. The occupational profile of workers varied significantly by residential status, and migration was associated with a gendered movement away from agriculture to non-agricultural occupations, predominantly in the services sector.

Keywords Labor market · Employment · Workforce participation rate · Occupation · Feminization of agriculture · Migration · Odisha

1 Introduction

This chapter studies the labor market in Odisha to discuss key dimensions of the work and employment scenario in the state. While most of the population of Odisha lives in rural areas, the labor market in Odisha has seen low employment growth in

N. Ramamurthy
Independent Researcher, Hyderabad, India

A. Datta (✉)
Indian Institute of Technology, Hyderabad, India
e-mail: amritadatta@la.iith.ac.in

A. Datta and S. I. Rajan (eds.), *Migration, Livelihoods and Gender*, International Perspectives on Migration, https://doi.org/10.1007/978-981-95-5465-2_7

the agriculture sector and negative employment growth in the manufacturing sector (Padhi & Panda, 2021). Employment growth has been high only in a few services subsectors, including construction (ibid), where wages are low, and the conditions of work are precarious. It is little surprise, therefore, that Odisha consistently ranked among the worst states—in the years 2005, 2012, 2019, and 2022—in the Employment Condition Index[1] (Institute for Human Development [IHD] & International Labour Organization [ILO], 2024).

It is concerning that the workforce participation rates for men and women declined from 81.8% and 28.1% in 2005 to 71.8% and 20.8% in 2022, respectively (IHD & ILO, 2024). Though the share of casual workers declined from 36.2% to 25.9%, it continues to be higher than the all-India average of 22.3%. The average monthly wages for casual workers at Rs 6581 continue to remain significantly lower than all-India (Rs 8421), and there is a significant wage disparity between males (Rs 7119) and females (Rs 4438) (ibid). In a context of underdevelopment, low per capita income, and a lack of employment opportunities in the state, the labor market, thus, is characterized by an outmigration of workers.

Against this backdrop, this chapter presents the results of the Odisha Migration Survey (OMS)[2] in three broad areas: First, we examine the primary activity status of men and women. Second, we look at the work status, which is derived from the primary activity status, and determine the workforce participation rate in Odisha. Third, we present the occupational profile of Odisha workers. The analysis is disaggregated by individual-level variables such as migration status, age, sex, marital status, and other variables such as social group, wealth status, locality, and region.

2 Primary Activity Status

What are the activities undertaken by the working-age population in Odisha? Table 1 presents the results of the OMS for the primary activity status of men and women in the age group 15–64 years. At the aggregate level, it emerges from the survey data that domestic work/household chores are the most important primary activity status; nearly one-third of individuals in the age 15–64 report this as their primary activity status (Table 1). Casual wage labor is the second most important activity status, followed by own account (self-employed) work and student. In our analysis, a worker is defined as an individual reporting any one of the following six activity statuses: (i) self-employed (employer), (ii) self-employed (own account worker), (iii) regular wage in the public sector, (iv) regular wage in the private sector, (v) casual

[1] The India Employment Report (2024) created an Employment Condition Index comprising the indicators: percentage of workers employed in regular formal work, worker population ratio, proportion of casual workers, proportion of self-employed workers with income below the poverty line, average monthly earnings of casual workers, unemployment rate of youths with a secondary or higher level of education, and youth not in employment, education, or training.

[2] See Chap. 1 for details on methodology and data collection of the OMS.

Table 1 Primary activity status by sex, 15 to 64 years (%)

Primary activity status	Sex		
	Male	Female	Total
Self-employed (employer)	2.9	0.4	1.7
Self-employed (own account worker)	21.8	4.0	13.2
Regular wage in public sector	2.5	1.6	2.1
Regular wage in private sector	15.8	1.5	8.9
Casual wage labor	30.2	8.3	19.6
Unpaid family labor	4.7	4.1	4.4
Domestic work/household chores	2.3	63.6	32.0
Student	13.4	11.5	12.5
Retired/pensioner/too old to work	1.4	1.7	1.5
Unemployed	3.8	2.2	3.0
Other	1.1	1.0	1.0
Total	100.0	100.0	100.0

Source Odisha migration survey 2023, Households sample

wage labor, and (vi) unpaid family labor.[3] Among workers, casual wage labor is the most important reported activity status. This is followed by own account (self-employed) work and regular wage in the private sector. Only a minuscule proportion of the workers are employers (3.4%) or regular wage workers in the public sector (4.2%).

Table 1 disaggregates primary activity status by sex and compares the primary activities of men and women. From the survey data, it emerges that the distribution of activity status for males and females is quite different.

For women, domestic/household chores are the most important activity status, with more than six in 10 women reporting this as their primary activity status. For men, on the other hand, domestic work/household chores are not—at all—an important activity status; only about 2% men report this as their primary activity status.

For female workers, casual wage labor is the most important activity status, followed by unpaid family labor and own account (self-employed) work. In the case of male workers, too, we see that casual wage labor is the most important activity status. However, this is followed by own account (self-employed) work and regular wage work in the private sector.

The survey data on primary activity status revealed stark *gendered* differences. As nearly two-thirds of the women report domestic work as their primary activity, they are less likely to be workers, compared to men. In turn, the data indicates that men are 3.6 times more likely to have casual wage labor as their primary activity

[3] Individuals reporting the following primary activity statuses: domestic work, student, retired/pension/too old to work, unemployed, and unable to work due to physical and mental disabilities, are not considered workers.

status than women. They are 5.4 times more likely than women to report own account (self-employed) work and 10.5 times more likely to be in regular wage work in the private sector than females. Lastly, unpaid family labor is marginally higher among men than women.

2.1 Primary Activity Status and Working Age

Table 2 presents primary activity status (PAS) by five age categories—in the working age, 15 to 64 years—for males and females.

In the age group 15–24, young people are most likely to be in education. The gender difference is low, and nearly one in two people, both young men and women, are students. While the share of males and females in education may be similar in this age cohort, significant differences emerge when we disaggregate the second most important primary activity status by sex. Among males in the 15–24 age cohort, nearly 40% are workers, while nearly one in three women report domestic work as a primary activity status in this age cohort.

An analysis of the next age cohort of 25–34 years reveals even more stark gender differences: 90% of the men are workers, while only 21% of the women are so. Male workers are most likely to be engaged in casual wage labor, followed by regular wage in the private sector and self-employment. While women workers are also most likely to be casual wage workers, this is followed by self-employment and unpaid family labor. In this age cohort, women's participation in domestic duties peaks, with about three in four women reporting domestic work and household chores as their primary activity. For men, the corresponding figure is only 2.1%.

In the next age group, 35–44 years, the share of both male and female workers in private wage employment declines while that in self-employment increases. This needs to be understood with respect to the preponderance of youth—in wage employment—in migration streams. A similar pattern persists in the next age cohort of 45–54 years, with a shift of workers from wage employment to self-employment for both men and women.

In the last age cohort, 55–64 years, self-employment emerges as the most important activity status for men. Among all age cohorts, men are most likely to be self-employed at this life-stage. For female workers, casual wage labor is the most important activity status in this age cohort, followed by unpaid family work; self-employment is reported by only 4.3% of women as a primary activity status (compared to 38.7% men) in this age cohort. This reflects their more precarious work status compared to male workers.

For both male and female workers, casual wage work is the most important activity and peaks in the age group 35–44 years. In the later age cohorts, as their bodies deplete and they are unable to perform physically strenuous manual labor, there is a shift toward own account work (Table 2).

Table 2 Primary activity status by age and sex

Primary activity status	Male						Female					
	15–24	25–34	35–44	45–54	55–64	Total	15–24	25–34	35–44	45–54	55–64	Total
Self-employed (employer)	0.3	2.3	3.5	4.7	5.3	2.9	0.1	0.5	0.6	0.5	0.7	0.4
Self-employed (own account worker)	5.2	19.0	27.8	33.1	33.5	21.8	2.3	4.3	4.6	5.5	3.6	4.0
Regular wage in public sector	0.5	3.4	3.1	3.3	3.0	2.5	0.5	1.5	2.3	2.9	1.1	1.6
Regular wage in private sector	11.0	26.9	20.1	13.0	5.3	15.8	1.7	2.5	1.3	1.1	0.7	1.5
Casual wage labor	18.2	33.9	35.8	34.9	32.1	30.2	4.9	8.4	11.7	9.7	6.8	8.3
Unpaid family labor	3.6	4.7	5.5	5.7	4.4	4.7	2.9	3.8	3.7	5.8	5.5	4.1
Domestic work/household chores	1.4	2.1	2.5	2.9	3.6	2.3	32.5	75.6	74.3	72.3	68.4	63.6
Student	50.0	2.6	0.0	0.0	0.0	13.4	47.8	1.1	0.1	0.1	0.0	11.5
Retired/pensioner/too old to work	0.0	0.0	0.1	0.4	9.0	1.4	0.0	0.1	0.5	0.8	10.3	1.7
Unemployed	9.3	4.4	0.7	0.5	1.5	3.8	6.7	1.8	0.4	0.2	0.3	2.2
Other	0.6	0.9	0.9	1.4	2.4	1.1	0.7	0.6	0.5	1.2	2.5	1.0
Total	100.0	100.0	100.0	100.0	100.0	100.0	100.0	100.0	100.0	100.0	100.0	100.0

Source Odisha migration survey 2023, Households sample

2.2 Primary Activity Status and Social Group

Table 3 presents primary activity status by social group and sex. Clear caste patterns emerge in this data. The most predominant work status of casual wage labor is most likely to be reported by Scheduled Caste (SC) and Scheduled Tribe (ST) workers and least likely to be reported by upper-caste and Other Backward Class (OBC) workers, among both men and women. Upper-caste women are the least likely to be casual workers (2.7%), while SC men (40.4%) are the most likely to be so.

On the other hand, upper-caste workers have a much higher probability of being in regular work, be it in the public or private sector. Compared to their SC counterparts, male upper-caste workers are 2.4 times more likely to be regular workers in the public sector—the gold standard of employment status in India. Interestingly, the corresponding figure for women at 1.3 times is significant and noteworthy, even though lower than that for male workers.

It can also be seen in Table 3 that among all social groups, upper caste men are most likely to be employers. Upper-caste and OBC men are also more likely to report self-employment as their primary activity status compared to SCs and STs. Overall, the data shows that gender intersects with caste in myriad ways; upper-caste women are at the top of the hierarchy, overrepresented in *better* activity statuses associated

Table 3 Primary activity status by sex and social group

Primary activity status	Male					Female				
	ST	SC	OBC	UC	Total	ST	SC	OBC	UC	Total
Self-employed (employer)	1.4	3.5	2.4	4.7	2.9	0.1	1.0	0.2	0.7	0.4
Self-employed (own account worker)	17.3	18.0	24.5	25.3	21.8	3.3	6.2	3.5	2.8	4.0
Regular wage in public sector	2.0	1.6	2.7	3.8	2.5	1.7	1.5	1.6	1.9	1.6
Regular wage in private sector	15.9	7.5	17.3	23.7	15.8	1.9	0.8	1.6	2.2	1.5
Casual wage labor	38.5	40.4	26.1	17.4	30.2	11.9	13.8	5.7	2.7	8.3
Unpaid family labor	4.5	5.6	5.4	1.8	4.7	3.8	7.6	3.1	2.1	4.1
Domestic work/ household chores	1.3	5.6	1.3	1.4	2.3	60.0	54.8	66.9	72.3	63.6
Student	12.9	12.6	13.4	15.0	13.4	11.9	10.2	12.0	11.5	11.5
Retired/pensioner/ too old to work	1.4	1.1	1.5	1.5	1.4	1.6	1.9	1.7	1.4	1.7
Unemployed	3.3	3.1	4.2	4.1	3.8	2.4	1.7	2.5	1.6	2.2
Other	1.3	1.1	1.0	1.1	1.1	1.2	0.6	1.1	0.7	1.0
Total	100.0	100.0	100.0	100.0	100.0	100.0	100.0	100.0	100.0	100.0

Source Odisha migration survey 2023, Households sample

with stable jobs, while SC and ST women, in particular, are at the bottom, with the most precarious work statuses, and fare much worse than upper-caste women.

Though a higher percentage of men report unpaid family labor as their primary activity compared to women, if we were to consider the share of unpaid family labor among workers, the share of female workers in unpaid family work (20.6%) is more than three times that of male workers in unpaid family work (6.0%).

While the gendered nature of domestic work/household chores is discussed in the previous section, there are significant variations by caste. It can be seen in Table 3 that the share of upper-caste women reporting domestic work as a primary activity is about 12 percentage points higher than that of ST women and 18 percentage points higher than the SC women's share.

2.3 *Primary Activity Status and Wealth Status*

In this section, we analyze the distribution of primary activity status based on the four wealth quartiles (Table 4).[4] Household wealth is clearly associated with outcomes in the labor market. It can be seen that persons in households in the lowest wealth quartile are most likely to be casual wage workers. As one moves up the wealth quartiles, the likelihood of being in casual wage labor reduces progressively. The survey results show that individuals in the lowest wealth quartile are 3.4 times more likely to be casual wage workers than individuals in the fourth (highest) wealth quartile. On the other hand, the pattern of regular wage work—in the public and private sector—is the converse. Persons in the lowest wealth quartiles are least likely to be regular wage workers. As one moves up the wealth quartiles, the likelihood of being a regular wage worker progressively increases. A person in the highest quartile is nearly 10 times more likely to report regular wage work in the public sector as their primary activity compared to a person in the first quartile. The share of self-employment, too, is highest among the highest quartile and the lowest among the lowest quartile. On the other hand, unpaid family labor is highest among the lowest quartile and is lowest in the highest quartile.

What about the primary activity statuses of domestic work and student? It is interesting to note that as we move up the wealth quartiles, the share of individuals reporting domestic work/household chores as their primary activity increases progressively. We have already seen how gendered this activity is in Sect. 2. The data clearly shows that higher wealth is associated with a greater share of individuals reporting domestic work/household chores as their primary activity. As expected, the share of students is the highest in the richest wealth quartile and decreases as we move to the poorest wealth quartile. Overall, from Table 4, it is evident that individuals in the higher wealth quartiles (Q3 and Q4) have activity statuses associated with more and better opportunities in education and employment, compared to individuals in the lower (Q1 and Q2) wealth quartiles.

---

[4] See Chap. 1, Endnote 7, for details on the construction of wealth quartiles.

Table 4 Primary activity status by wealth quartile

Primary activity status	Q1 (lowest)	Q2	Q3	Q4 (highest)	Total
Self-employed (employer)	2.1	2.2	0.7	1.7	1.7
Self-employed (own account worker)	11.3	12.7	13.3	15.4	13.2
Regular wage in public sector	0.5	1.2	1.6	4.9	2.1
Regular wage in private sector	3.8	8.4	11.0	12.2	8.9
Casual wage labor	31.2	21.5	17.5	9.1	19.6
Unpaid family labor	6.1	4.5	4.8	2.5	4.4
Domestic work/household chores	28.9	31.5	32.8	34.5	32.0
Student	9.6	12.7	13.3	14.0	12.5
Retired/pensioner/too old to work	2.0	1.0	1.3	1.9	1.5
Unemployed	2.8	3.3	2.8	3.0	3.0
Other	1.7	1.0	0.9	0.8	1.1
Total	100.0	100.0	100.0	100.0	100.0

Source Odisha migration survey 2023, Households sample

3 Work Status

3.1 Work Status and Migration

We now discuss work status disaggregated by sex and residential status (Table 5). We saw earlier that casual wage labor is the most commonly reported primary activity status by both male and female workers in Odisha. On average, nearly four in 10 workers are casual wage workers. However, there are significant differences by residential status. Resident workers are more likely to be casual wage workers compared to migrant workers. At the aggregate level, migrant workers are most likely to be regular wage workers in the private sector, followed by casual wage labor. The share of casual labor in the migrant workforce is higher for women than for men (Table 5).

It can be seen in Table 5 that the share of regular wage workers—in both the private and public sectors—is higher for migrants than for residents. Migrant male workers are more than three times more likely to be in wage work in the private sector compared to resident male workers, while migrant female workers are 4.8 times more likely to be in wage work in the private sector compared to their counterparts who do not migrate. Migration thus offers access to regular wage work, which is generally associated with job stability and higher incomes.

Residents, on the other hand, are more likely to be self-employed and be engaged in unpaid family labor. The latter is a particularly important activity status for resident female workers, as more than one in five reports this. In comparison, the share of female migrant workers in unpaid family labor is inconsequential.

Table 5 Work status by sex for migrants and residents, 15–64 years

Work status	Male			Female		
	Resident	Migrant	Total	Resident	Migrant	Total
Self-employed (employer)	4.4	1.1	3.7	2.2	2.5	2.2
Self-employed (own account worker)	31.7	13.6	28.0	20.4	13.1	20.0
Regular wage in public sector	2.8	4.9	3.2	7.9	12.7	8.2
Regular wage in private sector	14.1	44.3	20.3	6.3	30.3	7.7
Casual wage labor	40.2	32.9	38.7	41.4	38.5	41.3
Unpaid family labor	6.7	3.3	6.0	21.8	2.9	20.7
Total	100.0	100.0	100.0	100.0	100.0	100.0

Source Odisha migration survey 2023, Households sample

In addition, the share of women in public wage work is higher for both migrant and resident women, compared to men. This may be on account of social norms that make it acceptable for women to work in the public sector.

3.2 *Work Status and Social Group*

Table 6 shows the distribution of the six work statuses by the four social group categories. Clear caste patterns emerge in the results. SC workers are least likely to be self-employed, as employers or own account workers, while upper-caste workers are most likely to be so. Further down the social group and caste hierarchy, the data shows that OBC men have a higher probability of being self-employed when compared to both ST and SC men. A similar pattern is observed for regular wage in the public—as well as private—sector, where the share of upper-caste men is significantly higher than the OBCs and SCs, and in particular, the STs, whose share in regular wage work is abysmally low. On the other hand, in the case of casual wage labor, we see that both ST and SC men are overrepresented when compared to upper-caste men. In the case of unpaid family labor, we see that its share is the highest among ST men and the lowest among upper-caste men, which indicates the intersection of male and caste privilege. Overall, in the case of men, upper castes are overrepresented in better work statuses such as employer and regular wage work, while the SCs and STs are overrepresented in precarious work statuses such as casual wage work and unpaid family labor.

Caste patterns are striking in work status distribution for females, too. The data shows that among the females, the share of own account workers is the highest among the upper-caste women, and it is the lowest for SC women, followed by OBC and ST women. Similarly, upper-caste women are overrepresented in regular wage work, be it in the public or the private sector, in comparison with OBC, SC, and ST women, in that order. However, in the case of casual work, the opposite picture

Table 6 Work status by social group and sex, age 15–64 years

Work status	SC		Total	ST		Total	OBC		Total	UC		Total
	Male	Female		Male	Female		Male	Female		Male	Female	
Self-employed (employer)	1.8	0.5	1.5	4.6	3.2	4.2	3.1	1.3	2.8	6.1	5.7	6.1
Self-employed (own account worker)	21.8	14.7	20.2	23.5	20.1	22.5	31.2	22.4	29.8	33.0	22.5	31.7
Regular wage in public sector	2.5	7.4	3.6	2.1	4.8	2.8	3.5	10.3	4.6	5.0	15.1	6.3
Regular wage in private sector	20.0	8.4	17.5	9.8	2.6	7.8	22.0	9.9	20.1	30.9	17.8	29.2
Casual wage labor	48.3	52.3	49.2	52.7	44.8	50.6	33.3	36.2	33.7	22.7	21.8	22.5
Unpaid family labor	5.6	16.7	8.0	7.3	24.6	12.1	6.9	19.8	8.9	2.4	17.1	4.2
Total	100.0	100.0	100.0	100.0	100.0	100.0	100.0	100.0	100.0	100.0	100.0	100.0

Source Odisha migration survey 2023, Households sample

emerges. Among the women, the share of casual wage labor is the highest among SCs, followed by STs, OBCs, and it is the lowest among upper-caste women. The table also reveals that unpaid family labor is highest for ST women when compared to OBC and upper-caste women. Thus, work status is associated with caste and social group, and it intersects with gender. Together, a disaggregated analysis by caste and gender shows how social hierarchy translates into work status outcomes, with the SC and ST women being the worst off.

4 Workforce Participation Rate

The workforce participation rate (WPR) is calculated based on two definitions of work—narrow and wide. In the narrow definition, the following five work statuses are included: (i) self-employed (employer), (ii) self-employed (own account worker), (iii) regular wage in the public sector, (iv) regular wage in the private sector, and (v) casual wage labor. In the wide definition, a sixth activity status of unpaid family labor is added. The inclusion of unpaid family work in the concept—and definition—of work is particularly important in the context of Odisha, where agriculture is the most important source of employment, and, typically, a large number of women tend to be unpaid family workers in the agricultural sector. A definition that does not accommodate unpaid family work, in turn, excludes women—and men—who are engaged in activities in the realm of work.

We analyze the workforce participation rate by sex and migration status using the narrow and wide definitions. At first, we will provide aggregate analysis, subsequently disaggregated by sex, and we shall also do a comparative analysis between resident and migrant workforce participation rates. The survey data shows that the workforce participation rate is higher for migrants than for residents; both migrant men and migrant women have higher WPRs than their resident counterparts. When disaggregated by sex, we observe that the workforce participation rate is substantially higher for men in comparison to women. When we use the wide definition, the workforce participation rate, for both resident women and men, increases by more than four and five percentage points, respectively (Table 7).

Table 7 Workforce participation rate by sex for migrants and residents, 15–64 years

Workforce participation rate	Resident			Migrant			Total		
	Male	Female	Total	Male	Female	Total	Male	Female	Total
WPR, narrow definition	69.9	15.4	41.5	89.3	28.8	78.5	73.3	15.9	45.5
WPR, wide definition	75.0	19.7	46.2	92.3	29.6	81.1	78.0	20.1	50.0

Source Odisha migration survey 2023

4.1 Workforce Participation Rate and Marital Status

We now analyze the workforce participation rate based on marital status. Here again, we discuss the WPR using the narrow and wide definitions. There are five marital statuses—(i) never married, (ii) married, (iii) widow/widower, (iv) divorced, and (v) separated. For each of these categories, we discuss the workforce participation rate and also analyze it disaggregated by sex.

We have seen earlier that male workforce participation rates are significantly higher than female workforce participation rates. Here, we first discuss the results for the narrow WPR. We can see in Table 8 that this is true across all categories disaggregated by marital status. However, it is noteworthy that married male workers have the highest workforce participation rates, while married female workers have the lowest WPRs. This indicates gendered norms—the male breadwinner model—at play.

However, if women are separated, divorced, or widowed, their WPRs tend to be significantly higher, suggesting a disruption of work and care arrangements in the household and highlighting the economic pressure on women to provide for themselves and/or their families, with divorced women being the most vulnerable. The data also shows that widowers tend to have a significantly lower WPR than married men. This could be because, in the absence of their wives, social reproduction and care may be constrained in widowers' households, in turn, adversely affecting their ability to participate in the workforce.

The "never married" category is overrepresented by young people, and a significant proportion of them are in education. Thus, the male WPR here is lower than that of other categories of marital status. For "never married" females, though WPR is much lower than that of "never married" men, it is higher than that of married women. The share of workers, using the narrow definition, is higher among "never married" women than married women. This suggests that some women leave the workforce—quit their jobs or stop *working*—after they are married.

Table 8 Workforce participation rate by sex for marital status, 15–64 years

Workforce participation rate	Never married		Married		Widow/ widower		Divorced		Separated	
	Male	Female	Male	Female	Male	Female	Male	Female	Male	Female
WPR, narrow definition	46.4	14.6	88.5	13.9	68.7	36.9	83.3	57.9	87.8	50.0
WPR, wide definition	50.1	17.3	93.7	18.5	73.4	41.1	88.9	59.6	89.8	51.9

Source Odisha migration survey 2023, Households sample

In the wide definition of WPR, similar patterns as discussed above prevail. For divorced and separated women who have high WPRs and are less likely to be in traditional family systems, the share of workers doing unpaid family labor is significantly lower than that of married women.

Thus, the data clearly shows that marriage mediates workforce participation, but its outcomes diverge by sex. Marital status plays out very differently for men and women: While married men are most likely to be workers, married women arc least likely to be so. In the absence of a spouse, men are less likely to be in the workforce while women are more likely to be so. And, this is far more pronounced for women than men, and among women, it is more so for divorced and separated women than widows (Table 8).

4.2 *Workforce Participation Rate and Age*

In this section, we examine the workforce participation rate based on sex and age categories, taking into account both the narrow and wide definitions. Let us discuss the narrow WPR first. For both men and women, the WPR follows an inverted U curve. It first increases and then decreases with age. It can be seen that WPRs are the lowest—for men and women—in the age group 15–24. This is due to a high proportion of young people being in education in this age cohort. WPRs sharply increase for men and women in the age cohort 25–34, and they peak in the age cohort 35–45. Why may this be so? For men, the male breadwinner model—the need and compulsion to provide for their families at this life stage, along with masculinized work-dominated migration streams may explain this. Women in this age cohort, in addition to economic compulsion, possibly, are less constrained by childbirth and care responsibilities of young children (unlike women in the age cohort 25–34), and are able to join the workforce (Table 9).

At the aggregate level, the wide WPRs show a similar pattern as the narrow WPRs discussed above. While considering this definition, the share of unpaid family

Table 9 Workforce participation rate by age and sex

Age	Narrow WPR		Total	Wide WPR		Total
	Male	Female		Male	Female	
15–24	35.1	9.5	23.3	38.7	12.3	26.5
25–34	85.4	17.1	51.1	90.1	20.9	55.3
35–44	90.3	20.6	55.2	95.8	24.3	59.8
45–54	89.0	19.6	55.8	94.7	25.4	61.6
55–64	79.1	12.9	47.8	83.5	18.4	52.7

Source Odisha migration survey 2023, Households sample

workers among female workers is significantly higher than that among male workers, across all age cohorts, particularly in the youngest and older age cohorts.

4.3 Workforce Participation Rate and Social Group

We now look at the workforce participation rate disaggregated by sex and social group. By social group, it is evident that SCs have the highest WPR under the narrow definition. The WPR is higher than average for STs and SCs and lower than average for persons in the OBCs and upper caste groups. While using the wide definition, we see that SCs have the highest WPR, and it is followed by STs, OBCs and upper castes, in that order.

When we consider the narrow WPR definition among the females, we see that the WPR is highest among the SC women. ST women also have a relatively high WPR, while OBC and upper-caste women have lower than average WPRs. The table indicates a clear hierarchy by caste and social group that is significantly pronounced for women; the lower the social group, the higher the WPR. A similar pattern is found using the wide WPR definition (Table 10).

4.4 Workforce Participation Rate by Wealth Status

Table 11 provides the workforce participation rate for each of the four wealth quartiles, disaggregated by sex. At the aggregate level, there is a significant difference in the WPR between the poorest and richest quartiles. It can be seen that WPR is the highest for the bottom wealth quartile, and it declines as we move from the bottom to the top quartiles. Disaggregated by sex, this pattern holds for both male and female WPRs.

However, the variations in WPR are significantly higher for women than for men; women in the lowest quartile have a WPR that is about 2.4 times that of women in the highest quartile, while for men, this difference is only 5 percentage points more (Table 11).

5 Occupation

The analysis of occupation is based on the resident and migrant status of both men and women. In the OMS questionnaire, the occupation list has 81 codes, and for the purpose of this analysis, we have consolidated them into five broad categories: (i) agriculture and allied activities, (ii) manufacturing and mining, (iii) construction, (iv)

Table 10 Workforce participation rate by sex and social group

WPR	Male					Female					Total				
	ST	SC	OBC	Upper	Total	ST	SC	OBC	Upper	Total	ST	SC	OBC	Upper	Total
WPR, narrow	75.2	71.0	73.1	75.0	73.3	19.0	23.3	12.7	10.2	15.9	47.6	47.7	43.9	44.3	45.5
WPR, wide	79.7	76.6	78.5	76.8	78.0	22.8	30.8	15.8	12.3	20.1	51.8	54.3	48.2	46.2	50.0

Source Odisha migration survey 2023, Households sample

Table 11 Workforce participation rate by wealth status

Wealth quartile	Male WPR	Female WPR	Total WPR
Q1 (lowest)	79.3	31.6	55.0
Q2	78.7	19.9	50.5
Q3	78.5	15.7	48.9
Q4 (highest)	75.6	13.2	45.8

Source Odisha migration survey 2023, Households sample

services, and (v) others. Agriculture and allied activities consist of the following occupation codes: agriculture, animal husbandry, collection of forest produce, and fisheries. Manufacturing and mining constitute the following occupation codes: manufacturing worker, mining, quarry worker, shoemaker, and small-scale industry located in households. Construction has the following occupation codes: construction worker, site agent, site supervisor, crane operator, and mason. Services comprise 62 occupation codes, which are further classified into nine sub-categories: legal, finance and accounting, engineering and managerial, transport, hotel and hospitality, trade and repair, health and education, public service, village service, and other services. Lastly, the "others" category is diverse, comprising the following occupations: money lender, politician, graphic designer, cable operator, and others.

The OMS results indicate that agriculture is the most important occupation for residents, followed by services and construction. Nearly 45% of resident workers are in the agricultural sector, one-third work in a wide range of services, and about one in five workers are employed in the construction sector (Table 12). Within services, employment in the trade and repair services sector is high, followed by transport and health and education sectors.

In the case of migrants, we find that a majority—more than one in two—of the workers are engaged in occupations in the services sector. This is followed by employment in construction and the manufacturing and mining sector, in which 18% and 17% of migrant workers, respectively, are employed. Agriculture does not emerge as a leading occupation for migrant workers; while more than one in 10 migrant workers are employed in agriculture, migrants are nearly four times less likely than residents to work in agriculture.

When disaggregated by sex, the data reveals that among the residents in the agriculture and allied sector, the share of female employment is nearly 20 percentage points higher compared to that of males. This suggests the feminization of agriculture in Odisha. On the other hand, in non-agricultural occupations, such as services, construction, mining, and manufacturing, which are typically male-dominated occupations, it is observed that the share of male employment is higher than that of female employment. Men have diversified into a range of non-agricultural occupations while women workers predominantly remain—or are stuck—in agriculture.

There is occupational segregation by sex. Within the service sector, among both residents and migrants, the share of female employment is higher in the health and education sectors, whereas male employment is higher in trade and repair services.

Table 12 Distribution of occupation by migration status and sex, age 15–64 years

Occupation	Resident			Migrant		
	Male	Female	Total	Male	Female	Total
Agriculture and allied	40.4	59.6	44.5	11.0	18.6	11.5
Manufacturing and mining	1.8	1.8	1.8	17.5	5.2	16.6
Construction	21.3	11.1	19.2	18.6	11.9	18.1
Services						
Legal and accounting	1.6	0.7	1.4	2.6	2.1	2.5
Engineering and managerial	0.8	0.4	0.7	3.8	5.7	3.9
Transport	5.7	0.1	4.5	4.8	0.5	4.5
Hotel and hospitality	1.4	2.9	1.7	9.5	1.5	9.0
Trade and repair	15.3	6.3	13.3	17.7	21.6	18.0
Health and education	2.1	8.7	3.5	2.1	22.7	3.5
Public services	0.3	0.1	0.2	2.4	1.5	2.4
Village services	1.5	0.5	1.3	1.0	1.0	1.0
Other services	7.3	7.5	7.4	8.3	7.7	8.3
Others	0.5	0.4	0.4	0.6	0.0	0.0
Total	100.0	100.0	100.0	100.0	100.0	100.0

Source Odisha migration survey 2023, Households sample

Again, in transport, the share of male employment is higher compared to the share of female employment, among both migrant and resident workers.

5.1 Occupation and Work Status

Table 13 provides the distribution of occupation by work status. This allows us to disaggregate and assess the *nature* of work undertaken within each occupation. Occupations that offer a regular wage are most likely to be preferred, while those with a preponderance of casual wage and unpaid work are least likely to be preferred. It can be seen that for agriculture and allied occupations, a majority of workers are engaged in casual labor and are self-employed. Unpaid family work also emerges as important in agriculture. Construction appears as one of the most precarious occupations, as 86% of the workers in this occupation are employed as casual laborers.

On the other hand, in manufacturing and mining, we see that a regular wage in the private sector is the most important work status. In the services occupations, we see that legal and accounting, engineering and managerial, transport, hotel, and hospitality provide high rates of employment with regular wage in the private sector. These are among the *good jobs* or the *better occupations*, which are likely to offer a regular wage and higher incomes too.

Table 13 Occupation by work status

Occupation	Self-employed (employer)	Self-employed (own account worker)	Regular wage in public sector	Regular wage in private sector	Casual wage labor	Unpaid family worker	Total
Agriculture and allied activities	6.2	36.1	0.0	0.0	37.0	20.6	100.0
Manufacturing and mining	0.4	18.7	0.8	64.5	14.5	1.1	100.0
Construction	0.1	1.5	0.3	12.6	85.5	0.0	100.0
Services							
Legal and accounting	1.2	3.9	18.8	75.8	0.3	0.0	100.0
Engineering and managerial	0.4	0.8	12.9	85.8	0.0	0.0	100.0
Transport	0.1	12.3	1.6	65.0	21.1	0.0	100.0
Hotel and hospitality	0.0	21.7	6.2	59.1	13.0	0.0	100.0
Trade and repair	4.1	52.5	1.3	22.7	17.6	1.8	100.0
Health and education	4.6	11.3	63.7	19.6	0.8	0.0	100.0
Public services	0.9	0.0	99.1	0.0	0.0	0.0	100.0
Village services	0.7	52.4	0.4	4.4	39.6	2.6	100.0
Other services	1.6	17.8	6.0	29.1	42.0	3.6	100.0
Others	1.0	13.4	6.2	55.7	23.7	0.0	100.0

Source Odisha migration survey 2023, Households sample

5.2 Occupation, Age, and Sex

The analysis on occupation is based on sex and age categories. For the purpose of our analysis, the working-age population (15–64 years) is distributed in five categories. Among both male and female workers, the likelihood of being employed in agriculture and allied activities increases as we move from the younger age cohorts to the older age cohorts. Men in the age group 55–64 years are more than twice as likely to work in agriculture compared to those in the age group 15–24 years. For women, this likelihood is relatively lower at 1.3 times (Table 14). This *gender* difference can be understood due to the feminization of agriculture discussed earlier in this chapter. In all age cohorts, more than one in two women work in agriculture.

In contrast to agriculture, where the older population is more likely to be employed, occupations like construction and trade and repair services have a higher share of

Table 14 Distribution of occupation by sex and age categories

Occupation	Male					Female				
	15–24	25–34	35–44	45–54	55–64	15–24	25–34	35–44	45–54	55–64
Agriculture and allied activities	26.9	24.9	33.1	42.6	55.8	52.2	53.1	59.9	59.3	65.6
Manufacturing and mining	8.1	5.4	3.2	2.8	2.1	2.5	1.9	1.0	2.7	2.1
Construction	26.4	21.8	22.3	19.2	14.8	13.7	11.6	10.4	10.0	10.7
Services										
Legal and accounting	1.0	2.4	2.0	1.6	1.2	1.3	1.7	0.3	0.3	0.4
Engineering and managerial	1.2	2.4	0.9	0.7	0.6	1.3	1.7	0.2	0.1	0.0
Transport	5.5	8.1	6.9	4.1	1.4	0.0	0.1	0.2	0.0	0.0
Hotel and hospitality	4.2	3.2	2.4	2.2	1.6	1.5	2.5	2.9	3.6	3.3
Trade and repair	17.2	17.1	16.1	14.5	12.4	9.9	8.1	6.1	5.9	5.5
Health and education	1.0	2.1	2.1	2.5	2.6	8.5	10.3	9.9	10.2	5.5
Public services	0.4	1.2	0.8	0.3	0.1	0.2	0.2	0.1	0.1	0.0
Village services	0.9	1.5	1.5	1.9	1.3	0.2	0.6	0.6	0.5	0.6
Other services	6.8	8.1	8.1	7.3	6.0	8.4	7.9	7.9	7.0	6.3
Others	0.5	0.6	0.5	0.4	0.3	0.3	0.4	0.6	0.3	0.0
Total	100.0	100.0	100.0	100.0	100.0	100.0	100.0	100.0	100.0	100.0

Source Odisha migration survey 2023, Households sample

young workers. As we move to the higher age cohorts, the share of—both male and female—workers declines in construction. This can be explained due to the hard labor required in some of these occupations. For male workers, this is also evident in manufacturing and mining, and service occupations such as "hotels and hospitality" sector. For female workers too, at the aggregate level, there is a youth domination in employment in the services sector, where the age cohorts 25–34 years and 15–24 years have a higher share of workers compared to the older age cohorts. However, it can be seen in the most important services of health and education, where women are employed, their likelihood of employment does not vary much across the age cohorts.

Thus, overall, the data reveals considerable variations in occupations by sex and age. Women are more likely to be in agricultural occupations, and older women even more so. Men, on the other hand, are more likely to be in the services and construction sectors, and both younger men and women are more likely to be in occupations in these sectors compared to men and women in the older age cohorts, respectively.

5.3 *Occupation, Sex, and Social Group*

We now analyze the distribution of occupations by social groups. Distinct occupational patterns—by caste and gender—emerge from the survey data. SCs and STs, both men and women, are overrepresented in agriculture, while the upper castes and OBCs are underrepresented in agriculture. In a similar vein, STs are most likely to work in the construction sector, closely followed by SCs, and then the OBCs and the upper castes. The pattern is the same for men and women. Among SC males, agriculture is the most important occupation, followed by construction. Three-fourths of all SC male workers and about three-fifths of all ST male workers can be found in these two occupations. The occupational profile of OBC and upper-caste men is more diversified, with these castes being overrepresented in occupations in the services sector. The caste differences are stark: Upper-caste men are seven times more likely to be in the legal and accounting professions and 10 times more likely to be in engineering and managerial positions than SC men (Table 15).

At the aggregate level, women have a less diversified occupational profile than men, but when we disaggregate by social group, significant differences emerge. While nearly six in 10 female workers are employed in agriculture, this varies significantly by caste and social group. Like their male counterparts, upper-caste women are least likely to work in agriculture or construction and are most likely to be employed in the services sector. On the other hand, SC and ST workers are underrepresented in occupations in the services sector. The inequality between castes in being employed in *better* occupations is higher among female workers than among male workers. Upper-caste women are 15 times more likely than SC women to be in legal and accounting professions and 27 times more likely to be in engineering and managerial occupations. While female employment in manufacturing and mining-related occupations is low, ST women are most likely to be employed in this sector. As is expected, ST and SC women workers are far more likely to be employed in the construction sector than upper-caste or OBC women.

Disaggregated by sex, we find that females across all social groups tend to have a higher probability of being employed in agriculture and allied occupations when compared to men. When it comes to analyzing manufacturing and mining occupations, we see that the likelihood of men in these occupations is higher compared to women across the social categories. A similar pattern is observed in construction and service occupations.

Table 15 Occupation by sex and social group

Occupation	Male					Female					Total				
	ST	SC	OBC	UC	Total	ST	SC	OBC	UC	Total	ST	SC	OBC	UC	Total
Agriculture and allied	33.8	49.9	34.8	21.2	35.9	56.4	70.0	51.2	35.9	57.7	38.7	55.5	37.4	23.0	40.1
Manufacturing and mining	4.6	2.3	5.1	4.0	4.2	3.0	1.3	2.0	2.5	2.0	4.2	2.0	4.6	3.8	3.7
Construction	26.5	25.5	17.7	16.8	20.9	12.2	12.2	9.9	8.7	11.1	23.4	21.8	16.5	15.8	19.0
Services															
Legal and accounting	0.9	0.5	2.1	3.5	1.8	0.6	0.2	0.9	3.0	0.8	0.9	0.4	1.9	3.4	1.6
Engineering and managerial	0.6	0.3	1.4	3.0	1.2	0.5	0.1	0.8	2.7	0.7	0.6	0.2	1.3	3.0	1.1
Transport	6.2	4.8	5.5	6.3	5.6	0.1	0.1	0.1	0.0	0.1	4.9	3.5	4.6	5.5	4.5
Hotel and hospitality	2.6	0.7	3.1	4.3	2.7	1.7	1.1	5.3	3.5	2.8	2.4	0.8	3.5	4.2	2.7
Trade and repair	13.4	7.9	18.6	21.0	15.6	5.8	4.6	9.3	10.9	7.0	11.7	7.0	17.2	19.7	13.9
Health and education	1.7	0.8	2.3	4.0	2.1	8.3	4.4	11.4	22.5	9.3	3.2	1.8	3.8	6.4	3.5
Public services	0.4	0.7	0.6	0.9	0.6	0.1	0.1	0.2	0.0	0.1	0.3	0.5	0.5	0.7	0.5
Village services	1.3	0.5	0.9	4.4	1.5	1.7	0.2	0.1	0.5	0.5	1.4	0.4	0.8	3.9	1.3
Other services	7.7	5.6	7.5	9.8	7.5	9.1	5.7	8.1	9.2	7.5	8.0	5.7	7.6	9.7	7.5
Others	0.3	0.5	0.4	0.8	0.5	0.6	0.1	0.5	0.7	0.4	0.4	0.4	0.4	0.8	0.5
Total	100.0	100.0	100.0	100.0	100.0	100.0	100.0	100.0	100.0	100.0	100.0	100.0	100.0	100.0	100.0

Source Odisha migration survey 2023, Households sample

Table 16 Distribution of occupation by rural and urban locations

Occupation	Rural	Urban	Total
Agriculture and allied	45.3	12.1	40.1
Manufacturing and mining	3.9	2.7	3.7
Construction	17.7	26.1	19.0
Services			
Legal and accounting	1.2	3.5	1.6
Engineering and managerial	1.0	2.0	1.1
Transport	4.2	6.3	4.5
Hotel and hospitality	2.7	2.9	2.7
Trade and repair	12.4	22.0	13.9
Health and education	3.3	4.9	3.5
Public services	0.5	0.6	0.5
Village services	1.3	1.4	1.3
Other services	6.2	14.5	7.5
Others	0.3	1.1	0.5
Total	100.0	100.0	100.0

Source Odisha migration survey 2023, Households sample

5.4 *Occupation in Rural and Urban Areas*

Table 16 disaggregates occupation by rural and urban locations. Notably, less than half of the rural workforce is engaged in agricultural occupations. The table indicates that the share of agriculture and allied occupations is considerably higher in rural locations, compared to urban locations. On the other hand, as expected, both services and construction occupations are more likely to be in urban locations than rural. Within services, we see that occupations such as legal and accounting services, transport, and trade and repair are more concentrated in urban locations. Occupations such as engineering/managerial, hotel and hospitality, and public services are also marginally higher in urban locations.

6 Conclusion

This chapter presented the labor market and employment scenario in Odisha based on data from the OMS. A key limitation of the chapter is that it covered only the primary activity and work status and did not capture secondary work and employment of individuals, which is widely prevalent in the context of a rural and agrarian society. Having said that, the chapter first analyzed the activity and work statuses of individuals, followed by their workforce participation rates and occupations, disaggregated by sex, age, social group, wealth quartile, and residential status. The labor market is characterized by precarity, with more than two-thirds of the workers being casual wage laborers and own account workers, while *only* less than a quarter are in regular wage work. The upper castes are overrepresented in better work statuses, such as employer and regular wage work, while the SCs and STs are overrepresented in precarious work statuses, such as casual wage work and unpaid family labor. Workforce participation rates vary significantly by sex, social group, and residential status. Male WPRs are significantly higher than the female WPRs, migrants have a higher WPR than residents, and WPRs are higher for individuals in marginalized communities such as the SCs and STs, and those in the lower wealth quartiles.

The India Employment Report (IHD & ILO, 2024) highlighted that Odisha, along with Bihar, Jharkhand, Madhya Pradesh, and Uttar Pradesh, is among the less economically developed states in the country. This has placed workers in a disadvantageous position while impacting employment outcomes and leading to a narrow range of job opportunities. This is evident in the OMS results, which show that about 40% of all workers were employed in agriculture, and nearly 20% worked in the construction sector. However, occupational diversification is also gendered; while men have been able to access a broader range of non-agricultural occupations through migration, there has been a feminization of agriculture. Thus, the chapter highlights that along with labor market inequalities characterized by caste, gender, and region, migration plays a significant role in work and employment outcomes in Odisha.

References

Institute for Human Development (IHD) & International Labour Organization (ILO). (2024). India employment report 2024: Youth employment, education, and skills. IHD & ILO. https://www.ilo.org/publications/india-employment-report-2024-youth-employment-education-and-skills

Padhi, B., & Panda, S. (2021). Employment and economic growth dynamics in Odisha, India. *Journal of Public Affairs, 21*(2), e2168.

Chapter 8
Rural Livelihoods and Income

Amrita Datta, Nandini Ramamurthy, Iswarya Priya Jagannathan, and Fahin Faras

Abstract In the context of a changing rural economy and society, this chapter studies the role of agriculture, non-agriculture, and remittances among livelihoods undertaken by households in rural Odisha. Based on data from a primary survey and qualitative case studies, we examine the distribution of household income and explore how individuals and households combine multiple sources of livelihoods and income. The study finds that local non-agriculture emerges as the most important source of income, followed by agriculture, migrant remittances, and government transfers. Nearly one-third of households have migrants, but contrary to the mainstream migration and development literature, we find that households with migrants have lower incomes than households without migrants, indicating the distress-oriented nature of migration from rural Odisha. Further, we develop livelihood-and income-based household typologies to find that the *type of livelihood* matters: income levels and distribution of income vary significantly among agriculture-based households, non-agriculture-based households, remittance-based households, and government transfer-based households. The qualitative case studies, embedded in the analysis of household-based livelihood typologies, complement the survey data to better understand the processes of livelihood creation and diversification in rural Odisha.

Keywords Migration · Household livelihoods · Rural livelihoods · Income · Rural development · Migration and development · Odisha · India

A. Datta (✉) · I. P. Jagannathan · F. Faras
Indian Institute of Technology, Hyderabad, India
e-mail: amritadatta@la.iith.ac.in

N. Ramamurthy
Independent Researcher, Hyderabad, India

A. Datta and S. I. Rajan (eds.), *Migration, Livelihoods and Gender*, International Perspectives on Migration, https://doi.org/10.1007/978-981-95-5465-2_8

1 Introduction

Migration, in diverse contexts, contributes to generating alternative livelihood and income opportunities. Migration patterns vary—by individual characteristics such as gender and education and household and community characteristics such as caste and class—which, in turn, have differential impacts (Breman, 1996; Datta, 2020; Haberfeld et al., 1999; Sucharita & Rout, 2020). Migration may be *distress-oriented*, suggesting the impoverished state of rural households due to structural inequalities, climate change, and social hierarchies (Bellampalli & Yadava, 2023; Sreelakshmi, 2021). *Coping migration* is a mechanism that allows households to smooth consumption and manage risk, while *accumulative migration* allows for the accumulation of assets, savings, and investments (Deshingkar & Farrington, 2009). Over time and under favorable circumstances, coping migration streams may become *accumulative* (ibid.*)*. In the context of seasonal migration induced by chronic poverty and livelihood insecurity, development interventions in the source region have the potential to enhance local livelihoods and reduce distress and seasonal migration (Nienkerke et al., 2023). Studies point that long-term and permanent migration make migrants better off than seasonal and short-term migration, indicating that the type of migration matters (Datta, 2020; Srivastava, 2020). Moreover, comparing migrant households with non-migrant households is a commonly used method to examine the influence of migration (Qin, 2010).

Within the context of the rural livelihoods framework, migration and remittances contribute to a diversified portfolio of individual and household livelihoods in the source region (Ellis, 2000). There is an established migration and development literature that presents micro-evidence on the development outcomes of remittances. This literature shows that remittances lead to increases in income and consumption (Haberfeld et al., 1999; Taylor et al., 2003) and contribute to poverty reduction (Adams & Page, 2005; Lokshin et al., 2010; Murrugarra & Herrera, 2011; Sabates-Wheeler et al., 2008). Remittances also positively impact agricultural productivity and rural development (Kapri & Ghimire, 2020; Orozco & Jewers, 2019). In sum, this literature argues that remittances contribute significantly to economic development in the source regions.

The Indian rural landscape has been characterized by a *stalled*—a *ruptured*—rural transformation. Official statistics show that an increasing number of rural households are resorting to a combination of agricultural and non-agricultural activities for their survival (Abraham, 2024; Binswanger-Mkhize, 2013). Recent micro studies highlight the reliance of rural individuals and households on a multiplicity of livelihoods through labor migration, along with self-employment and wage employment in the non-farm sector (Choithani et al., 2021). In the emergent non-farm economy, however, social hierarchies and differential incomes persist (Jodhka, 2023; Jodhka & Kumar, 2017). While labor migration, on the one hand, can provide better employment opportunities and higher wages, it can also expose migrants to increased vulnerability through exploitation and abuse (Singh & Basu, 2020). For instance, the *Dadan* system of advance-based, contractor-mediated labor migration has existed for long, and it is characterized by high degrees of exploitation, unfreedom, and bondage (Acharya, 2021; Mishra, 2020). In Odisha, outmigration is due to low-agricultural productivity and a lack of non-farm employment opportunities (Mitra & Pradhan, 2016). Poor households engage in seasonal migration to supplement their inadequate incomes from local agricultural and non-agricultural sources (Sharma et al., 2014). In Odisha, in the post-liberalization period, the share of households receiving remittances rose sharply, suggesting an increased dependence on migration and remittances (Tumbe, 2011). In particular, migration streams are male-and youth-dominated, as there is a loss of interest in traditional work (NLUO, 2020).

Against this backdrop, this study on livelihoods and income in rural Odisha explores the following research questions: (i) What is the role of agriculture, non-agriculture, and remittances among multiple livelihoods undertaken by rural households? (ii) What is the distribution of household income from various sources? (iii) How do households and individuals combine multiple livelihoods in a changing rural landscape? To address these questions, a comprehensive module was developed to map household livelihoods and undertake an income accounting exercise. This module was administered to 506 households from 17 localities (villages) spread across 11 districts in the second phase of the Odisha Migration Study 2023. These households are a subset of 15,000 households interviewed in the first phase of the study in 2023.[1] The 11 districts under study—Balangir, Bargarh, Gajapati, Ganjam, Kalahandi, Koraput, Khordha, Nabarangpur, Nuapada, Rayagada, and Subarnapur—are districts declared by the Odisha government as migration-prone.

The rest of the chapter is organized as follows: Section 2 discusses the theories of sustainable livelihoods and livelihood diversification. Section 3 details the methodology and sample of the study. Section 4 presents migration and income details of the sample households, focusing on the incidence of household and individual migration and the levels and distribution of household income, disaggregated by migration status and social group. Section 5 discusses four distinct household livelihood typologies of agriculture-, non-agriculture-, remittance-, and government transfer-based households, along with a discussion on the pandemic and return migration. Section 6 concludes.

2 Sustainable Livelihoods and Livelihood Diversification: A Theoretical Approach

The idea of sustainable livelihoods emerges from capability, equity, and sustainability approaches (Chambers & Conway, 1991), for creating tangible and intangible resources for rural households. Since its introduction in the 1990s, the sustainable livelihoods approach has become a mainstay in development studies and practice (Natarajan et al., 2022). The origins and theoretical foundations of sustainable livelihoods debates lie in Sen's (1985) capability approach, where the focus is on

[1] See details in Chap. 1.

individuals as the locus for development (Scoones, 2009). Sustainable livelihoods approaches critique the conventional frameworks and analyses that heavily rely on production, employment, and poverty (Chambers & Conway, 1991). Since rural households combine several strategies to obtain a living, it is critical to further explore the determinants and pathways of rural livelihoods and diversification.

There has been a decline in agriculture, and processes of deagrarianization are underway in rural India (Datta, 2016; Jodhka, 2023). Increasing input costs, along with unsustainable extraction of natural resources, induce climate and environmental changes, making income from agriculture unsustainable (Taylor, 2015). In the context of the state retreating its support for agriculture, this creates a scarcity of livelihood options, increases precarity, and makes rural households vulnerable to livelihood shocks, making them unable to meet their basic needs for survival (Bhandari & Grant, 2007; Hietala & Singh, 2014). In such a context, migration may enable rural households to build sustainable livelihoods, allowing them to cope with stress and shock and maintain or enhance their capabilities (Mistri & Das, 2020).

In the livelihoods literature, diversification strategies are an important component in understanding the work, employment, and well-being of rural households. Ellis (1998) defined livelihood diversification as "the process by which rural families construct a diverse portfolio of activities and social support capabilities in their struggle for survival and in order to improve their standards of living" (p. 4). On the one hand, studies provide empirical evidence indicating a positive impact of diversification on rural households (Babatunde & Qaim, 2010; Ellis, 2000). However, critics (Katchova, 2005; Zhao & Barry, 2014) document the negative impacts of diversification. Peng et al. (2022), in a study in China, suggest diversification is profitable when rural households are capable of transitioning to non-farm income, alienating from land-based livelihoods for market-oriented activities. In the context of Nepal, Gautam and Andersen (2016) find that livelihood diversification into high-return non-farm sectors enhances household well-being. At the same time, caste and ethnicity mediate access to these sectors; thus, the authors argue that returns of livelihood diversification are unequally distributed in the local economy.

Furthermore, the COVID-19 pandemic highlighted the limits of livelihood diversification in using migration as a core strategy to build resilience (Samaddar, 2020; Sinha et al., 2022). Although the theoretical discussion on livelihoods has had largely positive connotations, recent studies foregrounded in structural perspectives emphasize precarities and vulnerabilities associated with rural livelihood diversification (Griffin et al., 2024; Natarajan et al., 2022; Porst & Sakdapolrak, 2018). It is against this backdrop that we examine household livelihoods and income in rural Odisha.

3 Methodology

This chapter is based on data collected as part of the second phase of the Odisha Migration Study from 506 households in 11 districts of Odisha. The 11 districts—Balangir, Bargarh, Kalahandi, Nuapada, Subarnapur, Ganjam, Gajapati, Rayagada,

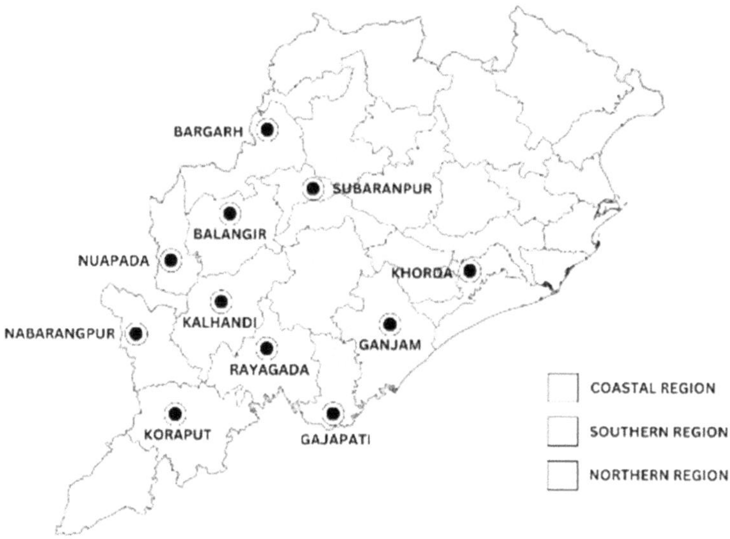

Fig. 1 The regions of Odisha and study districts. *Source* District map, Government of Odisha

Koraput, Nabarangpur, and Khordha—were purposively selected as they have been identified as migration-prone by the government of Odisha (see Fig. 1). The 506 households of the Odisha Migration Study Phase 2 are a subset of a larger representative sample of 15,000 households that were interviewed in Phase 1.[2]

For Phase 2, the sample size of the study was predetermined at 500. In the 11 aforementioned districts, rural localities with the highest migration rates in the Odisha Migration Study Phase 1 were selected for data collection. Within each district, the number of localities (and households) was selected based on their probability proportionate to the sample size in Phase 1. By this process, a total of 17 localities in 11 districts were selected. Locality and district-wise details of the household sample are given in Table 1.

It may be noted that seven of the 11 study districts belong to the poorest and most deprived southern region of Odisha, while one district is part of the relatively backward northern region. The remaining three districts in the sample are from the relatively advanced coastal region. Thus, the sample is biased toward the relatively poor and backward regions of the state.

A module was developed to capture household livelihoods and income through various agricultural and non-agricultural sources. Data on remittances and government transfers was also collected. Work and employment details of all household

[2] The first phase of the study, the Odisha Migration Survey (OMS), consisted of a quantitative survey conducted in all 30 districts of Odisha. The survey used a stratified multistage random sampling with a sample size of 15,000 households spread over 500 rural and urban localities, with 30 households in each locality. See Section 7 in Chap. 1 for details.

Table 1 Distribution of sample households by districts and villages

District	Locality (Village)	Number of households
Balangir	Babejuri	30
	Dangapata	30
Bargarh	Agalpur	30
	Jujgaon	30
Gajapati	Kutama	30
Ganjam	Gangadahani	30
	Kandharanipada	28
	Paikapada	30
Kalahandi	Balagaon	29
	Jariguma	29
Khordha	Bhenkatarayapur	30
Koraput	Balel	30
	Konga	30
Nabarangpur	Gadabaguda	30
Nuapada	Ganiary	30
Rayagada	Beruguda	30
Subarnapur	Samarchipa	30
Total		506

Source Odisha migration study 2023, Phase II, Household sample, Income and livelihood module

members were meticulously collected to map and better understand rural household livelihood portfolios and diversification.[3] In addition, 24 qualitative case studies were undertaken in the districts of Ganjam and Kalahandi for a nuanced understanding of *how* individuals and households make their employment decisions, choose their livelihood portfolios, and what sense they make of their income and livelihood sources in the context of a changing rural economy and society.

[3] The module was piloted in April 2023 in Kalahandi. After the pilot, the module was suitably modified and finalized for data collection. A small team of experienced field investigators was trained in administering the module. Data was collected from May to August 2023.

Table 2 Incidence of migration by household income quintile (% households)

First quintile (Poorest)	33.7
Second quintile	34.7
Third quintile	39.6
Fourth quintile	30.7
Fifth quintile (richest)	32.4
Total	34.2

Source Odisha migration study 2023, Household livelihood and Income module

4 Migration and Income

4.1 Migration

In this study, a migrant was defined as someone who was or had been away from the village in the reference period of one year preceding the survey. Thus, households with migrants,[4] also referred to as migrant households, were those households that had one or more members who were away from the village at any given time in the previous year. It can be seen that about one in three households was a migrant household (Table 2).

Migration is a widespread phenomenon, spread across all income groups (Table 2). At the same time, it can be seen that there are variations in the incidence of migration by income quintile groups. Migration is relatively lower for the poorest households in the first quintile, increases progressively for the second and third quintiles, and then decreases for the fourth quintile, again rising marginally in the fifth quintile of the wealthiest households. Thus, the data suggest that there is no linear relationship between migration rate and the level of household income.

By social group, the incidence of migration at the household level was the highest among Scheduled Caste (SC) households, followed by Other Backward Class (OBC) households. Migration was relatively lower among Scheduled Tribe (ST) and upper-caste households (Table 3).

Migration from Odisha is predominantly for work. At an aggregate level, the share of migrant workers to total workers is almost 20%. In other words, nearly one in five workers in the sample is a migrant. Migration for work is overwhelmingly male-dominated; nearly nine in 10 migrant workers are male (Table 3).

[4] The demographic composition of migrant and non-migrant households varied to some extent. The average household size was 4.6 for migrant households compared to 4.1 for non-migrant households. There was little difference in the average age of individuals in migrant households (31.6 years) compared to those in non-migrant households (31.3 years). Similarly, 50.1% of individuals were married in migrant households, compared to 49.6% in non-migrant households. However, on average, members in migrant households were less educated (average, 9.4 years of schooling) compared to those in non-migrant households (average, 10.4 years of schooling).

Table 3 Migration patterns

Social Group	Households with migrants (%)	Migrants among workers (%)	Males among migrant workers (%)
Scheduled caste	44.6	27.5	87.3
Scheduled tribe	22.0	12.8	85.7
Other backward class	40.8	22.8	91.3
Upper caste	20.8	16.0	87.5
Total	34.2	19.8	89.1

Source Odisha migration study 2023, Household livelihood and Income module

The duration of migration, i.e., the number of months a migrant is away from the village, varies significantly across the sample of migrant workers (Fig. 2). A majority of migrant workers migrate for a duration of six months or less. The share of migrant workers going out of the village for a duration of less than three months (10.1%) and greater than 10 months (15.6%) is low. The duration of migration peaks at six months, and nearly three-quarters of all workers are away for four to nine months. Migrant workers of rural Odisha typically combine multiple livelihoods in destination and source regions.

Where do migrant workers go? Migration to other states of India is the most common form of outmigration from rural Odisha; 93% of migrant workers are inter-state migrants. The remaining 7% of migrants migrate within Odisha to other districts.

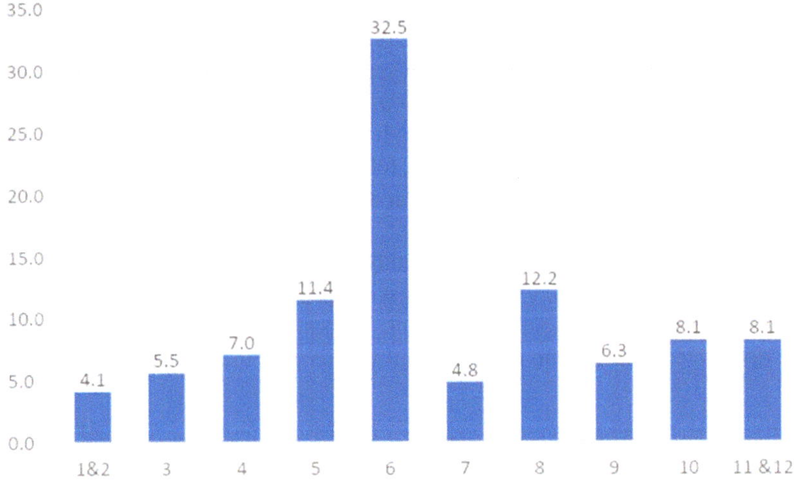

Fig. 2 Title: Number of months away in the last one year (% migrant workers). Legend, X Axis: Number of months away in last one year. Legend, Y Axis: % migrant workers. *Source* Odisha migration study 2023, Household livelihood and Income module

There was hardly any international migration in the sample households. For inter-state migration, Gujarat is the most common destination; more than one-fourth (26.6%) of migrant workers had gone to Gujarat in the previous year. This is followed by Telangana (18.5%), Tamil Nadu (15.1%), Karnataka (11.8%), Andhra Pradesh (9.2%), and Maharashtra (8.1%). Other destinations include Kerala, Uttar Pradesh, Jammu and Kashmir, and Delhi. A majority of migration (about 80%) is to urban destinations, and the most popular migrant destinations are Surat, Tiruppur, Coimbatore, Bengaluru, and Hyderabad.

4.2 Income

We use a four-fold classification to better understand income from various sources in the sample households (Table 4). To estimate the household income, we first mapped *all* work and livelihood activities undertaken by individuals in the sample households in the last year. For **agriculture and allied activities**, net income from self-employment was estimated by subtracting the total value of input from the total value of output for each production activity undertaken by the household or its members in the reference period of one year. Wage income was recorded. A similar exercise was undertaken to estimate household income from **non-agricultural activities**. Remittances include only that portion of migrant income that is sent back to the rural household and not the total income earned by the migrant at the destination. Income from **government sources** includes the total value of government transfers (including Krushak Assistance for Livelihood and Income Augmentation (KALIA), pensions, scholarships to students, etc., and wage income from casual labor in government programs such as the scheme under the Mahatma Gandhi National Rural Employment Guarantee Act (MGNREGA).

Table 4 Broad sources of household income and their components

Source of income	Component
Agriculture and allied activities, local	Self-employment in agriculture and allied activities
	Casual labor in agriculture and allied activities
	Salaried in agriculture
Non-agricultural activities, local	Self-employment in non-agriculture
	Casual labor in non-agriculture
	Salaried in non-agriculture
Remittances from migration	Remittances
Government sources	Government transfers
	Casual labor in govt programs (MGNREGA)

Source Odisha migration study 2023, Household livelihood and Income module

Table 5 Mean household income by income group in the last year

Income quintile	Mean average annual income (Rs)
First quintile (poorest)	37,686
Second quintile	64,881
Third quintile	83,040
Fourth quintile	1,07,986
Fifth quintile (richest)	2,25,854
All households (N = 504)	1,03,647

Source Odisha migration study 2023, Household livelihood and Income module

Before moving to the distribution of income sources, we look at the mean income by household migration status, income quintile, and social group. The mean annual income was Rs 1,03,647. At the aggregate level, households with migrants have a lower income (Rs 99,162) than households without migrants (Rs 1,05,992). That migrant households are worse off compared to non-migrant households in terms of income suggests adverse incorporation of such households into precarious migration streams. This is contrary to the mainstream migration and development literature, where migrant households have higher levels of income and consumption compared to non-migrant households (Choithani, 2022; Datta, 2022).

Table 5 shows the mean average income by quintiles. It can be seen that there is considerable income inequality in rural Odisha. The average income in the richest quintile is equal to six times that of the poorest quintile. This inequality can also be seen in the difference between the mean income (Rs 1,03,647) and median income (Rs 82,000).

Household income varies considerably by social group (Table 6). ST households have the lowest mean income, followed by the OBC and the SC households. The upper castes have the highest incomes. Thus, absolute incomes mirror social hierarchies, with the upper castes at the top and the STs at the bottom. In the next section, we examine the distribution of income sources in the survey households.

Table 6 Mean household income by social group in the last year

Social group	Mean average annual income (Rs)
Scheduled caste	1,10,146
Scheduled tribe	90,045
Other backward class	1,09,531
Upper caste	1,16,952
All households (N = 504)	1,03,647

Source Odisha migration study 2023, Household livelihood and Income module

4.3 Income Sources

Table 7 shows the distribution of household income for both migrant and non-migrant households. Overall, the share of income from agriculture and allied activities in total income is nearly 30%. Among total agricultural income, the share of income from self-employment in agriculture (73%) is significantly higher than that of labor in agriculture (27%). Income accruing to non-agriculture emerges as the most important source of income in the sample households. Here, unlike agriculture, salaried and labor incomes are predominant, while the share of income from self-employment is relatively low. Remittances contribute only 14.3% to total income. This is quite low and remittances are not among the more significant sources of income in rural Odisha, even though 34.2% of the sample households have migrant members. In fact, the share of income from government sources—income from government transfers and labor income from government programs such as the MGNREGA scheme—is higher than remittances at the aggregate level. This shows the importance of government assistance for rural households.

Box 1 Production in Agriculture and Allied Activities
Agriculture in Odisha is dominated by rice monocultures. In the sample households, paddy is the major crop, grown predominantly in the kharif season. If irrigation is available, it is also grown by households in the rabi season. Other than paddy,

Table 7 Distribution of household income in households with and without migrants (in rupees)

Source of income	Migrant households	Non-migrant households	All households
1. Self-employment in agriculture and allied activities	9736	27,755	21,570
2. Casual labor in agriculture	7815	8364	8176
3. Self-employment in non-agriculture	6228	9628	8461
4. Casual labor in non-agriculture	11,019	17,383	15,198
5. Salaried in non-agriculture	8405	22,825	17,875
6. Remittances	43,121	0	14,802
7. Casual labor in govt programs (MGNREGA)	824	2521	1938
8. Government transfers	11,529	16,247	14,628
9. Other	486	1269	1000
10. Total	99,162	1,05,992	1,03,647

Source Odisha migration study 2023, Household livelihood and Income module

mandia (finger millet) and biri, and mung (pulses) are commonly grown. While rice and millet production is predominantly for sale in the market, the bulk of pulses are used for self-consumption. Overall, there is little diversification. A very small number of sample households grow other crops (kolath, chana, kadal, maize) or vegetables (brinjal, tomato, pumpkin, bean, vurubuti). Vegetable cultivation, though lucrative, is undertaken by very few households as it is labor-intensive. Fruit production is even more limited—only one household reported growing mangoes. Thus, income from agriculture is dominated by proceeds from the sale of the paddy crop (Table 8).

Table 8 Agricultural production, Main crops

Main crops	Number of households engaged in cultivation	Average household production (in kg)	Share for self-consumption (%)	Share sold in the market (%)
Paddy kharif	316	2688	18.9	81.1
Paddy rabi	65	2844	4.1	96.1
Mandia (finger millet), kharif	72	219	24.7	75.3
Biri and mung (pulses), rabi	24	148	64.1	35.9

Source Odisha migration study, 2023. Household livelihood and Income module

The forest is an important source of livelihood for rural, particularly tribal households. Nearly 20% of the households collected wood and bamboo, predominantly for sale in the market. The proceeds from these, again, were very low.

Livestock ownership was quite limited. About 15% of the sample households owned livestock of any kind—chicken, goat, sheep, pig, bull, ox, and cow. Chickens and goats were most commonly owned, and in the sample households, the former had been predominantly used for market production, while the latter for self-consumption.[5] Six sample households owned bulls, used in cultivation, though it was understood that these are slowly disappearing from the rural landscape. Four sample households owned cows, and the average annual production of milk was 988 liters of milk per household, of which a majority (90.3%) was sold in the market.

Disaggregated by migration status, we find that households without migrants have higher household incomes compared to households with migrants (Table 7). This indicates that migrant households are worse off than non-migrant households. This is striking, not in resonance with the mainstream migration and development discourse based on empirical studies that find that migration is associated with improved—consumption and income—welfare outcomes. On the other hand, among non-migrant households, local non-agriculture emerges as the most important source of income, comprising 44% of total income. Here, the maximum income accrues to salaried work

[5] Forty-six households owned chickens (79.8% of the production was sold in the market); 30 households owned goats (68.8% of the production was sold in the market).

(43%), followed by casual labor (37%), and self-employment (20%). This is followed by income from agriculture and allied activities (34%). Non-migrant households are also more reliant on income from government sources (17.7%) compared to migrant households (12.5%). Income from government sources includes government transfers and wages from employment under MGNREGA, though the share of the latter in total income is low. Thus, the data shows that the distribution of income sources varies considerably by the migration status of the household. Though migrant households have lower incomes than non-migrant households, they excessively rely on remittances to support themselves; remittance income comprises 44% of total income in such households. The characteristics of households that are predominantly dependent on remittance income are explored in the next section.

Box 2 Non-Agricultural Enterprises in Sample Households

The share of income accruing to self-employment in non-agriculture is overall quite low (8.2%) and, as expected, lower for migrant households compared to non-migrant households. Less than 10% of the sample households engaged in non-agricultural self-employment or entrepreneurial activity. Retail shops, street vending, and tailoring/sewing enterprises comprised the majority of non-agricultural enterprises. It can be seen in Table 9 that there is a substantial variation in the profits in these enterprises.

Table 9 Enterprise details of sample households

Nature of enterprise	Frequency	Percent	Mean annual profit (in Rs)	Range (in Rs)	
				Min	Max
Tailoring/sewing	6	13.0	26,293	6000	75,500
Auto driving	3	6.5	99,000	84,000	1,20,000
Kirana store	4	8.7	1,13,506	97,750	1,48,400
Shop (cloth, medical, barber, liquor, photo)	12	26.1	2,26,387	10,745	16,61,000
Street vendors	9	19.6	64,907	1460	1,20,000
Handicraft (bamboo, carpentry, clay pots)	4	8.7	1,05,500	20,000	3,10,000
Restaurant/hotel	3	6.5	1,52,167	36,500	2,40,000
Coaching center	4	8.7	37,650	4200	96,000
Veterinary	1	2.2	96,000	0	0
Total	46	100.0	1,02,379		

Source Odisha migration study 2023, Household livelihood and Income module

Thus, overall, there are very few enterprises, and the majority of households are engaged in non-agricultural own account work in combination with other livelihoods.

What about the distribution of income sources by social group? We saw earlier that aggregate incomes were the lowest for ST households, followed by the OBC, SC, and upper-caste households. The distribution of income, too, follows a caste pattern. The share of income in agriculture and allied activities is the highest for STs, who have the lowest overall income. Conversely, upper-caste households derive the least share of income from agriculture and allied activities, and their average incomes are the highest among all social groups. We will further see in the next section that *agricultural-based households* tend to have the lowest average incomes.

On the other hand, a higher share of non-agricultural income is associated with higher levels of income. Here too, nearly three-fourths of the income in upper-caste households accrues to non-agriculture, whereas the corresponding figure is less than one-fourth (22.5%) for ST households. When we further disaggregate by type of activity within non-agriculture, STs are also most likely to do casual labor, while the upper castes are most likely to be salaried or engaged in entrepreneurial work, both associated with higher wages and stable incomes. Non-agricultural enterprises are very limited in the sample households; only 9% of the households reported own account non-agricultural work (see Box 2 for details).

The share of remittances in total income in SC and ST households is higher than average (Table 10). It was also seen earlier that migrant households among SCs and STs had lower mean incomes than non-migrant households. Together, these results show that SC and ST households are excessively dependent on remittances, and suggest that the migration is more likely to be distress migration, not accumulative migration.

The share of government transfers is by far the highest for ST households, followed by OBC, SC, and upper-caste households. Government transfers, by way of entitlements from the Public Distribution System (PDS), pensions of various kinds, educational scholarships, midday meals, etc., are important to all communities but are critical for the STs, who derive nearly one quarter of their income from government sources.

5 Households by Livelihood Typologies

Rural households practice multiple livelihoods for income generation. In this section, we explore household typologies defined by their primary sources of livelihoods. Based on the livelihood or income source from which a household derives its highest share of income, we classify it as agriculture-based, non-agriculture-based, remittance-based, or government transfer-based. Table 11 presents the distribution of the sample by these four distinct household typologies. It can be seen that agriculture-based households are the most common household type; more than a third of all households are agriculture-based. However, average incomes are significantly lower for agriculture-based households. On the other hand, non-agriculture-based households comprise nearly a third of the overall sample, but their average income is substantially higher than the overall mean household income.

Table 10 Distribution of annual household income by social group (in rupees)

	Scheduled caste	Scheduled tribe	Other backward class	Upper caste	All
1. Self-employment in agriculture and allied activities	13.6	33.2	17.4	6.8	20.8
2. Casual labor in agriculture	12.0	10.2	5.7	3.9	7.9
3. Self-employment in non-agriculture	2.9	1.9	12.1	20.2	8.2
4. Casual labor in non-agriculture	20.5	14.1	13.1	15.4	14.7
5. Salaried in non-agriculture	19.5	6.5	20.5	37.8	17.2
6. Remittances	19.8	10.1	16.0	5.4	14.3
7. Casual labor in govt programs (MGNREGA)	1.0	4.1	1.0	0.5	1.9
8. Government transfers	10.5	20.0	12.2	10.0	14.1
9. Other	0.0	0.0	1.9	0.0	1.0
10. Total	100.0	100.0	100.0	100.0	100.0

Source Odisha migration study 2023, Household livelihood and Income module

Table 11 Distribution of sample by type of household livelihood typologies (% of households) and mean annual income in rupees

Type of household	Sample households		Mean annual income in rupees
	Frequency	Percent	
Agriculture-based households	177	35.1	86,545
Non-agriculture-based households	167	33.1	1,45,610
Remittance-based households	99	19.6	87,762
Government transfer-based households	61	12.1	64,175
Total households	504	100.0	1,03,647

Source Odisha migration study 2023, Household livelihood and Income module

One in five sample households is remittance-based. We saw earlier that the incidence of migration is 34.2%. Thus, a majority (57%) of migrant households are remittance-based. However, on the whole, migration is negatively selected, and like agriculture-based households, remittance-based households also have significantly lower incomes than average. This suggests that context matters; migration and a remittance-based household livelihood strategy are not accumulative in the particular context of rural Odisha, as they may be in other contexts of migration in India or the Global South. The last category, government transfer-based households, is the smallest and the most precarious household category, with the lowest levels of income among all household categories. We have already seen earlier how low government transfers are in Sect. 4.3.

5.1 Agriculture-Based Households

Table 12 highlights the distribution of income sources in migrant and non-migrant agriculture-based households. Though 35% of sample households are agriculture-based, i.e., agriculture is their main source of income, on the whole, agriculture is far more extensively practiced—by 88.2% of the survey households. Agriculture is significant—socially, culturally, and economically—in rural Odisha. Yet, only 24.7% of the households derive their income *solely* from agriculture, in combination with government assistance, suggesting that agriculture-based households rely on diverse sources of income.

The incidence of migration (18.1%) is low in agriculture-based households. Migration here is evidently distress-oriented, and inadequate work in agriculture and the rural areas pushes individuals from such households to leave the village in search of work. These households that migrate are among the poorest in the sample and excessively rely on government programs to get by. Migration and multiple livelihoods and sources of income for this household typology are associated with lower household incomes.

That said, several individuals in the household case studies reported that agriculture could be lucrative with more support from the government or other sources. Take the case of 35-year-old Bikram Nahak. Since 2000, Bikram has been migrating—to Surat for four to five months every year to work in the power looms—as there is not

Table 12 Distribution of annual income in migrant and non-migrant agricultural-based households (in rupees)

Source of income	Migrant households	Non-migrant households	All households
Income from agriculture	43,076	63,656	59,935
Income from local non-agriculture	3213	8228	7321
Income from remittances	15,313	0	2768
Income from government programs	14,570	16,950	16,520
Total income	76,171	88,834	86,545

Source Odisha migration study 2023, Household livelihood and Income module

enough work in the village for him to make ends meet and support his five-member household.

Bikram has a keen interest in agriculture, which he has been practicing since his childhood. When he is not migrating, Bikram likes to work and spends his time on the household farm in the village. His family owns only 0.5 acres of land. He feels that if he could access more land, he would diversify beyond paddy cultivation (which his household currently undertakes) and start cultivating vegetables too. Bikram explains, with a twinkle in his eye:

> I like to work in the fields, in agriculture. If I could grow vegetables on my land, I could sell those and get money in a jiffy… I would like to lease in land, but I don't have the money. No one provides any help in agriculture…

Bikram genuinely likes working in agriculture. He would prefer to stay in the village and not migrate if he had the means to lease in land for cultivation.

5.2 *Non-Agriculture-Based Households*

Thirty-three percent of the sample households are non-agriculture-based. This household typology has the highest average annual income. Both salaried income and income from self-employment emerge as important in this category. A majority (77.2%) of these households are engaged in agriculture, and 22% of households have migrant members. While the rate of migration, like agriculture-based households, is lower than average, these households have the highest average incomes, and migration here offers a pathway to higher incomes and remittances (Table 13).

Non-agriculture-based households are positively selected for education and land ownership. Income from government programs is limited for such households. These results find resonance in findings from qualitative data and case studies that suggest that if local opportunities for work are available in the non-agricultural sector, workers are not pushed to migrate for low-paying jobs.

Table 13 Distribution of annual income in migrant and non-migrant non-agriculture-based households (in rupees)

Source of income	Migrant households	Non-migrant households	All households
Income from agriculture	16,050	11,869	12,795
Income from local non-agriculture	98,557	1,15,368	1,11,643
Income from remittances	28,351	0	6281
Income from government programs	10,264	12,976	12,375
Income from other sources	0	3231	2515
Total income	1,53,223	1,43,443	1,45,610

Source Odisha migration study 2023, Household livelihood and Income module

Table 14 Distribution of annual income in remittance-based households (in rupees)

Source of income	Amount
Income from agriculture	9727
Income from local non-agriculture	6698
Income from remittances	59,101
Income from government programs	11,387
Income from other sources	848
Total income	87,762

Source Odisha migration study 2023, Household livelihood and Income module

Several individuals in the case study households clearly articulated that they preferred not to migrate. One such person is Jagdesh Panda. Forty-eight-year-old Jagdesh is an auto driver, and his wife, Sarasbati (43), runs a petty shop in the front veranda of their house in Ganjam. Last year, Jagadesh's income from driving an auto-rickshaw was Rs 96,000, while Sarasbati's income from the shop was Rs 35,500. Jagadesh has never been interested in either working in agriculture or migrating for work. When he was younger, he used to help out on his family farm by driving a tractor. Later, seeing the demand for this, he started driving tractors for other people's farms in the village to earn a living. This led him to take an interest in driving. After his marriage to Sarasbati, he decided to buy an auto and drive it for a living. Jagadesh and Sarasbati are content with their livelihoods and earnings in the village and do not feel the need to migrate. They are keen on educating their children and do not want them to migrate for work. Sarasbati says, emphatically: "None of us has ever migrated, and we do not wish to migrate either. We were born here, and we will die here itself… we will never migrate."

5.3 *Remittance-Based Households*

We saw earlier that 34.2% of households have migrants, whereas 19.6% of households are remittance-based. Given that the mean annual income of remittance-based households (Rs 87,662) is lower than that of migrant households (Rs 99,162), the data suggests that households that heavily rely on remittances as a source of income[6] are worse off than households that are able to combine migration and remittances with other more lucrative livelihood options and income sources.

In other words, many migration streams are precarious, and this clearly emerged in our case studies. Take the case of 38-year-old Sabetre Samal's five-member household. Her 26-year-old son Jilesh is a migrant worker in Surat. Sabetre's rural household's *only* source of income is the remittance sent by Jilesh. Jilesh does not wish to

[6] In remittance-based households, more than two-thirds of the income accrues to remittance income (Table 14).

migrate but is compelled to do so to support his family, which, other than Sabetre, includes his 70-year-old grandmother and two younger siblings, who have dropped out of school. The household is landless, unable to engage in agricultural cultivation. The family is dependent upon Jilesh's remittances for their survival.

Sabetre's is also a female-headed household; her husband no longer lives with her. When he did, he was physically violent, rendering Sabetre incapable of working. In our study, it was observed that female-headed households are particularly vulnerable, and they have lower average incomes compared to male-headed households. This case study shows that the intersection of multiple vulnerabilities—such as adverse incorporation in migration, gender, class, landlessness, etc.—leads to worsening economic and social outcomes for individuals and households.

Jilesh's first migration was to Bengaluru as a garment worker, for a contract period of three years. Since he had lived within the factory premises, at the end of the contract, the company refused to pay wages, stating that it was adjusted toward expenses for his stay and food. Jilesh left that work, came back to the village, and then migrated to Surat along with his friends in search of a job. For the past five years, he has been working at a spinning mill in Surat, earning Rs 12,000 a month and remitting Rs 5000 to Sabetre every month. During the COVID-19 lockdown, Jilesh was forced to return to the village. After the pandemic, he did not want to go back to Surat. However, given the precarious situation of the household and the lack of employment opportunities in Ganjam, Sabetre convinced him to migrate again.

It is also not uncommon for migrants to experience exploitation, abuse, and deceit. Fifty-five-year-old Kishor Das and his wife, 40-year-old Janani, are return migrants who worked as live-in domestic servants for a family in Bengaluru. Kishor worked as their gardener, and Janani worked as their housemaid. When the couple started work, about two decades ago, their wages were fixed at Rs 5000 per month. They were offered food and shelter, and they did not receive any wages for three years. When the employer moved cities, he gave them a total of only Rs 60,000 after deducting money for three years of food and stay. This came as a big shock to the household, since they had expected that the amount would be much higher, enabling them to buy agricultural land in Ganjam. Dreams were shattered, and having no other contact or acquaintance in Bengaluru, Kishor and Janani were forced to return to Ganjam with their young sons, Deb and Ranjan.

Being landless, once back in Ganjam, the family found it hard to find any stable and well-paying source of employment. Janani resorted to doing casual labor in agriculture, while Kishor started migrating to Hyderabad and Kerala, doing odd jobs in construction and agriculture for two years. Now, being older, Kishor is not able to be as active and hence, he settled down as a security guard in a nearby brick kiln. Here, he works long hours, often staying overnight on the contractor's orders. There is no proper provision of food at the brick kiln, and Kishor has developed health issues as a result.

For Kishor and Janani, the fact that their sons were more interested in migrating than in studies is a source of disappointment. Deb ran away from home when he was 14 years old to work in a hotel in Hyderabad. Last year, Ranjan followed Deb.

Table 15 Distribution of annual income in government transfer-based households (in Rs)

Source of income	Amount
Income from agriculture	21,043
Income from local non-agriculture	5407
Income from remittances	1148
Income from government programs	36,577
Income from other sources	0
Total income	64,175

Source Odisha migration study 2023, Household livelihood and Income module

Currently, they work as housekeeping staff at the same hotel. While the sons collectively remitted around Rs 1,80,000 last year, their work is hard; they work for 12 to 14 hours a day, without any paid leave or benefits. Thus, even with high remittances, work at destinations can be precarious, and migrants themselves and their families may not wish for them to migrate. Janani worries about the health of their sons. Concern, worry, and anxiety emerge as the common emotions felt by those left behind, especially mothers of migrants.

Exploitative advance-based family migration systems[7] are prevalent in Odisha. In our sample, 26% of the migrant households were engaged in this type of migration to brick kilns. Brick kiln migration is seasonal in nature, and a poor kharif harvest accentuates this precarious stream of migration. Brick kiln migration is characterized by long working hours and hard labor. Concentrated in the two source districts of Balangir and Nuapada, these households migrate either within Odisha or to the neighboring state of Andhra Pradesh and other southern states of Telangana and Karnataka. The average household advance was Rs 23,417, and the average income of such households was even lower than that of remittance-based households at the aggregate level.

5.4 Government Transfer-Based Households

These are the worst-off households with the lowest average incomes. As 92% of households in this category are resident households, we do not attempt to disaggregate our analysis into migrant and non-migrant households separately (Table 15).

On average, these households derive a majority of their income (57%) from government programs. The livelihood combination, government transfers along with agriculture, is most commonly found in this household typology. Here, too, we

[7] In advance-based migration systems, contractors (sardars) pay a lumpsum amount as advance wages, typically to the entire family unit. The workers thus remain tied to the contractor at destination for the entire duration of their migration, as determined by the contractor.

see that the intersection of vulnerabilities compounds poor social and economic outcomes.

While the data shows that government transfers are positively targeted toward the most vulnerable populations, such as ST and female-headed households, it emerges from the case studies that some households are unable to access government programs meant for their benefit. For instance, 55-year-old Sumati Behera lives alone in a rented house and is incapable of working due to recurring joint pain. Her 60-year-old elderly husband is forced to migrate to Mumbai for work. Sumati is not aware of any government scheme that may benefit her household, apart from the Public Distribution System (PDS), from where she accesses rice. Lack of land or home ownership, coupled with little help from the government, compounds her vulnerabilities and makes Sumati fear the future. She laments: "My husband is also getting old, and I do not know for many more years he can work. Once he stops working, I am not sure how we are going to survive."

5.5 The Pandemic and Return Migration: Households that Successfully Combine Multiple Livelihoods

The COVID-19 pandemic led to significant return migration to the villages of Odisha from destinations all over the country. As the pandemic eased, workers typically went back to migrating again to make ends meet and support their households. Yet, it emerges from our data that some workers were able to stop migrating after the pandemic. Take the case of Dasarath Behera. Fifty-six-year-old Dasarath and his two sons, Param (25) and Barun (18), have stopped migrating for work after the pandemic. First, Param decided to put a halt to his migration after he married, as he did not wish to be separated from his wife. He found a job in a retail cloth store in the nearby town of Berhampur, where he commutes daily to work. Seeing Param, Dasarath stopped migrating as well and opened a small tea and snack shop that he operates with his wife. Barun, too, stopped migrating after he opened a *kirana* (grocery) store in the village, on Param's advice. The main motivation for the men to stop migrating was to be closer to their families and to be able to live in the village. In this case, the determination to stay in the village was matched by the ability to find local non-agricultural employment as well as raise resources—through savings accumulated during migration and loans—to start new enterprises in the village.

Another case pertinent to this discussion is that of Satya Sahu. After working in Mumbai as a mason for more than two decades, 42-year-old Satya decided not to go back to the megacity after the pandemic. Relying on the masonry skills he had learned in the city, Satya decided to become a mason-contractor in the village. Through his social networks, he has been able to generate a decent business locally and earn an income similar to what he earned in Mumbai. His family takes pride in his transition from survival-based migration to becoming a business owner. His wife

Lata reflects, "Our household is not so poor. He does not have to migrate anymore for us to survive. At least here, he is an owner. In Mumbai, he was just a worker."

It is evident from the data that non-agricultural households have the highest incomes. At the same time, it also emerges that in this household typology, households typically combine multiple sources of livelihoods and income to their advantage. The livelihood success stories of households that stopped migrating show that the local economy has the scope to create employment and livelihoods. However, such opportunities are not equally accessible to all; not everyone who wishes to stop migrating can do so. Lack of financial capital, human capital, and social networks—amid severe structural constraints—are considerable barriers in accessing non-agricultural work in rural areas.

6 Conclusion

The analysis in this chapter was based on data collected through a specially designed livelihood and income module that was administered to 506 households in 11 high-migration districts of Odisha. Mean annual household income was Rs 1,03,647, and when disaggregated by caste and tribe and income levels, it mirrored social hierarchies with the Scheduled Tribe households at the bottom, and the upper-caste households at the top of the income ladder. Households with migrants had a lower average income (Rs 99,162) than households without migrants (Rs 1,05,992), indicating that migrant workers were incorporated into precarious migration streams with low-paying jobs.

For rural households, local non-agricultural income emerged as the most important income source, followed by agriculture, government transfers, and migrant remittances. While a majority of the households were engaged in agriculture, yet, its share in household incomes was quite low. About one-third of the households had migrants, and migration spanned across social groups. Migration streams were male-dominated and peaked at six months in a year, with a majority of migrants combining work in *both* destination and source regions.

We developed livelihood and income-based household typologies to find that the *type of livelihood* mattered: income levels and distribution of income varied significantly among agriculture-based households, non-agriculture-based households, remittance-based households, and government transfer-based households. Non-agriculture-based households had the highest incomes, but there were significant barriers to accessing employment in this sector. Within this context, migration emerged as an important livelihood strategy that provides income and remittances, particularly to the poorer rural households. More than migration, however, government transfers were a lifeline for about a quarter of rural households that relied predominantly on income from government sources to sustain themselves.

Several implications for policy emerge from this chapter. First, there is a dire need for agricultural diversification, along with concerted interventions toward raising agricultural output, productivity, and profitability in the rice monocultures of Odisha.

This, in turn, would create employment and raise agricultural incomes. At the same time, a simultaneous push for local rural industrialization is important in a context where livelihoods in the local economy are dominated by services, particularly in retail and trade. It should be of concern to policymakers that households with migrants have lower incomes than households without migrants. Distress-oriented migration streams, such as those discussed in the study, need to be conceptually and critically incorporated into the mainstream literature to better understand and problematize linear migration and development discourses. While migration needs to be managed, and workers in precarious streams need safeguarding and support, it is the lack of livelihood opportunities in the local economy that is a major cause of outmigration from Odisha. Addressing the livelihood question through an emphasis on *both* local non-agricultural and agricultural development is critical for both inclusive growth and balanced development in rural Odisha.

Acknowledgments Data collection for the household survey of this study was meticulously undertaken by Ritesh Kumar Hans, Rakesh Kumar Ranabida, Parthab Bag, Anuradha Jena, and Priyanka Pallavi Hial.

References

Abraham, V. (2024). Ruptured rural transformation from non-farm to mixed households in rural India. *Economic and Political Weekly, 59*(50), 84–92.

Acharya, A. K. (2021). Caste-based migration and exposure to abuse and exploitation: Dadan labour migration in India. *Contemporary Social Science, 16*(3), 371–383.

Adams, R. H., Jr., & Page, J. (2005). Do international migration and remittances reduce poverty in developing countries? *World Development, 33*(10), 1645–1669.

Babatunde, R. O., & Qaim, M. (2010). Impact of off-farm income on food security and nutrition in Nigeria. *Food Policy, 35*(4), 303–311.

Bellampalli, P. N., & Yadava, N. (2023). Distress out-migration from rural India: Exploring livelihood realities and interventions to mitigate. *Journal of Human Rights and Social Work, 8*(3), 262–272.

Bhandari, B. S., & Grant, M. (2007). Analysis of livelihood security: A case study in the Kali-Khola watershed of Nepal. *Journal of Environmental Management, 85*(1), 17–26.

Binswanger-Mkhize, H. (2013). The stunted structural transformation of the Indian economy: Agriculture, manufacturing and the rural non-farm sector. *Economic & Political Weekly, 48*(26–27), 5–13.

Breman, J. (1996). *Footloose labour: Working in India's informal economy*. Cambridge University Press.

Chambers, R., & Conway, G. (1991). *Sustainable rural livelihoods: Practical concepts for the 21st century*. (IDS Discussion/Paper no 296). Institute of Development Studies.

Choithani, C. (2022). *Migration, food security and development: Insights from rural India*. Cambridge University Press. https://doi.org/10.1017/9781108885799.

Choithani, C., van Duijne, R. J., & Nijman, J. (2021). Changing livelihoods at India's rural–urban transition. *World Development, 146*, 105617.

Datta, A. (2016). Migration, remittances, and changing sources of income in rural Bihar (1999-2011): Some findings from a longitudinal study. *Economic and Political Weekly, 51*(31), 85–93.

Datta, A. (2020). Circular migration and precarity: Perspectives from rural Bihar. *The Indian Journal of Labour Economics, 63*(4), 1143–1163.

Datta, A. (2022). *Migration and development in India: The Bihar experience.* Routledge.

Deshingkar, P., & Farrington, J. (Eds.). (2009). *Circular migration and multilocational livelihood strategies in rural India.* Oxford University Press.

Ellis, F. (1998). Household strategies and rural livelihood diversification. *The Journal of Development Studies, 35*(1), 1–38.

Ellis, F. (2000). *Rural livelihoods and diversity in developing countries.* Oxford University Press.

Gautam, Y., & Andersen, P. (2016). Rural livelihood diversification and household Well-being: Insights from Humla, Nepal. *Journal of Rural Studies, 44*, 239249.

Griffin, C., Sirimorok, N., Dressler, W. H., Sahide, M. A. K., Fisher, M. R., Faturachmat, F., & Clendenning, J. (2024). The persistence of precarity: Youth livelihood struggles and aspirations in the context of truncated agrarian change, South Sulawesi, Indonesia. *Agriculture and Human Values, 41*(1), 293–311.

Haberfeld, Y., Menaria, R. K., Sahoo, B. B., & Vyas, R. N. (1999). Seasonal migration of rural labor in India. *Population Research and Policy Review, 18*, 471–487.

Hietala, R & Singh, R.B. (2014). Livelihood security in changing socio-economic environment: Summary and policy recommendations. In Livelihood security in northwestern Himalaya: Case studies from changing socio-economic environments in Himachal Pradesh, India. (pp. 249–257), Spinger.

Jodhka, S. S. (2023). *The Indian village: Rural lives in the 21st century.* Aleph.

Jodhka, S. S., & Kumar, A. (2017). Non-farm economy in Madhubani, Bihar: Social dynamics and exclusionary rural transformations. *Economic and Political Weekly, 52*(25–26), 14–24.

Kapri, K., & Ghimire, S. (2020). Migration, remittance, and agricultural productivity: Evidence from the Nepal living standard survey. *World Development Perspectives, 19*, 100198.

Katchova, A. L. (2005). The farm diversification discount. *American Journal of Agricultural Economics, 87*(4), 984–994.

Lokshin, M., Bontch-Osmolovski, M., & Glinskaya, E. (2010). Work-related migration and poverty reduction in Nepal. *Review of Development Economics, 14*(2), 323–332.

Mishra, D. K. (2020). Seasonal migration and unfree labour in globalising India: Insights from field surveys in Odisha. *Indian Journal of Labour Economics, 63*(4), 1087–1106. https://doi.org/10.1007/s41027-020-00277-8

Mistri, A., & Das, B. (2020). *Environmental change, livelihood issues, and migration.* Springer.

Mitra, A., & Pradhan, B. K. (2016). *Migration, remittances, and changing patterns of livelihood: evidence from western Odisha villages* (Working Paper/No. 363). Institute of Economic Growth.

Murrugarra, E., & Herrera, C. (2011). Migration choices, inequality of opportunities, and poverty reduction in Nicaragua. In E. Murrugarra, J. Larrison, & M. J. Sasin (Eds.), *Migration and poverty: Towards better opportunities for the poor* (pp. 101–122). The World Bank.

Natarajan, N., Newsham, A., Rigg, J., & Suhardiman, D. (2022). A sustainable livelihoods framework for the 21st century. *World Development, 155*, 105898.

Nienkerke, I. M., Thorat, A., & Patt, A. (2023). From distress migration to selective migration: Transformative effects of agricultural development on seasonal migration. *World Development Perspectives, 29*, 100483.

NLUO. (2020). *Social mapping of migrant workers in Odisha.* Labour and ESI Department, Government of Odisha.

Orozco, M., & Jewers, M. (2019). *The impact of migrants' remittances and investment on rural youth.* IFAD.

Peng, W., Robinson, B. E., Zheng, H., Li, C., Wang, F., & Li, R. (2022). The limits of livelihood diversification and sustainable household Well-being, evidence from China. *Environmental Development, 43*, 100736.

Porst, L., & Sakdapolrak, P. (2018). Advancing adaptation or producing precarity? The role of rural-urban migration and translocal embeddedness in navigating household resilience in Thailand. *Geoforum, 97*, 35–45. https://doi.org/10.1016/j.geoforum.2018.10.011

Qin, H. (2010). Rural-to-urban labour migration, household livelihoods, and the rural environment in Chongqing municipality, Southwest China. *Human Ecology, 38*, 675–690.

Sabates–Wheeler, R., R. Sabates, & A. Castaldo. (2008). Tackling poverty–migration linkages: Evidence from Ghana and Egypt. Social Indicators Research, 87(2), 307–328.

Samaddar, R. (2020). *The postcolonial age of migration*. Routledge.

Scoones, I. (2009). Livelihoods perspectives and rural development. *Journal of Peasant Studies., 36*, 171–196.

Sen, A. (1985). A sociological approach to the measurement of poverty: A reply to professor Peter Townsend. *Oxford Economic Papers, 37*(4), 669676.

Sharma, A., Kulkarni, R., & Khandelwal, R. (2014). *Studies, stories and a canvas: Seasonal labour migration and migrant workers from Odisha*. Centre for Migration and Labour Solutions.

Singh, C., & Basu, R. (2020). Moving in and out of vulnerability: Interrogating migration as an adaptation strategy along a rural–urban continuum in India. *The Geographical Journal, 186*(1), 87–102.

Sinha, S., Narain, N., & Bhanjdeo, A. (2022). Building back better? Resilience as wellbeing for rural migrant households in Bihar, India. *World Development, 159*, 106031.

Sreelakshmi, A. (2021). *Distress migration: A case study of KBK districts in Odisha*. The Peninsula Foundation. Retrieved December 10, 2024, from https://www.thepeninsula.org.in/2021/11/07/distress-migration-a-case-study-of-kbk-districts-in-odisha/

Srivastava, R. (2020). *Vulnerable internal migrants in India and portability of social security and entitlements*. (Working Paper/No. 2, Centre for Employment Studies Working Paper Series). Institute for Human Development.

Sucharita, S., & Rout, L. (2020). Determinants of seasonal migration of Jharkhand: An empirical investigation. *Journal of Public Affairs, 20*(3), e2070.

Taylor, J. E., Rozelle, S., & De Brauw, A. (2003). Migration and incomes in source communities: A new economics of migration perspective from China. *Economic Development and Cultural Change, 52*(1), 75–101.

Taylor, M. (2015). *The political ecology of climate change adaptation: Livelihoods, agrarian change and the conflicts of development*. Routledge.

Tumbe, C. (2011). *Remittances in India: facts and issues* (Working Paper/No. 331). Indian Institute of Management.

Zhao, J., & Barry, P. J. (2014). Income diversification of rural households in China. *Canadian Journal of Agricultural Economics, 62*(3), 307–324.

Chapter 9
Youth Aspirations and Attitudes Toward Agriculture

Amrita Datta, Haripriya Narasimhan, and Subhadarshee Nayak

Abstract This chapter, based on qualitative research, explores youth aspirations and attitudes toward agriculture in the context of smallholder rainfed cultivation in a high-migration region of Odisha. It finds that despite harsh structural realities of farming being adversely impacted by climate variability, water scarcity, increasing input costs, and declining agricultural profits, young people value agriculture for the food security it provides. Farming is not just an activity but is considered an occupational, social, and cultural identity, despite monetary income from farming being meager in comparison to income from remittances or local non-farm incomes. Young people value land, and those with land consider themselves fortunate and committed to cultivation. Even if they migrate, young people remain involved in agriculture. Migration does not supplement agriculture; instead, it complements agriculture. Male youth migration has led to an increase in women's work in farming; in the absence of men, young women have a heavier workload and take on more farm tasks, including farm management. Among youth migrants across social classes, the desire to remain in the village, or eventually return to the village, is very strong. For young migrants, including highly educated migrants and those earning comfortable incomes in destination regions, the imagination of their future remains tied to the village, closely linked with agriculture. At the same time, youth cultures of temporary migration are widespread—a rite of passage, particularly for those who are less educated—due to an aversion to agriculture at a young age, and the lack of employment options in source regions.

Keywords Rural youth · Agriculture · Migration · Livelihoods · Aspirations · Agrarian change · Odisha

---

A. Datta (✉) · H. Narasimhan
Indian Institute of Technology, Hyderabad, India
e-mail: amritadatta@la.iith.ac.in

H. Narasimhan
e-mail: haripriya@la.iith.ac.in

S. Nayak
Collectives for Integrated Livelihood Initatives, Baripada, Odisha, India
e-mail: sdnpintu@gmail.com

A. Datta and S. I. Rajan (eds.), *Migration, Livelihoods and Gender*, International Perspectives on Migration, https://doi.org/10.1007/978-981-95-5465-2_9

1 Introduction

In recent decades, there has been a decline in youth involvement in agriculture across diverse agrarian settings in the Global South (Rigg et al., 2019; Thompson et al., 2019; White, 2020). As young people exit agriculture to work in local non-farm occupations or migrate to the cities, there are significant implications for rural households and livelihoods (IFAD, 2019; FAO, 2018; Wiggins, 2016). In the context of our research, smallholder rainfed farming in the eastern Indian state of Odisha is characterized by outmigration due to low-agricultural productivity and a lack of non-farm opportunities (Mishra 2020; Mitra & Pradhan, 2016; Sharma et al., 2014).

Results from the Phase 1 survey of the Odisha Migration Study show that workers in the age-group 15–34 years are significantly less likely to be engaged in agriculture compared to older workers in rural Odisha (see Chap. 7 for details). There exists a dominant narrative that agriculture has a "generation problem," and young people don't like to work in agriculture due to the hard work, declining profits, and uncertainties associated with agriculture (Leavy & Hossein, 2014; White, 2020). Instead, they prefer to migrate. Against this backdrop, the broad objective of this study is to explore youth aspirations and attitudes toward agriculture in a high-migration region of rural Odisha. Our qualitative research unpacks the linear narrative that suggests that young people are not interested in working in agriculture. We prioritize youth perspectives and find that empirical reality is complex and nuanced, and it does not fit the binaries of interest or disinterest, aspirations or the lack of aspirations toward agriculture. Instead, drawing on the concept of youth as a social construction and a structural framing of aspirations and livelihoods, we find that the analytical lenses of the family and the household, generation, gender, and structural factors like caste and land mediate young people's relationship with agriculture and the rural.

The rest of the chapter is organized as follows. In the next section, we briefly discuss the conceptual frames of youth, aspirations, and livelihoods used in the study. Then, we present the research method, sample characteristics, and research sites. This is followed by our results—the key themes that emerge from our research: education and youth aspirations; agriculture as hard labor; the structural constraints youth face in agriculture; food security and livelihoods; land; sharecropping and new farmers; gender and the feminization of agriculture; and migration and agriculture. Last, we conclude with some policy implications.

2 Conceptual Frames: Youth, Aspirations, and Livelihoods

2.1 *Youth*

Notwithstanding the conceptualization of youth as a social construct, studies focusing on young people predominantly use biological age-based definitions to define youth. The United Nations defines "youth" as a category of persons belonging to the age-group 15 to 24 years (UNDESA, 2013). The Government of India, in its National Youth Policy, 2014, defines youth as individuals aged 15–29 years, while acknowledging that "youth is a more fluid category than a fixed age-group" (Government of India, 2014, p. 9).

These aforementioned age categories for the youth are considered appropriate for conventional youth studies focusing on transitions from childhood to adulthood, education to work, etc. On the other hand, studies that focus on youth in agriculture (Srinivasan & White, 2024; Mohanty & Lenka, 2023; Elias et al., 2018) use an expansive definition of youth that goes up to 35 or even 45 years. This is done to better understand the process of becoming a farmer amid the multiple livelihoods—non-farm work, migration, and agriculture—pursued by young people and the transitions into agriculture that may typically happen later in one's youth. In our study, we follow this latter approach and define youth as individuals between 15- and 35-years-old. In particular, this also allows us to tell the stories of *new farmers*, those who have taken to working in agriculture in their thirties on account of a myriad of circumstances in rural Odisha.

2.2 *Aspirations*

While aspirations are fairly well-studied in education and migration, literature on aspirations is still emerging in farming and agriculture (Nandi & Nedumaran, 2021). Simply put, aspirations refer to what an individual wants to achieve or do in their life. In the context of our study, we draw on the concept of "opportunity space" (Leavy & Smith, 2010; Leavy & Hossein, 2014) to argue that aspirations are bounded by a person's opportunity space.

> Aspirations are influenced by and evolve in response to many factors including peer effects, role models, personal interests, media etc. as well as their expectations. These expectations tend to be formulated within a person's 'opportunity space', involving reasonable assessments of what is possible within their geographical, socio economic, and policy context, and given their own qualities and characteristics. (Leavy & Hossein, 2014, p. 7).

Thus, we subscribe to the view that aspirations are socially determined, and people form aspirations by seeing them within their cognitive window (Genicot & Ray, 2017). Appadurai (2004) argues that certain sections of society, for instance, the poor and marginalized, have a limited capacity to aspire. The capacity to aspire,

> is not evenly distributed in any society... the relatively rich and powerful invariably have a more fully developed capacity to aspire… the better off you are (in terms of power, dignity, and material resources), the more likely you are to be conscious of the links between the more and less immediate objects of aspiration… (Appadurai, 2004, p. 68).

In the context of our research, in line with the above, aspiration failure may be seen not as a cause, but a consequence of poverty (Dalton et al., 2015). To sum up, conceptually, our work views aspirations as socially determined, bounded by an individual's opportunity space and the capacity to aspire. In the framing of aspirations, therefore, we use analytical lenses, beyond the individual, of the family and the household, livelihoods, generation, gender, and thus, lean toward structural and "political-economy perspectives" that mediate young people's relationship with agriculture and the rural (White, 2020, p. 59).

2.3 Livelihoods

This study draws on the livelihoods literature, particularly the concepts of livelihood diversification (Ellis, 2000; Ellis, 1998) and sustainable livelihoods (Chambers & Conway, 1991). We use the seminal definition of livelihoods below and lean toward a structural framing of livelihoods and rural development (Natarajan et al., 2022).

> A livelihood comprises the capabilities, assets (stores, resources, claims, and access) and activities required for a means of living: a living is sustainable which can cope with and recover from stress and shocks, maintain or enhance its capabilities and assets, and provide sustainable livelihood opportunities for the next generation; and which contributes net benefits to other livelihoods at the local and global levels and in the short and long term. (Chambers & Conway, 1991, p. 6).

Rural households diversify their livelihoods, i.e., they construct a diverse portfolio of activities and social support capabilities in their struggle for survival and in order to improve their standards of living (Ellis, 1998, p. 1). Livelihood strategies may include agriculture intensification and/or extensification, livelihood diversification, and migration (Scoones, 2009; Scoones, 1998). However, a livelihood is considered sustainable "when it can cope with and recover from stresses and shocks, maintain or enhance its capabilities and assets, while not undermining the natural resource base" (Chambers & Conway, 1991, p. 6).

These concepts are helpful in understanding the multiple livelihoods pursued by our research participants and their households. Yet, they fall short of critically engaging with the structural conditions that join the dots of multiple livelihoods within the household. Why do households withdraw from specific livelihoods or enter new ones? Is the incorporation into new livelihoods on favorable or adverse terms for the individual, the household, and the family? To address these questions, as emerging from our empirical study, it is "necessary to see farming not as a singular occupation but instead as part of livelihood complexes" (Rigg et al., 2019, p. 306), along with a focus on structural perspectives in the framing of rural livelihoods (Natarajan et al., 2022).

3 Method and Sample Characteristics

This chapter is based on interviews conducted with 44 research participants from two villages in Ganjam district in Odisha. The rationale for the selection of the district and sample size is as follows. At the outset, this sub-study of the Odisha Migration Study wanted to explore the youth-agriculture nexus in the context of high migration. Given this objective, based on the results of the Phase 1 survey, Ganjam district was purposively selected as it had the highest number of estimated current outmigrants.[1] The sample size was not predetermined; data collection was undertaken following the principle of saturation in qualitative research. The villages under study, Mujagada and Kandharanipada, are a subset of villages from where household data was collected in Phase 1 of the Odisha Migration Study.

Purposive sampling was used for the selection of our research participants. We prioritized youth who were farmers or belonged to farming households, young women, and sharecroppers, in the selection of our sample. Thus, our sample is dominated by Other Backward Class (OBC) and Dalit youth who currently practice farming and/or belong to households engaged in agriculture.[2] We also included older people in our sample and interviewed them to understand their perspectives on youth in agriculture.

Our semi-structured interview schedule captured respondents' demographic details, experiences of working in agriculture and allied activities, details of agricultural production, perceptions and attitudes toward agriculture, and their imagination of the future of agriculture. This was followed by migration details of the respondent and their family members and questions on the impact of migration on agriculture. Last, we covered aspirations, focusing on education, livelihoods, income, politics, media, communication, and mobility.

It can be seen in Table 1 that the sample was evenly distributed between males and females. Our respondents' educational attainments vary significantly. About a third of the respondents are migrants, and a majority are married. Two social groups—backward classes and Dalits—dominate our sample, and occupationally, a majority of the respondents are farmers with a history of cultivation in their families. More than three-quarters of the respondents owned land, and nearly half leased in land. A majority of our respondents had learnt agriculture from their parents or family members, or simply by observing others. The role of formal agricultural training was limited in our research sites. Though more than a third of all respondents currently owned livestock, this had greatly reduced in recent years due to the lack of space and resources to care for the livestock. Nevertheless, most respondents considered agriculture their main household livelihood, even though it was a primary source of

[1] The Odisha Migration Survey (OMS) estimated 4,21,928 current migrants for Ganjam district in 2023. Chapter 3 for details.

[2] Mohanty and Lenka (2023) report the exodus of upper caste youths from agriculture in rural Odisha. This was found in our research sites as well, and as we prioritized interviewing young people *in* agriculture, our sample does not include upper caste youth.

household income for less than a third of the respondents. This point deserves further elaboration.

The disaggregated livelihoods income data clearly shows that agriculture is *not* the primary source of income in the majority of households. Economically, households derive a majority of their income from sources other than agriculture. Yet, socially and culturally, a majority of our research participants *consider* agriculture to be the main livelihood of the household (Table 1). That the majority of our research participants consider agriculture to be their *main livelihood,* even when it is not the primary source of household income, shows their affinity to agriculture, and that they deeply identify themselves as *cultivators* or *farmers.*

4 Research Sites

4.1 Mujagada

Mujagada village is located in the Bhanjanagar block in Ganjam district of Odisha. Agriculture is one of the main occupations of the inhabitants here. Rice is the major crop of the village, cultivated as a *kharif* crop. Though there is a large water reservoir near Bhanjanagar, irrigation facilities have not reached the farmers of Mujagada; in fact, agriculture is largely rainfed in the village. Apart from cultivating rice, some farmers who have access to irrigation also cultivate vegetables. The nearest market for these farmers is Bhanjanagar, located 13 kilometers from the village. Mujagada is also surrounded by forests, which makes agricultural fields susceptible to being damaged by wild animals, a problem fairly common in forest regions of the state.

Mujagada is a large village. According to the 2011 Census, there were 1009 households in Mujagada, and the total population of the village stood at 4443. In the village, 25% of the households are Dalit households, 14% are Adivasi households, and the rest are clubbed as "Other" caste groups. The literacy rate is 71% (male literacy 82% and female literacy 60%). There is one government high school in the village. For further education, i.e., Class 12 and higher education like BA or BSc, young boys and girls have to commute to Bhanjanagar. The village is well connected by road through public and private buses.

4.2 Kandharanipada

Kandharanipada is a village located in the Beguniapada block of Ganjam district in Odisha. The nearest town is Kodala, around 8 kilometers away from the village. Most households in the village depend on agriculture. Rice is the major crop in the village, as only a few farmers have irrigation facilities to grow vegetables, particularly after harvesting paddy. The nearest market for them is Kodala, which is an urban location.

Table 1 Details of research participants

	Number	Percent
Research participants	44	100%
Sex		
Male	25	56.8%
Female	19	43.2%
Age		
15–35	21	47.7%
35–45	12	27.3%
45+	11	25.0%
Education		
Illiterate	12	27.3%
Primary school	8	18.2%
Middle school	10	22.7%
Secondary school	3	6.8%
Higher secondary	6	13.6%
Degree and above	5	11.4%
Migration status*		
Migrant	6	13.6%
Non-migrant	29	65.9%
Return migrant	9	20.5%
Marital status		
Not married	14	31.8%
Married	27	61.4%
Widowed	3	6.8%
Social group		
OBC	28	63.6%
SC	15	34.1%
ST	1	2.3%
Occupation		
Farmer	29	65.9%
Non-agricultural worker	5	11.4%
Migrant worker	4	9.1%
Student	4	9.1%
Unemployed	2	4.5%
Relationship with farming		
Currently practicing agriculture	34	77.3%
Practiced agriculture in the past	2	4.5%
Never practiced agriculture, family is currently farming	7	15.9%

(continued)

Table 1 (continued)

	Number	Percent
Never practiced agriculture, family practiced farming in the past	1	2.3%
Learnt farming from		
Father/mother	19	43.2%
Other relatives	2	4.5%
Father-in-law/mother-in-law	2	4.5%
Observing others in the field	4	9.1%
Any agricultural training attended	5	11.4%
Land and livestock (household-level)		
Own land (%)	34	77.3%
Average size of own land (in acres)	2.8	
Leased in land (%)	21	47.7%
Average size of leased in land (in acres)	1.7	
Own cultivation + leased in cultivation	14	31.8%
Livestock (%)		
Currently owns livestock	15	34.1%
Agriculture is the primary source of household income	14	31.8%
Agriculture is considered the Main livelihood of the household	28	63.6%

*Current migrants here refers to individuals who had migrated in the reference period of the past 12 months, while return migrants were individuals who had migrated in the past, but had been in the village in the reference period of 12 months; and non-migrants refers to individuals who had never migrated

Kandharanipada is a small village. According to the 2011 Census, there were 359 households, and the total population of the village was 1585 in 2011. Kandharanipada is also a multi-caste village. Dalit households comprised around 18% of the total population of the village, while the rest comprised OBCs and the upper castes. There were no Adivasi households in this village. The literacy rate of the village was 69% (male literacy 75% and female literacy 63%). Boys and girls go outside their village to attend high school and college. The nearest college is in Kodala.

Both villages have a long history of outmigration. Currently, the most prominent migration streams from the villages are to the power mills in Surat, Gujarat, and various destinations in southern India, such as Andhra Pradesh, Tamil Nadu, Telangana, and Kerala. In fact, the Ganjam-Gujarat migration corridor is one of the densest migration corridors in India; more than 5% of Ganjam's population works in Gujarat (Tumbe, 2018).

5 Results

5.1 Education and Aspirations

In our study sites, the aspirations of young people varied considerably by their educational status. Individuals who had completed at least a bachelor's degree or had attended professional training (for example, a polytechnic course) aimed to get employed in a public sector job and did not prefer to practice agriculture. Such individuals, particularly from economically well-off families, preferred to wait for their opportunities and prepare for competitive exams for public sector employment. Twenty-five-year-old KB has completed a BSc degree in Chemistry. Currently unemployed, KB prefers not to work in agriculture even though his father practices agriculture on their family farm.[3] KB has applied to different job vacancies but has not heard back. Although the educated prefer to get employed in the public sector or salaried jobs in the private sector, there is a sense of aspirational failure in KB's narrative. He laments that though "now is the time (for him) to work, there are limited opportunities… the lack of jobs and poor infrastructure in the state lead to young people migrating outside for work." In the future, he might migrate or work in his father's business.

JN, a young Dalit woman, is the first person in her family to graduate from college. JN aspires to be a teacher but has found it hard to get a job. She explains, "Knowledge and skill are not enough to get employment. For every job, we must appear for the entrance exam. To get a job, we need to have manpower and money power. Those who have money get jobs easily." JN is currently unemployed and cannot imagine not being a teacher. From a young age, her parents shielded her from agriculture and encouraged her to study. JN's mind has been so set on becoming a teacher that she cannot think of doing anything else, such as starting a business or helping her father in agriculture. The cases of JN and KB show the "aspiration-achievement gap" experienced by young people, where the promise of their education in securing formal employment remains unfulfilled (Elias et al., 2018, p. 82).

In the consideration of pursuing agriculture as an occupation in a context where smallholder cultivation dominates in our research sites, DS, a 28-year-old man with education up to Class 5, points out, "The elders of our village have an interest in agriculture and farming, but today's generation is not like that. They want to study and do a job and get settled."

In our research sites, smallholder cultivator families are making massive financial and emotional investments in their children's education as a pathway for a better future. It is thus hardly surprising when KB mentions, "If an educated person is found farming, people would comment: You have pursued studies, so why are you into farming? Go outside and earn; how much can you possibly earn by farming?"

[3] As KB *waits it out* for a government job, he is fine with giving a helping hand at the family enterprise—a retail store that sells utensils.

This resonates with studies in the literature that find that "education is seen as a way of escaping agriculture rather than as being complementary to good farming" (Agarwal & Agarwal, 2017, p. 15). Thus, "youth aspirations in rural areas are often not built around farming, but around strategies for a way out of agriculture" (Narayanan et al., 2024, p. 236). In the literature, higher education is associated with a greater dislike for farming and is seen as a pathway out of agriculture (Agarwal & Agarwal, 2017). At the same time, youth is a heterogeneous category, and young people have diverse perceptions and aspirations of agriculture (Sunam, 2020). Ramesh Sunam, based on a village study in rural Nepal, finds that while well-off youth "look for futures outside agriculture, young people from poor backgrounds continue to see farming as highly important to their livelihoods" (Sunam, 2020, p. 74).

In our research sites, too, for young people, there exists a powerful narrative of success: study hard and do a respectable job. Success is thus framed as outside the village and outside of agriculture. At the same time, those who drop out or fail to get into professional education prefer to migrate and get employed in private companies. Compared to their parents, they are more educated. Their preferred occupation, at this juncture in their lifecycle, is not agriculture. The preference for a salaried job is due to the economic security this brings vis-à-vis the uncertainty of income associated with agriculture (this is discussed further in the next section).

A salaried job is the first choice among the less educated. Such jobs are hard to come by in the agrarian economy of the research sites. The prevalence of migration in the village and in the region plays an important role in encouraging the less educated youth to migrate. Social networks—either a friend, a fellow villager, or a family member—provide first-hand information about employment opportunities in destination regions. The expected salary also works as a pull factor for young people. Given the limited availability of land and employment opportunities in nearby towns, an average school dropout in the study villages prefers to migrate. Those who drop out *know clearly* that they have to migrate. After spending one or two years in the village, they take the help of their friends or family members and migrate. This is true for individuals across social groups if they have dropped out or discontinued studies. In other words, the youth culture of migration is widespread, often a rite of passage for those who are less educated. In fact, individuals with better educational status also migrate temporarily when the situation demands. For example, OP, an 18-year-old belonging to a landed farming family, took it upon himself to migrate to ease his family's financial burden when the family faced sudden economic hardship.

In our study sites, young people start migrating after they are done with their education. For a majority of our research participants, migration was an outcome of their education journey being cut short, due to a lack of resources and financial problems in the family. An aversion to agriculture at a young age means that young people leave the village for work. Migration outcomes for such individuals, who had to suspend their education and start working, are distinctly different from those who can complete their desired level of education. The latter are more likely to gain employment in higher-paying jobs and obtain a better foothold in the urban areas.

However, a firm urban foothold does not necessarily imply a desire to permanently leave the village. On the contrary, even among our highly educated research participants, life aspirations were attached to the rural. Take the case of 23-year-old SS, who recently received his engineering diploma degree and was immediately employed—through his professional networks—in a manufacturing job in Delhi. SS started working as a safety management officer with an automobile company eight months ago in the national capital.

During our fieldwork, SS was visiting his family in the village. SS's family owns no land. In the past, his father has been a sharecropper. The family currently owns a cow that is being taken care of by his father. Other livestock—goats—have been leased out as the family does not have the capacity to care for them. SS feels that agriculture is badly affected when youth migrate for work.

> It is affected because young people are not interested in learning farming. The mindset of people is to do the job and survive; they do not want to work in the fields. The parents, who are involved in farming, continue to farm on the land, but they want their children to stay away from home for work and use their money for cultivation and other purposes. (SS, 23-year-old migrant worker, Mujagada)

SS is determined to buy land in the village. He thinks buying land is a good idea as "we can produce food for ourselves". The land can also be used for commercial development, he explains. SS is clear that he would not cultivate this land himself; older family members or hired-in labor would do the job. While he is a young and successful migrant, he is not enamored by the bright lights of the city; he does not like to migrate. Despite being absorbed in regular employment in the country's national capital, he asserts that his future is in his village, closely intertwined with agriculture:

> Interviewer (I): *Where do you see yourself in the next 10 years?*
>
> SS: *I am confident that I will attain success in life. I want us to have our own land (in the village). I would like to settle in Odisha rather than migrate to other places.*
>
> I: *Why?*
>
> SS: *It would give a sense of ownership and pride.*
>
> I: *Why do you want to settle in Odisha?*
>
> SS: *The main reason is that I can look after my parents and also be involved in agricultural activities. I will be happy if I stay in Odisha.*

Thus, young people's motivations to migrate are complex, and we find that their work and livelihood priorities may shift in response to family demands and lifecycle needs.

5.2 *Farmer Identity*

> What is not to like (about agriculture)? We have to earn our own food. (GN, male, 19 years old)

KB is a 25-year-old man from the Kuruma caste (categorized as an Other Backward Class [OBC]). He has completed his graduation and is looking for jobs commensurate with his qualifications. His family owns about an acre of land (5 *bharanas*). His father and brother are involved in cultivation. His brother also works at a shop when not working in the field. KB is very clear that he will not pursue farming. He wants to seek jobs aligned with his education, in chemistry, medicine, or similar areas. He is also looking for jobs outside Odisha.

AP is 15 years old, from Surda caste (also, OBC). He is currently studying in Class 10. The family owns three acres of land. He has extensive knowledge of farming. He helps his father in preparing the land, seedling transplantation, transporting paddy, threshing, and packaging, among other things. He is very keen on continuing farming, even as he plans to apply for government jobs after his education. No one from his family has migrated. He has no plan to migrate either.

These two case studies depict the diverse views young people have about agriculture in Odisha. It will be difficult to describe agriculture as a "vocation" or "career." For them, agriculture is a part of their lives, always present. The articulations of the youth in our study, therefore, do not fall into a binary of whether one should practice agriculture in the future or not. While many respondents who are older farmers do argue that young people will not practice agriculture in the future and will move to cities in search of jobs, young people themselves do not rule out the possibility of taking up farming in a more long-term manner, past a certain age. And even when they are migrants in other cities of India, they do come back to help their parents and elders with the seasonal requirements of farming. So, to assume that young people are not at all interested in farming is not borne out by the data we have. In any case, young people start thinking about farming as a career only in their late teens and later (Srinivasan & White, 2024). Entry into farming is contingent upon individual and family circumstances, the availability of family land for cultivation, the overall basket of livelihoods at the household level, the opportunity cost of leaving migrant and/or non-agricultural work, among other factors.

The narratives emerging from the interviews speak to the ambiguities, concerns, worries, and questions youths have about maintaining a viable future for themselves and their families as they hold on to their lands and contemplate a way to both earn a reasonable income and sustain a living, and simultaneously maintain their identities as farmers.

Srinivasan and White (2024) contend that being a "farmer" is not just an occupation but an identity. In this context, it is interesting to look at some of the answers we received to the question, "Who is a farmer according to you?" BP, a 30-year-old widow, chuckled as she said, "A farmer means a poor man," reiterating the notion that farming is associated with poverty. For 15-year-old AP, a farmer is someone who "produce(s) something." To 60-year-old KR, "the person involved in agricultural work is known as a cultivator." He is a laborer and cultivates the land, he said.

Not only is a farmer a person who cultivates land, but he is also usually assumed to be male and in ownership of the land under cultivation. Though many respondents who had leased in land also identified themselves as farmers, owning land is seen as important to a farmer's identity. In addition, a farmer is also seen as someone who owns implements for cultivation. Many respondents felt that owning tractors and threshers is also crucial to being a farmer, especially a successful one.

Being dependent on the state, neighbors, or influential figures in the village is seen as a problem. One farmer mentioned that he desired to be "self-reliant." Based on the interviews, the following facilities were identified as necessary for a farmer to be successful: regular and secure water supply, land (preferably own), tractors or other machinery, a power tiller, and *no oxen*. The last condition implied that a successful farmer need not own draught animals like oxen but can afford to rent or buy a tractor, thresher, harvester, etc. In addition, knowledge of the seeds and the soil is also seen as pivotal to being a successful farmer. This comes from informal learning and apprenticeship, as well as training, the latter of which most of our respondents lacked.

5.3 Agriculture as Hard Labor

A salient point to have emerged from this qualitative study is the ways in which young people's attitudes to land, farming, and agriculture are described by others. Almost unanimously, respondents said that agriculture is hard work, which young people have a disdain for.

The quote from GN, mentioned at the beginning of this section, summarizes the broad view of many of our respondents. Agriculture is not something they dislike. Quite a few of them mentioned that they intended to keep the land and farm it for as long as possible. However, in this section, we want to highlight the myriad ways in which they approach agriculture as an activity.

A general assumption among older respondents and parents of young people was that agriculture is akin to manual labor, which the "educated" youth did not want to engage in. The excerpts given below capture the attitude succinctly.

> I can't say anything about the young generation because they don't have an interest in agriculture. The main reason is that agriculture needs more hours of labor and effort, but the young generation is interested in going outside and working for fewer hours to earn more money… They don't want to be involved in agriculture because now they are educated and they don't want to enter the muddy field. (SN, 55-year-old male farmer, father of a migrant youth)

> Today's generations are not attracted to agriculture because they don't enter the muddy fields. They go to an outside state to earn a good amount. In agriculture, there is no profit, so they are demotivated to pursue agriculture. (JD, 40-year-old female, new farmer)

DS, a 28-year-old sharecropper and migrant worker, said, "Earlier, people had an interest in agriculture and farming. But today's generation is not like that… they want to study and get a job and get settled…" When asked what the main reason was behind young people not accepting agriculture as an occupation, DS replied,

> People are no longer going to the fields with their parents… they are not observing the process… they are not learning…. I was working as a laborer; I have learned by practice… but children are not doing that. They only want to study and find a job.

We would like to expand on two main points emphasized by several respondents. One is the supposed aversion of young people to enter a "muddy field." Mud is often associated with dirt and filth—not seen as worthy of someone educated. It is considered the work of illiterate people or those incapable of doing anything else. Therefore, across the sample, we found this reference to the muddy field as a metaphor that, in itself, explains why young people are moving away from agriculture.

Aversion to mud is also a euphemism for a perceived aversion to hard work, which, the elder farmers believe, is quite common among the younger generation. Young people are seen as being lazy, just wishing to earn quick money by working as migrant workers in cities (regardless of how arduous that work typically is), and prefer "comfort" to sweat.

> Due to the lack of employment opportunities, several young generations migrate to the neighboring states to earn more money by working in cotton mills, prawn farming, etc. Agriculture is not affected by it because the younger generation remains away from agricultural activities. Agricultural work is not known to many people, and it is not a profitable business. So many people leave the village and go outside. As a result, the agricultural burden is borne by the remaining people. (LB, female, 35-year-old sharecropper)

SG is a 37-year-old widow, a new farmer with a teenage son. She does not expect her son to enter farming since he's studying. She, too, feels young people shun hard work and are just lazy. They look for "easier" jobs that urban areas are believed to provide. Yet, she does not really wish her sons to work in agriculture either. She says they (she and her husband) toiled so that her sons could have better lives. She is willing to educate her son for a few more years and then see if he gets a job or returns to farming. Their landholding is very little (just 0.8 acres), so she doubts whether it would be practical for both her sons to take up farming.

5.4 *Structural Constraints in Agriculture*

We saw in the earlier section that the youth, in general, do not see agriculture as their first-choice occupation. It is left to the people who stay back in the villages, particularly the elderly senior farmers. In this section, we discuss the constraints that discourage youth at our research sites from taking up agriculture as a full-time profession.

We found structural constraints like land size, irrigation facilities, and crop loss due to wild animal attacks in the study villages to be the most important deterrents to practicing agriculture. One of the common problems highlighted by older farmers and young people regarding agriculture in the study villages is the loss of crops due to wild animal attacks, particularly by elephants. The common crop across the two villages is rice, which is cultivated as a kharif crop. Both villages are surrounded by forests and have wild animals like elephants and wild boars that often enter fields and destroy standing crops. It not only affects them economically, but also discourages them from viewing agriculture as a viable occupation.

A senior farmer from Mujagada points out,

> The animals (elephants and wild boars) come and eat away at our crops. The government is also not helping us in any way. Help in the sense... when elephants come and eat our crops, people from the forest department come to drive the elephants back into the forest, but they do not give us any kind of monetary compensation for our loss. So, we receive no help from the government.

RG, a young farmer, points out, "When there is a natural disaster like floods, the crop gets destroyed. Moreover, farmers do not get adequate compensation for the losses, making their lives extremely difficult."

Other issues highlighted by young farmers were the limited availability of land and the lack of irrigation facilities. Ganjam is one of the most densely populated districts of Odisha. Hence, there is pressure on land for agriculture. The small size of the landholding limits the scope of growing commercial crops and the profitability of agriculture. Although the majority of farmers grow a single crop (rice), some of the farmers also grow vegetables. Due to a lack of proper water facilities, farmers hesitate to cultivate vegetables. RG explains,

> We depend on rain. Due to less rain, the land becomes very dry, and there are cracks on the land. The rainwater is also not distributed evenly. In some parts, it rains, and in other parts, it does not. If such things happen, we can't grow any crops.

On being asked what would facilitate or encourage them to practice agriculture as a full-time profession, the youth pointed out that they need irrigation facilities and sizable landholding. Furthermore, the idea of a successful farmer is also viewed as someone having a large landholding and irrigation. KS, a driver as well as a farmer, argues,

> There's the water—irrigation—problem as well. Because of this (water) scarcity, we have to wait for the availability of water. If there's some kind of pump system to facilitate water (supply), then it would be helpful for the farmers. Otherwise, a farmer can never be successful. If everything a farmer does is by paying other people, then what is he benefiting from?

The uncertainty in rainfall and irrigation/water supply were two points mentioned by *all* the respondents as problems in agriculture at present. A lot of the farmers found relying on rainfall a precarious dependence. SG said that because she lacked information regarding the weather, her produce was lost due to rain. Without proper storage facilities, crops are damaged in excessive rain. A key informant, NM, an 18-year-old young man from the Kondha community (ST), said, when asked if farming can be a primary occupation: "It completely depends on rain. In the year when it rains well, the yield is good. And if there's no proper rain, then the yield is not good that year."

For another key informant, RKS, agriculture is not a feasible form of livelihood due to the lack of water resources. He says,

> People who own large tracts of land can make a livelihood from farming. But for those like us, who have small holdings, it's difficult to earn a profit. And we are completely dependent on rainwater. There are no water sources like a dam, river, or pond for irrigation in our village.

For young people with little experience in dealing with the vagaries of the weather and the uncertainties of agriculture, it is especially hard. BD, a 38-year-old female farmer, explains, "See, now there is no water, the paddy gets burnt due to that. They (young people) feel dejected. So, they don't feel like coming to the fields."

5.5 *Agriculture: Food Security and Livelihoods*

Despite the difficulties associated with agriculture, young people in our research sites see agriculture as important—socially and culturally—and as a part of their everyday lives. Even as they say time and again that the economic rewards from agriculture are not always guaranteed, our research participants could not imagine giving up on agriculture. A dominant view expressed by the youth centers on the food security they get from cultivating rice; it provides them with food and nourishment. In conversations about the future of agriculture, the most common response was that if the youth gave up agriculture, there would be food shortages and inflation. In turn, the farming communities would have to buy at higher prices what they could grow on their own. It emerged that though the Public Distribution System (PDS) has helped them reduce their dependency on the market for food grains, it has not been enough to meet all their food requirements. Agriculture, at least, ensures that they have food on their plate. Further, the food they get from the market is also expensive and not always readily available.

SN explains,

> It (agriculture) is important because I own land… if I do not cultivate, it will remain unused. When I cultivate and work for six months, I store rice for a year. Procuring rice from my field is more essential than buying it in the market. If I do not cultivate, then owning land is in vain.

Thirty-year-old sharecropper BP, when asked if she wished to lease in more land for farming, replied, "Yes, of course; otherwise, what will I eat?" In a similar vein, the quote by GN earlier summarized succinctly: "What is not to like (about agriculture)? We have to earn our own food."

Thus, our research participants saw their own cultivation as a means to household food security—something they valued greatly. Despite widespread access to food grain through the PDS, our research participants relied on their farms to feed themselves and their family members. And, they had firm intentions to continue doing so in the future. Thus, while the economic rewards of farming were low, agriculture was considered important for food security. The historical context of hunger, scarcity, and famine in the region (Mohanty, 2022) embedded in the collective psyche of the people may explain the deep attachment to land and cultivation and attitudes of self-reliance toward food security.[4]

"Farmer First" Many youths' common response to the question about the main occupation of the household was agriculture, even when the young person was a migrant with a salaried job. In our research sites, we saw that the "farmer" identity, attachment to land, and affinity toward agriculture go hand in hand. As detailed in Chap. 8, rural households combine multiple livelihoods. Farming is a seasonal activity, and for smallholder cultivators, monetary income from farming is quite meager in comparison to income from remittances or local non-farm incomes. But, because farming provides food grains *all year long*, and it is something they have been doing for generations, occupationally, they consider themselves farmers *first.* Their farming identity is very strong. In our sample, though agriculture was the primary source of household income for 14 (31.8%) research participants, 28 (63.6%) research participants considered agriculture as their main livelihood.

Take the case of JG, who is an ASHA worker, and her husband is a seasonal migrant to Surat. Both, individually, earn a higher income from their respective non-agricultural occupations than they do collectively from farming. Yet, JG unambiguously considers farming as their main source of livelihood. She explains, "Our main work in the village is farming *(chasi)*, and additionally, we are into other professions... If our income from farming were sufficient, he (the husband) would not have to migrate."

Elsewhere in rice-growing regions of southern India and Indonesia, Huijsmans et al. (2021) find a similar predicament where land holdings are often too small for cultivators to rely fully on farming. Along with small holdings, smallholder rainfed agriculture is fraught with risk and uncertainty. Yet, despite uncertain and low incomes and structurally adverse conditions in agriculture, our research participants—young and old—consider themselves farmers first. OP, echoing JG, explains: "It doesn't matter if there is profit or loss in agriculture. Agriculture is the main livelihood of our family."

5.6 *Land*

Land is valued, and those who have land—no matter how small their land tracts may be—consider themselves fortunate and are committed to cultivation. Even if they migrate, young people remain involved in agriculture. An overwhelming majority of young workers in our sample contributed to agriculture in one way or the other—either by returning to the village during cultivation to work on their farms and/or by sending remittances to financially support cultivation. Thus, in our research sites, migration did not supplement agriculture; instead, it complemented agriculture.

There is a clear class dimension within the farming community. For those with small and marginal landholdings, being able to cultivate their land—or lease in

[4] For a historical account of the migration-famine nexus, see Mohanty (2022).

land for cultivation—was not only a matter of pride, but also provided a sense of accomplishment. Rural households aspired to own more land. Those with large tracts of land wished to purchase even more land for cultivation, as well as for commercial purposes. The desire to own land among sharecroppers is very strong. However, among the landless and the resource-poor, land has always been so out of reach that they don't imagine or expect to purchase it. For instance, when 30-year-old KG was asked if she wanted to purchase land in the future, she replied, "I have no money for this, so I cannot dream about it." This resonates with Appadurai (2004), who argues that the poor and marginalized have "limited capacity to aspire." From the lens of class, these findings are similar to other studies in South Asia. Based on a village study in Nepal, Sunam (2020) finds that for youth in well-off families, land had a social and cultural value. On the other hand, poorer youth considered land to be significant for household and food security (Sunam, 2020).

A deep attachment to land at the research sites was evident. Not one research participant intended to sell their land in the near future. The sale of land was associated with dire economic distress and financial problems, such as healthcare expenses if someone was critically ill, a daughter's dowry or marriage, and children's education. Land was seen both as an asset and a safety net. Despite the hardship and declining profitability faced in cultivation, 29-year-old ND explains, "This is our ancestral property. Even if we don't continue farming, we will not sell it. What if we need it in the future?"

5.7 Sharecropping and "New" Farmers

In our research sites, sharecropping was quite prevalent. In our sample, 14 (31.8%) of our research participants, in addition to their own cultivation, leased in land for sharecropping, while seven (16.8%) were exclusively sharecroppers (see Table 1).

In line with Mohanty and Lenka (2023), we find that sharecropping provides access to land, contributes to food security, and is preferred over migration. At the same time, sharecroppers experience multiple barriers in the market, such as the lack of access to formal credit and the inability to sell their produce at the remunerative *mandi*[5] price. Often, they were locked in unfavorable land lease arrangements[6] that had the potential to cause extreme distress, for instance, in the case of crop failures.[7]

In our sample, we also have women in their thirties who are *new farmers.* These women started practicing agriculture late in life—typically after marriage—and often practiced a combination of their own cultivation and sharecropping. Other empirical studies also discuss young farmers in the context of a late(r) entry to agriculture (Srinivasan & White, 2024; Mohanty & Lenka, 2023). Srinivasan and White (2024) argue that "most youth do not become farmers when they are chronologically young" (p. 6). Focusing on this category does not allow us to study individual trajectories *into* agriculture, after young people may have returned to the rural areas from their migration journeys. They view becoming a farmer as a process, rather than an event, and for most young people, entry into farming follows work across different places and sectors, often some non-agricultural, urban work (Srinivasan & White, 2024).

In a similar vein, based on village studies in Odisha, Mohanty and Lenka (2023) find that, on the whole, agriculture is greying. At the same time, young people from erstwhile landless households are able to access land and farming through sharecropping. The following excerpt from an interview with a 26-year-old farmer from the SC community in their study captures this caste-class dynamic of agriculture and migration.

> For generations, we were landless agricultural laborers and farmed the lands of higher castes. We have witnessed how agriculture changed their fortunes. Now their children have shifted to cities for lucrative careers. For them, farming may be the last resort, but for us, it is a new hope. (Mohanty & Lenka, 2023, p. 17)

Take the case of KG, who is a 35-year-old widow. She is a *new farmer* who, after her husband's death, moved to her natal village and started leasing in land for cultivation. "I have had knowledge about agriculture since my childhood, as I learned it from my parents," she explains.

KG currently leases in 0.8 acres of land and grows paddy in the kharif season. She plants the saplings, weeds out the grass, and reaps the crops. For the preparation of land, application of fertilizers and pesticides, and harvesting and threshing, she hires labor. Typically, she borrows cash from the landlord to purchase inputs—seeds,

---

[5] *Mandi* here refers to an agricultural market where prices for specific crops are regulated by the government. In Odisha, the government offers a minimum support price for paddy to farmers cultivating paddy on their own land. As sharecroppers do not farm on their own land, they are unable to sell their paddy produce at the mandi. They have to resort to selling it in the open market, where the sale price is relatively lower.

[6] Sharecropping is the dominant form of leasing arrangement in the research sites, wherein the total output is shared by the landlord and the sharecropper in a ratio of 1:1. Typically, input costs are borne by the sharecropper. Seldom do landlords provide seeds and fertilizers to the sharecropper. Other forms of leasing arrangements, such as fixed rent, were not prevalent in the research sites.

[7] Mohanty and Lenka (2019) find that one of the leading causes of farmer suicides in Odisha is the inability of sharecroppers to repay the money owed to their landlords. Typically, this happens in the case of crop failure. In our sample, four research participants referred to farmer suicides, of which three specifically mentioned indebtedness due to specific crop failures.

fertilizers, pesticides, payment for agricultural labor—and repays the loan after the sale of the paddy crop.

Last year, she produced 11.2 quintals of paddy, of which half was given to the landlord as their share. Of her own share of the remaining half (5.6 quintals), KG kept 3.2 quintals for self-consumption and sold 2.4 quintals in the market. Being a sharecropper, KG is unable to sell her produce directly at the mandi and has to rely on traders for the sale of her crop.[8] She also grows *mung* and *urad* (pulses), entirely for self-consumption. In the past, she has independently sharecropped on as much as three acres of land. In recent years, she has had to scale down the size of her farm due to her commitment toward her Indira Awas Yojana housing allotment, for which she has taken a loan.

She does not consider herself a farmer. KG's views are embedded in a paradigm where invisibilization of women's work by women themselves continues to be a persistent feature in agriculture and beyond, in the Global South (Hirway & Jose, 2011; Agarwal, 1994). In addition, male-and technology-dominated discourses of agriculture and development define KG's worldview of what a farmer is supposed to be.

For her, a farmer is

> The person who cultivates their land and who possesses some agricultural tools like tractors and power tillers. But we don't have anything. We do agriculture for our family's survival... The farmer who becomes financially strong and protects his crop from wild animals is a successful farmer.

She does not consider agriculture a profitable activity. She explains, "We invest a lot but earn very less... A good harvest depends on luck and chance... But I cannot imagine leaving agriculture as it is our only source of survival."

5.8 *Gender and the Feminization of Agriculture*

It emerged from the Phase 1 survey of the Odisha Migration Study that in the agriculture and allied sectors, the share of female employment is higher compared to that of males, and this pattern is more pervasive among the youth (see Chap. 7 for details). This suggests the feminization of agriculture in Odisha and resonates with other studies in eastern India, for instance, in Bihar and West Bengal (Datta, 2022; Pattnaik et al., 2018). This feminization of agriculture needs to be understood in the context of male-dominated migration, which may be accumulative or distress-driven. However, as noted in Chap. 1, over time, coping, or distress-driven migration streams can also turn "accumulative" (Deshingkar & Farrington, 2009).

Against this backdrop, the conversation below, between GN (male, 19 years old) and the interviewer, highlights the gendered nature of outmigration and agricultural work.

[8] Legally, crops can be sold at the mandi *only* by the landowners. Sharecroppers, or those who lease in land, thus, are not able to sell their harvest at the mandi.

I: *What does the youth from your village do?*

GN: *Most of the boys migrate for work, and the girls help in farming.*

I: *Why do the youths prefer to migrate for work?*

I: *Those who work in the fields need to wait for six months to generate income. But those migrating for work are paid weekly.*

Migration from our research sites was male-dominated, masculinized. As in other contexts in India, men were able to migrate and access non-agricultural occupations, while women's mobility—geographical and occupational—was constrained (Narayanan, 2024; Datta, 2022). With heavy male outmigration from our research sites, the burden of cultivation disproportionately fell on the women *left behind*. Survey data from Phase 1 of the Odisha Migration Study corroborates this and points toward a feminization of agriculture in rural Odisha. Take the case of 29-year-old ND. Her husband, SD (36), is a Surat migrant.[9] He started migrating *after* marriage to support his family of six members: his parents, wife, and two daughters (11 and 9). As a result, ND had to take over managing their agricultural land of 0.4 acres, divided into two plots, of which only one is irrigated.

The family produces about 5–5.5 quintals of paddy, which is used solely for self-consumption. ND has been managing the family farms for the past nine years. During paddy cultivation, she has to go to the fields every other day to supervise the farm work. Some tasks take more time compared to others. At the time of weeding, she has to be in the fields from 6 a.m. to 11 a.m. On other days, when only irrigation has to be checked, it doesn't take much time. Water scarcity is a serious concern; she wants the government to assist in the provision of irrigation. She prefers the convenience of a borewell since it operates as a private asset and thus is easily managed. "If we have a borewell, we can do our work on our own. Canal water, on the other hand, requires help (cooperation) from others," she explains. There is also the issue of the availability of ploughing machines that need to be rented. The machinery is not readily available when required, and the machine owners often delay the work, she laments.

Yet, ND is quick to mention:

> I don't know anything (about farming). I only hire people to do the work and instruct the workers. Whatever (notional) profit is earned after harvesting goes back to paying them (the laborers). Only because I have land of my own, I am continuing the work (farming)... But there is no profit.

While SD sends back remittances to support cultivation, he does not return to the village for farming. It does not make sense for him to come. In fact, it is necessary for him to stay in Surat and work to be able to remit, as wages for farm workers have increased in the village. "Only if he earns there can we pay them (the workers) here (in the village)," says ND, explaining their financial predicament. She feels she is

[9] In the past, ND accompanied her husband to Surat, but she returned as it was not financially viable for her to stay there. She explains, "In my village, if someone has a lot of income, then only they can sustain their family there (in Surat). You cannot live there with your family on a minimal income."

able to manage just fine in his absence. The only issue is with water and machinery, according to her.

It emerged from several other interviews like ND's that earlier, men used to regularly return to the village in the agricultural season for cultivation. Lately, as workers' wages have increased in rural Odisha, remittances from the city are becoming necessary to pay for the high labor costs in the village.[10] Women continue with cultivation themselves, along with other family members, and also by hiring laborers. Cultivation is considered sacrosanct and *does not stop*, despite the decreased availability of men than earlier.

ND does not wish to acquire more land for farming: "We spend more than what we get in return from farming; what is the point?" On the other hand, she has no intention of selling her land either.

> This is our ancestral property. Even if we don't continue farming, we will not sell it. What if we need it in the future? Farming cannot improve the financial standard of my family. But I will not abstain from farming. As long as we have these fields, we will continue farming.

For ND, a successful farmer is someone:

> Who has an abundance of land, one who can work efficiently, and has all kinds of availability of resources. A successful farmer is also someone smart, has good management skills, does not focus only on one crop; farms multiple crops and vegetables too, and has deep knowledge about farming.

This case study of ND exemplifies the feminization of agriculture as a consequence of male outmigration. Yet, the sex segregation of agricultural tasks continues; women are not involved in ploughing, land preparation, or tilling, and men are not involved in sowing, reaping, gathering, or plucking. Thirty-five-year-old JG, who cultivates her family farm, explains, "If someone asks for a kilo of vegetables, a man will not pluck them and give them. It would be a woman's task."

Interestingly, we observed that in our research sites, the mechanization of agriculture—the use of land tillers, tractors, and harvesters—has reduced men's tasks in agriculture. In turn, the loss of agricultural work in the rural areas is cited as one of the reasons for male migration. For women, tasks have remained the same, as the mechanization of women's tasks in agriculture has not happened in a substantive manner. Sowing, weeding, and transplanting continue to be labor-intensive female tasks. At the same time, in the absence of men, women have to do more work and get more involved in agriculture. They are responsible for everyday farm management—hiring labor, paying labor, arranging money for inputs, buying inputs, etc. In line with the findings of Pattnaik and Lahiri-Dutt (2022), we observe that the preparatory work undertaken by women on family farms in a range of agricultural tasks is immense. This often goes unreported and unrecorded in conventional data collection exercises by researchers and policymakers.

---

[10] At the time of fieldwork in 2023, the daily wage for casual labor in the survey sites varied from Rs 200 to 250. A *Surat migrant* typically earns Rs 10,000–12,000 every month, of which, significant proportions are remitted for the sustenance of the rural household.

In our research sites, gender intersects with generation, and the burden of agricultural work falls disproportionately on *older women*. Thirty-eight-year-old BD manages her family farm of 1.2 acres, while her husband and four sons migrate for work. BD is a *new farmer*, as is evident by her description of her entry into agriculture:

> I: *For how many years have you been engaged in farming?*
>
> BD: *My mother-in-law used to do the work. After her death, I have been working for six-seven months.*
>
> I: *How did you learn farming? Who taught you?*
>
> BD: *By going to the fields, watching others work in the fields.*
>
> I: *Did your mother-in-law teach you?*
>
> BD: *No, I did not go there while she was alive. It was only after her death that I went to the fields.*
>
> I: *What all works are you doing in the field?*
>
> BD: *Preparing the fields, sowing all these...*

Prior to this, BD had no experience with farming. Earlier in the year, her husband returned to the village for land preparation, sowing, and applying fertilizers. "He comes and does all the work; I take care of the rest. If he is not there, we (can) hire people to do this work. But we face a lot of problems," she explains.

This resonates with JKG, who elaborates that in the absence of their husbands in the village, "The woman gets more involved, and she does not get the support that she gets while her husband is at home. She arranges money and other things, and she performs various tasks (related to agriculture)…".

NP, a 38-year-old sharecropper and daily wage laborer, when asked about the impact of migration on agriculture, feels, "A man should be there at home to lift heavy stuff, but now we (women) are doing everything."

Similar sentiments are echoed by 24-year-old DN, a young Dalit man:

> Women and mothers are doing more work now. They cut the crop, wash it; it is all done by the mothers. With the use of tractors, mothers continue farming using the help of labor, and the farming goes on… Mothers are responsible for housework and farming, as the males will go out, leaving the land. So, mothers have to do farming no matter what, as food is the outcome, so it's inevitable.

These findings echo micro-studies in the literature—across diverse geographies in India dominated by rice monocultures—that male outmigration leads to an increase in women's work on family farms and as sharecroppers. Women have a heavier workload and take on more farm tasks, including farm management, in the absence of men (Pattnaik & Lahiri-Dutt, 2020; Datta & Mishra, 2011; Paris et al., 2005). A recent study based on nationally representative data finds that in households with seasonal or short-term migration, women are more likely to be major decision-makers on farms (Chandrasekhar et al., 2022). Thus, migration plays a critical role in the feminization of agriculture, including the feminization of farm management.[11]

---

[11] For an alternative perspective, see Pattanaik et al. (2018). For a discussion on the debate on managerial feminization and labor feminization, see Gartaula, et al. (2010).

5.9 Migration and Agriculture

5.9.1 Why Do Young People Migrate?

Migration and agriculture are closely intertwined. In our interviews, the lack of adequate work in agriculture emerged as the fundamental reason for migration from rural areas. As discussed in the previous section, young people interested in practicing agriculture are confronted with the harsh structural realities of farming being adversely impacted by climate variability, irrigation water scarcity, increasing input costs, and declining agricultural profits. The lack of irrigation facilities is the single most important factor that constrains agricultural potential in our research sites. Despite the existence of a canal irrigation system, farming continues to be predominantly rainfed, and most farmers have not been able to transition from single to double cropping. At the same time, the mechanization of agricultural activities has reduced the demand for labor, especially male labor. On the other hand, the demand for casual labor elsewhere in India has opened new opportunities for young people.

It is against this context that 19-year-old GN, a final-year BA student from Mujagada, explains why young people migrate:

> The income generated in three months by working outside, in companies, is equal to the income generated from farming in six months. Young people find it easier to work outside than in the fields. So, they prefer to migrate for work.

5.9.2 Do Young People Like to Migrate?

It emerged from the interviews with young people that labor migration is not their preferred livelihood option. The predominant migration stream in the region is seasonal and distress-oriented, closely linked with the agricultural calendar. After the crop harvest, a majority of young men migrate to the power mills in Surat. The Ganjam-Surat migration stream is male-and youth-dominated, a part of household livelihood strategies to make ends meet. In the literature, such streams are aptly referred to as survival or coping migration, distinctly different from accumulative kinds of migration that are associated with higher skills and income and job security (Deshingkar & Farrington, 2009).

Indeed, as the livelihoods and income study of the Odisha Migration Study shows in Chap. 8, households with migrants, paradoxically, have a lower income than households without migrants. This suggests the adverse incorporation of migrant households into precarious streams. It is no surprise, thus, that young people express their discomfort and displeasure with such migration, shunning it when there is an option of doing so.

Among youth migrants—across social classes—the desire to remain in the village, or eventually return to the village, is very strong. For young migrants, including highly educated migrants[12] and those earning comfortable incomes in destination regions, the imagination of their future lies in the village, closely linked with agriculture.

We now discuss the case of KG, whose husband's untimely death pushed her into agriculture. It also led to her son SG dropping out of school in Class 6, and eventually migrating to Surat with his uncle two years ago. SG works at a power loom mill in Surat, earning about Rs 8000 per month. He has asked KG to migrate to Surat so that they can work together and repay the loan taken for house construction. KG, however, is not keen on migrating to Surat. Her son has not visited the village in the last two years. Sometimes, he sends money for cultivation. "We never force him to send money because he is young," KG explains. Her account of her son's involvement in agriculture highlights the complexities of young people's relationship with agriculture and the rural.

I: *Does the young generation have any interest in agriculture?*

KG: *No, I have no idea about the young generation. My son is not interested in agriculture because he is working outside and earning more.*

I: *Do you think that the young generation should be involved in agriculture?*

KG: *Yes, our children should support us in agricultural activities.*

I: *If your son wants to pursue agriculture, how should you guide him?*

KG: *He should first know how to cultivate land. Two years back, when he was here, he helped me with various agricultural activities. He was also taking care of the poultry.*

I: *Is the younger generation from your village doing agricultural work?*

KG: *The younger generation is not involved in agriculture because they are migrating to Delhi, Surat, Bombay, or other cities.*

I: *Does your son accept agriculture as a profession?*

KG: *Yes, he thinks that it is the source of our livelihood, but he has not come home for the last two years.*

I: *Is your son associated with agriculture?*

KG: *He knows about it, but we have no idea what he would do in the future.*

I: *Do you want to involve your son in agriculture?*

KG: *When he comes, he visits the agricultural field and brings us food. This shows that he has an interest in agriculture.*

At the outset, KG claims straightaway that SG is not interested or involved in agriculture. Upon probing, it emerges that in the past, he has worked in agriculture, and currently, while being away, he sends remittances that are critical to sustaining agriculture in the village. She then argues that he may indeed be interested in agriculture. This conversation shows that perceptions regarding young people's association with agriculture cannot be captured in binaries: *interested* or *uninterested* and *farms* or *does not farm*. These choices and decisions, apart from being a function of household livelihoods, generation, gender, and structural factors like land (as discussed earlier) are also nested in wider social and economic realities such as the availability of non-farm employment, the quality of jobs in the non-agricultural sector, attitudes toward rural workers in urban destinations, etc.

---

[12] As we saw in the case of SS in the earlier section on aspirations.

6 Conclusion

In this chapter, we explored youth aspirations and attitudes toward agriculture in the context of smallholder rainfed cultivation in a high-migration region in eastern India. Drawing on the concept of youth as a social construction and a structural framing of aspirations and livelihoods, we found that the aspirations of young people varied considerably by their educational status. At the first instance, there existed a powerful narrative of success for young people—to study hard, and do a respectable job; success was thus spatially located outside the village, and outside of agriculture. Agriculture was considered hard work and dirty work, not a preferred occupation for the youth. At the same time, young people interested in practicing agriculture were confronted with the harsh structural realities of farming being adversely impacted by climate variability, water scarcity, increasing input costs, and declining agricultural profits. The lack of irrigation facilities was the single most important factor that constrained agricultural potential in the research sites.

Despite these structural constraints, young people valued agriculture for the food security it provided. Because farming provided foodgrains all year long, and they had been farming for generations, occupationally, they considered themselves farmers first. Young people's farming identity was quite strong, despite farming being a seasonal activity, and for smallholder cultivators, monetary income from farming was quite meager in comparison with the income from remittances or local non-farm incomes. In our sample, agriculture was the primary source of household income for only 14 (31.8%) research participants, but as many as 28 (63.6%) research participants considered agriculture their main livelihood.

Young people valued land, and those with land—no matter how small their land tract might have been—considered themselves fortunate and committed to cultivation. Even if they migrated, young people remain involved in agriculture. All young migrants in our sample contributed to agriculture in one way or the other—either by returning to the village during cultivation to work on their farms and/or by sending remittances to financially support cultivation. Thus, in our research sites, migration did not supplement agriculture; instead, it complemented agriculture.

Male and youth migration led to an increase in women's work on family farms, and as sharecroppers, women had a heavier workload and had to take on more farm tasks, including farm management. We also interviewed *new farmers*; individuals, mostly women in our sample, who took up agriculture later in life due to a myriad of circumstances. Migration was closely intertwined with the feminization of agriculture and an increased burden on women.

Sharecropping provided access to land and food security and was preferred over migration, especially among the older youth. At the same time, sharecroppers experienced multiple barriers in the market, such as the lack of access to formal credit and the inability to sell their produce at the remunerative mandi price. Often, they were locked in unfavorable land lease arrangements that had the potential to cause extreme distress, for instance, in the case of crop failures.

Migration was not the preferred choice of young people. Among youth migrants—across social classes—the desire to remain in the village, or eventually return to the village, was very strong. For young migrants, including highly educated migrants and those earning comfortable incomes in destination regions, the imagination of their future lied in the village, closely linked with agriculture. At the same time, youth cultures of temporary migration were widespread, a rite of passage, particularly for those who were less educated. An aversion to agriculture at a young age and the lack of employment options in source regions played a significant role in shaping this pattern.

In the context of these empirical findings, we have some policy recommendations. First, government intervention needs to address structural issues, such as the provision of irrigation, which will help this region transition from single to multiple cropping and allow for crop diversification. In turn, this would enhance not only food and nutritional security, but also the commercialization of agriculture and an increase in farming incomes. Second, given the widespread prevalence of sharecropping, access to land needs to be institutionalized. This will help young farmers directly access formal credit and agricultural markets (mandis). Third, recognition of young women as farmers is critical for them to be able to access credit and agricultural inputs and become successful farmers. Fourth, agricultural extension and training for women need to be prioritized, particularly in the context of high male migration and feminization of agriculture. Fifth, the role of agriculture and the value of farming in society need to be enhanced.[13] Ultimately, the agricultural sector has the potential to provide work and employment to rural youth in a context where young people prefer to stay in rural areas if decent livelihood options are available.

References

Agarwal, B. (1994). *A field of ones own: Gender and land rights in South Asia.* Cambridge University Press.

Agarwal, B., & Agrawal, A. (2017). Do farmers really like farming? Indian farmers in transition. *Oxford Development Studies, 45*(4), 460–478. https://doi.org/10.1080/13600818.2017.1283010

Appadurai, A. (2004). The capacity to aspire. In V. Rao & M. Walton (Eds.), *Culture and public action* (pp. 59–84). Stanford University Press.

Chambers, R., & Conway, G. (1991). *Sustainable rural livelihoods: Practical concepts for the 21st century* (IDS Discussion Paper No. 296). Institute of Development Studies, Sussex, UK.

Chandrasekhar, S., Sahoo, S., & Swaminathan, H. (2022). Seasonal migration and feminization of farm management: Evidence from India. *Feminist Economics, 28*(1), 86–113. https://doi.org/10.1080/13545701.2021.1976808

Dalton, P. S., Ghosal, S., & Mani, A. (2015). Poverty and aspirations failure. *The Economic Journal, 126*(590), 165–188. https://doi.org/10.1111/ecoj.12210

Datta, A. (2022). *Migration and development in India: The Bihar experience.* Routledge.

Datta, A., & Mishra, S. K. (2011). Glimpses of women's lives in rural Bihar: Impact of male migration. *The Indian Journal of Labour Economics, 54*(3), 457–477.

[13] One of the ways to do this is to meaningfully include farming in the school curriculum.

Deshingkar, P., & Farrington, J. (Eds.). (2009). *Circular migration and multilocational livelihood strategies in rural India*. Oxford University Press.
Elias, M., Mudege, N., Lopez, D. E., Najjar, D., Kandiwa, V., Luis, J., Yila, J., & others. (2018). Gendered aspirations and occupations among rural youth, in agriculture and beyond: A cross-regional perspective. *Journal of Gender, Agriculture and Food Security, 3*(1), 82–107.
Ellis, F. (1998). Household strategies and rural livelihood diversification. *The Journal of Development Studies, 35*(1), 1–38.
Ellis, F. (2000). *Rural livelihoods and diversity in developing countries*. Oxford University Press.
FAO. (2018). *The state of food and agriculture 2018: Migration, agriculture and rural development*. Retrieved January 10, 2025, from https://openknowledge.fao.org/server/api/core/bitstreams/0106019d-2529-4f93-b9e5-cce52bee33c3/content
Gartaula, H. N., Niehof, A., & Visser, L. (2010). Feminisation of agriculture as an effect of male out-migration: Unexpected outcomes from Jhapa district, eastern Nepal. *International Journal of Interdisciplinary Social Sciences, 5*, 565–577.
Genicot, G., & Ray, D. (2017). Aspirations and inequality. *Econometrica, 85*(2), 489–519. https://doi.org/10.3982/ecta13865
Government of India. (2014). *National youth policy 2014*. Department of Youth Affairs, Ministry of Youth Affairs and Sports.
Hirway, I., & Jose, S. (2011). Understanding womens work using time-use statistics: The case of India. *Feminist Economics, 17*(4), 67–92. https://doi.org/10.1080/13545701.2011.622289
Huijsmans, R., Ambarwati, A., Chazali, C., & Vijayabaskar, M. (2021). Farming, gender, and aspirations across young peoples life course: Attempting to keep things open while becoming a farmer. *European Journal of Development Research, 33*(1), 71–88. https://doi.org/10.1057/s41287-020-00302-y
IFAD. (2019). *Creating opportunities for rural youth. 2019 rural development report*. International Fund for Agricultural Development. Retrieved January 10, 2025, from https://www.ifad.org/documents/38714170/41190221/RDR2019_Overview_e_W.pdf/699560f2-d02e-16b8-4281-596d4c9be25a
Leavy, J., & Hossain, N. (2014). *Who wants to farm? Youth aspirations, opportunities, and rising food prices*. IDS Working Papers, (439), 1–44. https://doi.org/10.1111/j.2040-0209.2014.00439.x
Leavy, J., & Smith, S. (2010). Future farmers: Youth aspirations, expectations and life choices. *Future Agricultures Discussion Paper, 13*, 1–15.
Mishra, D. K. (2020). Seasonal migration and unfree labour in globalising India: Insights from field surveys in Odisha. *The Indian Journal of Labour Economics, 63*(4), 1087–1106. https://doi.org/10.1007/s41027-020-00277-8
Mitra, A., & Pradhan, B. K. (2016). *Migration, remittances, and changing patterns of livelihood: Evidence from western Odisha villages*. Working Paper No. 363. Institute of Economic Growth.
Mohanty, B. B., & Lenka, P. K. (2019). Small farmers' suicide in Odisha. *Economic & Political Weekly, 54*(22), 51–59.
Mohanty, B. B., & Lenka, P. K. (2023). For them farming may be the last resort, but for us it is a new hope: Ageing, youth and farming in India. *Journal of Agrarian Change., 23*(4), 771–791. https://doi.org/10.1111/joac.12538
Mohanty, B. (2022). *A haunting tragedy: Gender, caste and class in the 1866 famine of Orissa*. Manohar.
Nandi, R., & Nedumaran, S. (2021). Understanding the aspirations of farming communities in developing countries: A systematic review of the literature. *The European Journal of Development Research, 33*(4), 809–832.
Narayanan, S. (2024). I had to bear this burden: Youth transcending constraints to become farmers in Madhya Pradesh, India. In S. Srinivasan (Ed.), *Becoming a young farmer: Young people's pathways into farming: Canada, China, India and Indonesia* (pp. 277–301). Springer International Publishing.

Narayanan, S., Vijayabaskar, M., & Srinivasan, S. (2024). The youth dividend and agricultural revival in India. In S. Srinivasan (Ed.), *Becoming a young farmer: Young peoples pathways into farming: Canada, China, India and Indonesia* (pp. 221–251). Springer International Publishing.

Natarajan, N., Newsham, A., Rigg, J., & Suhardiman, D. (2022). A sustainable livelihoods framework for the 21st century. *World Development, 155*, 105898. https://doi.org/10.1016/j.worlddev.2022.105898

Paris, T., Singh, A., Luis, J., & Hossain, M. (2005). Labour out migration, livelihood of rice farming households and women left behind: A case study in eastern Uttar Pradesh. *Economic and Political Weekly, 40*(25), 2522–2529.

Pattnaik, I., & Lahiri-Dutt, K. (2020). What determines women's agricultural participation? A comparative study of landholding households in rural India. *Journal of Rural Studies, 76*, 25–39.

Pattnaik, I., & Lahiri-Dutt, K. (2022). Do women like to farm? Evidence of growing burdens of farming on women in rural India. *The Journal of Peasant Studies, 49*(3), 629–651.

Pattnaik, I., Lahiri-Dutt, K., Lockie, S., & Pritchard, B. (2018). The feminization of agriculture or the feminization of agrarian distress? Tracking the trajectory of women in agriculture in India. *Journal of the Asia Pacific Economy, 23*(1), 138–155. https://doi.org/10.1080/13547860.2017.1394569

Rigg, J., Phongsiri, M., Promphakping, B., Salamanca, A., & Sripun, M. (2019). Who will tend the farm? Interrogating the ageing Asian farmer. *The Journal of Peasant Studies, 47*(2), 306–325. https://doi.org/10.1080/03066150.2019.1572605

Scoones, I. (1998). *Sustainable rural livelihoods: A framework for analysis*. IDS working paper, 72. Brighton: IDS.

Scoones, I. (2009). Livelihoods perspectives and rural development. *The Journal of Peasant Studies, 36*(1), 171–196. https://doi.org/10.1080/03066150902820503

Sharma, A., Kulkarni, R., & Khandelwal, R. (2014). *Studies, stories and a canvas: Seasonal labour migration and migrant workers from Odisha*. Centre for Migration and Labour Solutions.

Srinivasan, S., & White, B. (2024). Young people's pathways into farming. In S. Srinivasan (Ed.), *Becoming a young farmer: Young people's pathways into farming: Canada, China*. Palgrave Macmillan.

Sunam, R. (2020). *Transnational labour migration, livelihoods and agrarian change in Nepal: The remittance village*. Routledge.

Thompson, E. C., Rigg, J., & Gillen, J. (2019). Introduction: Asian smallholders in comparative perspective. In E. C. Thompson, J. Rigg, & J. Gillen (Eds.), *Asian smallholders in comparative perspective*. Amsterdam University Press.

Tumbe, C. (2018). *India moving: A history of migration*. Penguin India.

United Nations Department of Economic and Social Affairs (UNDESA). (2013). *Definition of youth*. Retrieved January 10, 2025, from https://www.un.org/esa/socdev/documents/youth/fact-sheets/youth-definition.pdf

White, B. (2020). *Agriculture and the generation problem*. Practical Action Publishing.

Wiggins, S. (2016). *Agricultural and rural development reconsidered: A guide to issues and debates*. IFAD Research Series 01. International Fund for Agricultural Development.

Chapter 10
Male Migration and Left-Behind Women's Socioeconomic Outcomes

Gaurav Dhamija

Abstract Women's economic participation, physical mobility, and decision-making abilities foster inclusive development, reduce poverty, promote economic growth, and catalyze social progress. Using data from Phase II of the Odisha Migration Study 2023, this chapter studies the relationship between husbands' migration and socioeconomic outcomes of left-behind wives, especially in resource-constrained regions of Odisha characterized by high migration. Our analytical sample includes married women aged 18–49 with valid data on their employment, physical mobility, and decision-making autonomy. We first estimate the associations between husbands' migration and left-behind wives' employment, mobility, and autonomy. Then, we explore the heterogeneity of these relationships based on woman-, husband-, and household-level characteristics. The findings reveal a positive association between husbands' migration and left-behind wives' employment outcomes, though no association is observed with their physical mobility and decision-making autonomy. Moreover, we find substantial variation in the relationship between husbands' migration and wives' mobility across woman- and household-level characteristics. This evidence highlights that the complex relationship between husbands' migration and left-behind wives' socioeconomic outcomes cannot be generalized in a singular direction. On the one hand, distress-driven migration of husbands compels left-behind women to take up employment to sustain household livelihoods in their husbands' absence. On the other hand, this shift fails to translate into enhanced autonomy for these women due to the short-term nature of the migration.

Keywords Migration · Employment · Mobility · Decision-making autonomy · Odisha · India

G. Dhamija (✉)
Department of Liberal Arts, Indian Institute of Technology Hyderabad, Sangareddy, India
e-mail: gauravdhamija@la.iith.ac.in

A. Datta and S. I. Rajan (eds.), *Migration, Livelihoods and Gender*, International Perspectives on Migration, https://doi.org/10.1007/978-981-95-5465-2_10

1 Introduction

Globally, India ranks as the leading country of origin for international migrants (Singh, 2022). According to the World Migration Report (McAuliffe & Oucho, 2024), India has nearly 18 million individuals living abroad. Similarly, the number of internal migrants in India increased from 309 million in 2001 to 450 million recorded in the 2011 Census, marking a 45% rise (De, 2019). The Multiple Indicator Survey 2020–21 shows that nearly three out of 10 individuals in India are reported as migrants (Singh, 2024). The survey also reveals that 48.8% of male migrants migrate in search of better work opportunities (ibid.), often leaving their wives behind due to limited income, unstable employment opportunities, high living costs at migration destinations, and obligations to manage land or care for elderly parents in their places of origin (Lei & Desai, 2021). Given the emphasis on advancing women's socioeconomic outcomes as a catalyst for accelerated development in recent development literature (Duflo, 2012; Goulart et al., 2021), understanding the relationship between husbands' migration and the socioeconomic outcomes of left-behind wives becomes essential.

Out-migration of men changes the dynamics and structure of the household. This shift may improve left-behind wives' economic and social outcomes, including increased participation in the labor market, higher disposable income, physical mobility, and autonomy (Fakir & Abedin, 2021; Gulati, 1987; Luna & Rahman, 2019; Yabiku et al., 2010). Conversely, it may increase the burden of household responsibilities (Koirala, 2023; Paris et al., 2005), vulnerability, and stress (Gunnarsson, 2011; Heller & Kaushik, 2020). Recent empirical studies indicate that male migration can lead to a decline in women's participation in paid work (Binzel & Assaad, 2011 for Egypt; Khan & Valatheeswaran, 2016 for India; Lokshin & Glinskaya, 2009 for Nepal; Mendola & Carletto, 2012 for Albania; Mu & Van De Walle, 2011 for China; Rodriguez & Tiongson, 2001 for the Philippines). This reduction in labor force participation is often attributed to the inflow of remittances, which can raise the reservation wage of left-behind women, making them less likely to engage in paid work (Binzel & Assaad, 2011). Moreover, it can reduce their mobility and autonomy due to interventions by the extended family in the absence of husbands (De Haas & Van Rooij, 2010; Kaur, 2018). Thus, the relationship between the husband's migration and the wife's outcomes could be positive or negative. The variations in findings could be attributed to the diverse geo-social contexts, household structures, and the differences in research approaches and methodologies employed by various researchers (Ghimire et al., 2021).

The existing empirical literature examining the relationship between husbands' migration and the socioeconomic outcomes of left-behind wives in India is scarce. Furthermore, the few studies that do explore these relationships present mixed and somewhat inconsistent findings. For instance, using data from the nationally representative dataset India Human Development Survey 2004–2005, Desai and Banerji (2008) find that husbands' migration improves decision-making power among left-behind wives. Similar findings are reported by Singh (2018) using data from two villages in the northern state of Uttar Pradesh. On the contrary, Sinha et al. (2012)

use data from the National Family Health Survey 2005–2006 and report no significant difference in the decision-making power between left-behind wives and those living with their spouses. In line with Sinha et al. (2012), Ram Mohan et al. (2023) contradict the notion of higher decision-making power among left-behind wives using data from three districts in the state of Bihar.

In 2011, Odisha, with a total working population of 17.5 million, reported 1.54 million individuals as migrant workers (Census of India, 2011). The primary drivers of out-migration in Odisha include low agricultural productivity and limited non-farm employment opportunities (Mitra & Pradhan, 2016). Frequent droughts leading to loss of employment and income compel marginal farmers, landless agricultural laborers, and poorer sections of the society to migrate to more developed regions in search of employment as a coping mechanism (Tripathy, 2021). In the context of women's socioeconomic outcomes in Odisha, data from the fifth round of the National Family Health Survey (NFHS-5) reveal that 27.3% of currently married women reported employment within the 12 months preceding the Survey (International Institute for Population Sciences [IIPS] & ICF, 2021). While self-employment is predominant among women, their involvement in casual work activities (Senapati & Ojha, 2019) often leads to fluctuating incomes and exacerbates financial instability. Furthermore, 30.1% of currently married women indicated that they are allowed to travel alone, and 71.3% reported having some degree of decision-making power in household matters (IIPS & ICF, 2021).

Against this backdrop, this study draws on data from the Odisha Migration Study 2023, focusing on married women aged 18–49. It makes a fresh attempt to address two key questions: (1) What is the direction of the relationship between husbands' migration and wives' employment, physical mobility, and decisionmaking autonomy? and (2) Does this relationship vary across woman-, husband-, and household-level characteristics? Estimating the heterogeneity in the relationship between husbands' migration and wives' socioeconomic outcomes, alongside the average association, allows us to examine whether the direction of this relationship is consistent across different subgroups. This approach enables us to address not only the question, "Is there any association between husbands' migration and wives' socioeconomic outcomes?" but also to understand whether the change in socioeconomic outcomes of some wives due to husbands' migration differs from that of others.

The results of this study are interesting. The regression analysis suggests that, on average, the likelihood of current employment and employment in the last 12 months seems to be higher for wives of migrants than for the wives of non-migrants. However, there is no statistical difference in the mobility and autonomy of migrants' wives compared to non-migrants' wives. The heterogeneity analysis reveals that, while no significant association emerges between husbands' migration and wives' physical mobility in the overall sample, this relationship varies substantially across different subgroups of women. Specifically, the heterogeneity analysis shows that the husbands' migration is positively associated with the wives' mobility among younger women, women from smaller households, the poorest wealth category households, and the Scheduled Tribe (ST) background. Conversely, we observe a negative relationship between husbands' migration and wives' mobility among women from larger households and the richest wealth category households.

These findings align with existing literature, which shows that wives' employment often increases following their husbands' migration (Hondagneu-Sotelo, 1992; Paris et al., 2005). However, their participation is predominant in low-productivity agricultural work (Paris et al., 2005) and informal sector activities (Hondagneu-Sotelo, 1992). Moreover, these transitions are unlikely to foster significant women empowerment among left-behind wives, as decision-making autonomy regarding major expenditures often remains under the control of male family members (Jetley, 1987) due to the short-term nature of migration.

Our study engages with two primary strands of literature. First, it connects to the body of research that focuses on women's empowerment. The extensive literature on women's empowerment encompasses a broad range of topics, from the theoretical conceptualization and measurement of empowerment to the exploration of its determinants and consequences (see Priya et al. (2021) for a review of literature on women's empowerment in the last two decades). Second, our work is aligned with studies examining the association between husbands' migration and the socioeconomic outcomes of left-behind women in developing countries, including India (Datta & Mishra, 2011; Green et al., 2019; Khan et al., 2023; Khan & Valatheeswaran, 2016; Lei & Desai, 2021; Zachariah et al., 2001).

2 Data

We utilize a sample of married women surveyed during the second phase (Phase II) of the Odisha Migration Study[1] 2023. Phase II of the Odisha Migration Study 2023 focused on mixed-methods studies addressing livelihoods and income, gender and well-being, women's autonomy and mobility, and youth aspirations and attitudes toward agriculture. Quantitative studies specifically targeting household income, livelihoods, and women's economic and social empowerment were conducted in 11 districts identified as migration-prone by the Odisha government: Balangir, Bargarh, Gajapati, Ganjam, Kalahandi, Koraput, Khordha, Nabarangpur, Nuapada, Rayagada, and Subarnapur. A total of 17 rural localities, with the highest migration estimates based on Phase I data, were selected for household data collection in Phase II. All 506 households surveyed from these 17 localities in Phase I were subsequently chosen for data collection in Phase II.

A separate gender module was administered to households included in the income and livelihood survey that had married women aged 18 to 49 years. Among the 506 households, 346 had at least one married woman within the eligible age range, resulting in valid data collection from 244 married women across 227 households.

[1] Details related to the sampling strategy of Phase I of Odisha Migration Study 2023 are available in Chapter 1.

Table 1 Distribution of women by regions and districts

Regions	Districts	Number of women
Coastal	Khordha	16
Northern	Balangir	45
	Subarnapur	19
Southern	Ganjam	24
	Kalahandi	28
	Koraput	44
	Nuapada	29
Total		205

The interviews for these women were conducted between May and August 2023. The gender module also recorded the presence of family members during the survey. To improve the reliability and independence of respondents' answers, we have restricted the analytical sample to 205 married women who were surveyed alone. The distribution of districts for the women included in the analytical sample is available in Table 1.

2.1 Outcomes

We focus on a set of three socioeconomic outcome variables: (a) employment, (b) physical mobility, and (c) decision-making autonomy. First, women's current employment and employment in the last 12 months are used to measure their economic participation. Specifically, a woman's current (in the last 12 months) employment takes a value of one if she has done any work aside from her household activities during the past seven days (12 months) preceding the survey and zero otherwise.

Second, women's physical mobility is measured by their accessibility to places such as (i) grocery shops, (ii) places of worship, (iii) local health centers, (iv) places of recreation, (v) friends' or relatives' houses, and (vi) places located at short distances by train or bus. Specifically, we create a mobility index that takes a value of one if a woman can travel alone with or without permission to all six destinations, including places located at short distances by train or bus, and zero otherwise.

Third, women's decision-making autonomy is measured by their role in various decisions such as (i) cooking (what to cook or when to cook), (ii) purchasing small items (groceries), (iii) purchasing expensive items (television or fridge), (iv) purchasing land or property, (v) expenditure on a social function (marriage), (vi) women's health care, (vii) women's work (outside the home), (viii) timing of having children, and (ix) number of children the couple can have. Specifically, we create an autonomy index that takes a value of one if a woman has the sole or joint decision-making power in all nine decisions and zero otherwise.

2.2 *Covariates*

Our main explanatory variable is the husbands' migration status. The Odisha Migration Study 2023 categorizes the migration status of every household member into three groups: current migrants, return migrants, and non-migrants. Individuals are classified as current migrants if they are residing away from their village in the reference period of the last year. Notably, this classification of current migrants includes those migrants who are temporarily at home in their villages for festivals or other reasons. Individuals whose last residence differs from their residence in the village but currently residing in their village are categorized as return migrants. Those who have never left their village are categorized as non-migrants. We use this information to classify the husbands' migration status into migrants and non-migrants. Specifically, a husband's migration status takes a value of one if he is classified as a current or return migrant and zero otherwise.

We include a range of control variables, such as woman-, husband-, and household-level characteristics associated with their employment, mobility, and autonomy (Akter et al., 2024; Azra Batool et al., 2018; Banerji & Deshpande, 2021; Eswaran & Malhotra, 2011; Gupta & Yesudian, 2006; Samanta, 2020) in our regression models. Women's level characteristics include age (in years), education[2] (grades 0–3; grade 4 or higher), and marriage duration (in years). Husband-level characteristics include age (in years), education (grades 0–5; grade 6 or higher), and husband's status as the household head (yes; no). Household-level characteristics include household size (number of members), land ownership (yes; no), wealth quartile[3] (poorest; poor; rich; richest), social group (Upper Caste [UC]; Scheduled Caste [SC]; Scheduled Tribe [ST]; Other Backward Class [OBC]), and region (coastal, including Khordha district; northern, including Balangir and Subarnapur districts; southern, including Ganjam, Kalahandi, Koraput, and Nuapada districts).

---

[2] We use the median level of women's education (grade 3) and husbands' education (grade 5) to divide their respective education levels into two categories.

[3] Wealth index is constructed using Principal Component Analysis (PCA) on the ownership of 18 assets including tractor, agricultural machinery, non-agricultural machinery, four-wheeler vehicle, two-wheeler vehicle, bicycle or cycle rickshaw, basic mobile phone, smart mobile phone, color television, refrigerator, desktop computer, laptop, broadband internet connection, air conditioner, washing machine, microwave oven, radio, and bed. Following the Demographic and Health Survey approach, we further divide the wealth index into four quartiles after adjusting for sample weights and household size. Specifically, the households are categorized into poorest (quartile=1), poor (quartile=2), rich (quartile=3), and richest (quartile=4) households.

2.3 Statistical Analysis

To examine the association between wives' outcomes and husbands' migration status, we estimate the following Ordinary Least Squares[4] (OLS) regression model:

$$y_{ihr} = \beta_0 + \beta_1 \text{Migration}_i + \boldsymbol{\gamma X_{ih}} + \boldsymbol{\mu_r} + \in_{ihr} \quad (1)$$

Here, y_{ihr} denotes the status of current employment, employment in the last 12 months, mobility index, and autonomy index of woman i belonging to household h from region r, Migration$_i$ denotes the husband's migration status, X_{ih} denotes the vector of woman-, husband-, and household-level controls, μ_r indicates the region-specific dummies, and $\in_{ihr}$ is the error term that includes unobserved determinants of outcome variables. Robust standard errors are used in this analysis. Our parameter of interest is the coefficient β_1 which captures the association between the husband's migration status and the wife's current employment, employment in the last 12 months, mobility index, and autonomy index in different specifications. A positive (negative) value of β_1 indicates that the husband's migration status has a positive (negative) association with the outcome variable. To reduce the influence of confounding factors on the association between husbands' migration and wives' outcomes, we control for a range of woman, husband, and household characteristics. Region-specific dummies μ_r account for time-invariant region-level determinants of the outcome variables, including geographic characteristics such as soil type, latitude, longitude, altitude, and terrain ruggedness. Moreover, these dummies are likely to control for unobserved regional gender norms, which tend to remain stable over short periods (Afridi et al., 2025).

Next, we analyze whether the association between husbands' migration and wives' outcomes varies by woman-, husband-, and household-level characteristics using the following regression model:

$$y_{ihr} = \beta_0 + \beta_1 \text{Migration}_i + \boldsymbol{\gamma X_{ih}} + \boldsymbol{\alpha}\text{Migration}_i * \boldsymbol{X_{ih}} + \boldsymbol{\mu_r} + \in_{ihr} \quad (2)$$

Here, the husband's migration status, measured by Migration$_i$, is interacted with the vector of woman-, husband-, and household-level characteristics X_{ih} in separate specifications. The remaining variables are as described earlier in Eq. (1). The coefficient of interaction between migration status and the vector of woman-, husband-, and household-level characteristics captures the heterogeneity in the association between husbands' migration and wives' outcomes by various characteristics. Specifically, a statistically significant positive (negative) α indicates that the association between husbands' migration and wives' outcomes increases (decreases) with the increasing level of woman-, husband-, and household-level characteristics. However, it indicates the differential association for the comparison group relative to the reference group of a categorical characteristic. We compute the average marginal effect of husbands'

[4] Our results remain qualitatively unchanged with the logistic regression model. These results are available upon request.

migration across all categories of categorical characteristics, such as women's education, husbands' education, husbands' status as household head, wealth quartile, and social group. For continuous characteristics, we compute the marginal effects of husbands' migration at representative values. These characteristics include women's age, husbands' age, and household size. All analyses are conducted using Stata statistical software version 16.0 (StataCorp LLC).

3 Results

3.1 Sample Characteristics

Table 2 shows the distribution of the outcome variables, woman-, husband-, and household-level characteristics for the analytical sample as well as by the husbands' migration status. It shows that the average proportion of women who report being employed at the time of the survey is 37%, and the percentage of women who reported being employed in the last 12 months preceding the survey is 59%. Around 18% of the women report that they have the mobility to travel alone to all six destinations, while 37% report that they have some autonomy in the household decision-making of all nine decisions. Fifty-two percent have completed 0 to 3 years of education, the average age being 36.22 years, and the average duration of marriage is 16.66 years. The husbands' characteristics show that 40% are migrants[5]; their average age is 41.15 years. Thirty-two percent have completed 0 to 5 years of education, and 24% are the heads of the household. In terms of household characteristics, we find that the average household size consists of 4.69 members, and 69% of the households report the ownership of land, 27% (35%) belong to the poorest (poor) wealth category, 13% (28%) are from SC (ST) background, and 61% (31) are residing in southern (northern) region.

Compared to women married to non-migrant husbands, a higher proportion of women with migrant husbands have reported working in the past seven days {absolute difference: 32 percentage points (p.p.)} or the past 12 months (26 p.p.). They are more likely to travel alone (10 p.p.), belong to the poor wealth category (14 p.p.), have an OBC background (15 p.p.), and reside in coastal regions (7 p.p.). Additionally, women married to migrant husbands are younger (34.14 years vs. 37.63 years), have younger husbands (39.55 years vs. 42.24 years), and have completed fewer years of marriage (14.63 years vs. 18.04 years).

The distribution of the individual components of mobility and autonomy indexes is presented in Appendix Table 1. Compared to women married to non-migrant husbands, a higher proportion of women with migrant husbands can travel alone to grocery shops (12 p.p.), places of worship (11 p.p.), local health centers (15 p.p.), places of recreation (12 p.p.), friends' or relatives' houses (13 p.p.), and places

---

[5] Among the migrants, 14% are categorized as current migrants, while 26% are identified as return migrants.

Table 2 Distribution of variables of married women aged 18–49 years in 2024, Odisha

Variables	Proportion/mean				
	Overall	Migrant	Non-migrant	Difference	*p*-value
	(1)	(2)	(3)	(4)	(5)
Outcome variables					
Current employment					
Yes	0.37	0.55	0.24	0.32***	(0.00)
No	0.63	0.45	0.76	−0.32***	(0.00)
Employment in the last 12 months					
Yes	0.59	0.75	0.48	0.26***	(0.00)
No	0.41	0.25	0.52	−0.26***	(0.00)
Physical mobility index					
Yes	0.18	0.24	0.14	0.10*	(0.06)
No	0.82	0.76	0.86	−0.10*	(0.06)
Decision-making autonomy index					
Yes	0.37	0.31	0.40	−0.09	(0.20)
No	0.63	0.69	0.60	0.09	(0.20)
Main explanatory variable					
Husband's migration status					
Migrant	0.40	1.00	0.00		
Non-migrant	0.60	0.00	1.00		
Woman's characteristics					
Age (in years)	36.22	34.14	37.63	−3.49***	(0.00)
Education (grades)					
0–3	0.52	0.54	0.51	0.03	(0.63)
4 or higher	0.48	0.46	0.49	−0.03	(0.63)
Marriage duration (in years)	16.66	14.63	18.04	−3.41***	(0.00)
Husband's characteristics					
Age (in years)	41.15	39.55	42.24	−2.68**	(0.04)
Education (grades)					
0–5	0.32	0.29	0.34	−0.06	(0.41)
6 or higher	0.68	0.71	0.66	0.06	(0.41)
Household head					
Yes	0.24	0.27	0.23	0.04	(0.56)
No	0.76	0.73	0.77	−0.04	(0.56)
Household characteristics					
Household size	4.69	4.53	4.80	−0.26	(0.28)
Land ownership					
Yes	0.69	0.75	0.66	0.09	(0.17)

(continued)

Table 2 (continued)

Variables	Proportion/mean				
	Overall	Migrant	Non-migrant	Difference	p-value
	(1)	(2)	(3)	(4)	(5)
No	0.31	0.25	0.34	−0.09	(0.17)
Wealth quartiles					
Poorest	0.27	0.20	0.31	−0.11*	(0.09)
Poor	0.35	0.43	0.30	0.14**	(0.04)
Rich	0.22	0.28	0.19	0.09	(0.14)
Richest	0.16	0.08	0.20	−0.12**	(0.02)
Social group					
SC	0.13	0.13	0.12	0.01	(0.84)
ST	0.28	0.19	0.34	−0.14**	(0.02)
OBC	0.55	0.64	0.48	0.15**	(0.03)
UC	0.05	0.04	0.06	−0.02	(0.49)
Region					
Coastal	0.08	0.04	0.11	−0.07*	(0.07)
Northern	0.31	0.33	0.30	0.02	(0.74)
Southern	0.61	0.64	0.59	0.05	(0.49)
Observations	205	83	122	205	

*** $p < 0.01$, ** $p < 0.05$, * $p < 0.1$

located at a short distance (16 p.p.). Additionally, women with migrant husbands exhibit greater decision-making power for their healthcare (10 p.p.).

3.2 Regression Analysis

The average marginal effects (AMEs) of the husband's migration status for each of the four outcomes are presented in Figs. 1 and 2. The first specification shows the raw differences in outcomes due to the husband's migration status (Unadjusted Specification). Next, we include the vector of woman-, husband-, and household-level characteristics to reduce the influence of these confounding variables in the second specification (Adjusted Specification).

The findings based on the crude specification reflect large and significant positive associations between employment outcomes and the husbands' migration status (Fig. 1). Specifically, women married to migrant husbands seem to be more likely to engage in current employment (AME, 0.32; 95% CI, 0.18–0.49) and employment in the last 12 months (AME, 0.26; 95% CI, 0.13–0.39) than women married to non-migrant husbands. The findings from the second specification indicate that the

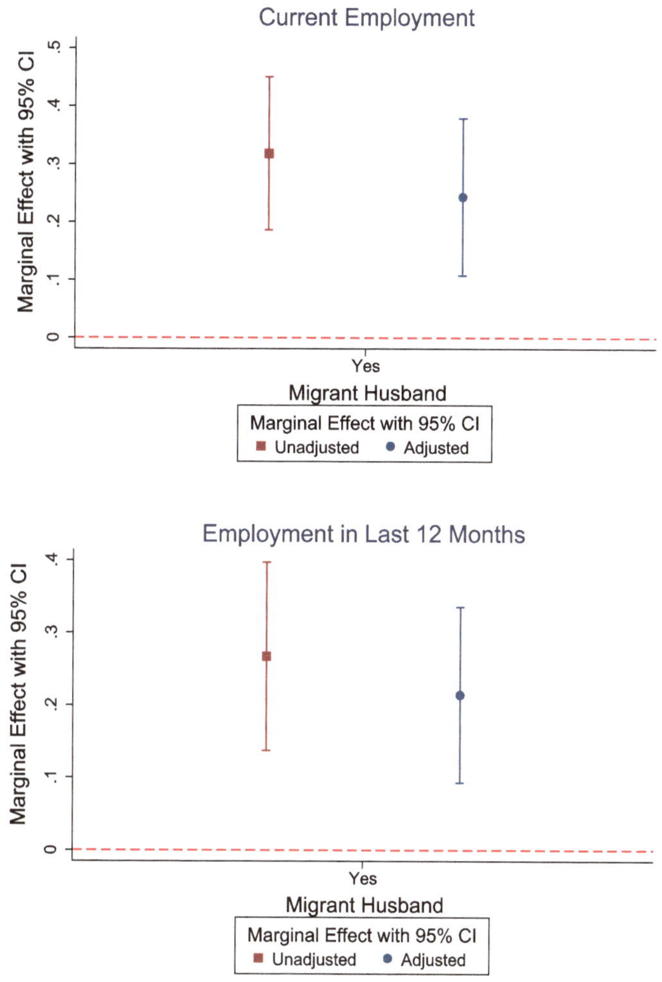

Fig. 1 Average marginal effects of husbands' migration on wives' employment

vector of woman-, husband-, and household-level characteristics explains a significant proportion of the association between employment outcomes and husbands' migration status. However, the positive associations persist for both the outcome variables: current employment (AME, 0.24; 95% CI, 0.11–0.38) and employment in the last 12 months (AME, 0.21; 95% CI, 0.09–0.34).

Cultural norms deeply rooted in Indian society perpetuate the idea of male dominance within the institution of marriage. Male migration often alters the distribution of workload within households (Burki, 1984), leading to the increased necessity for left-behind women to engage in economic activities. At the same time, this shift could be interpreted as a form of women's economic empowerment, particularly if

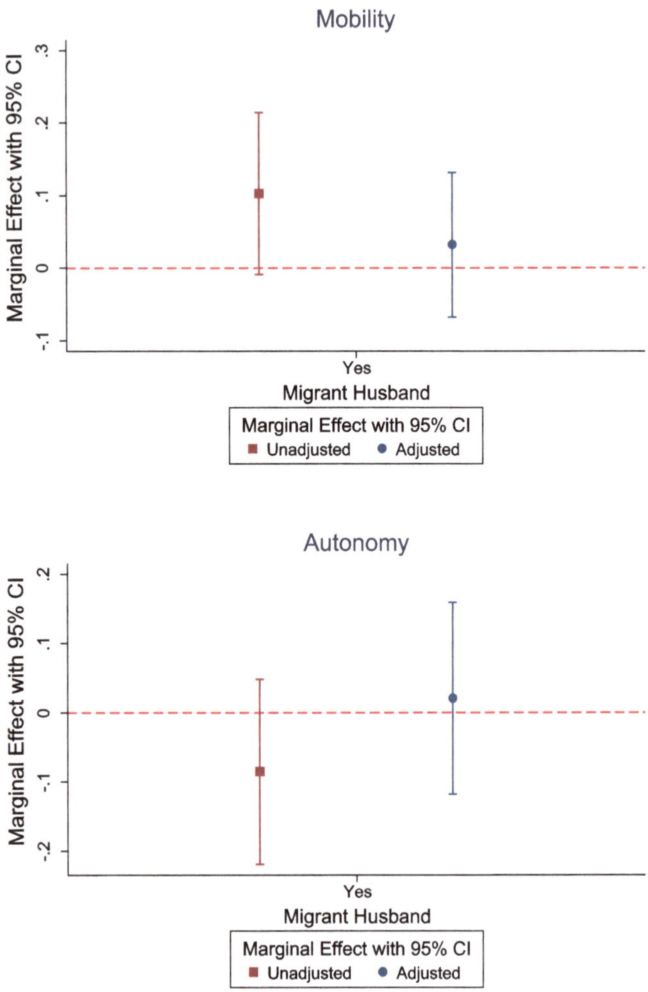

Fig. 2 Average marginal effects of husbands' migration on wives' physical mobility and decision-making autonomy

it enables them to gain control over their income. However, caution is warranted when drawing such conclusions. Pattnaik et al. (2018) highlight the potential risk of women's marginalization when their increased labor force participation occurs predominantly in agriculture, a sector where the viability as a sustainable livelihood source is steadily declining. Moreover, the rise in women's economic engagement is unlikely to substantially enhance their economic status if it is confined to low-skilled informal jobs. A tabulation of the type of occupations among left-behind wives in our analytical sample indicates that over 70% of those who reported working in the last seven days are employed in either the agricultural or construction sector.

The results of the regressions that examine the association between women's mobility index and husbands' migration status are presented in Fig. 2. The coefficients of migration status based on the adjusted and unadjusted specifications indicate a positive association between women's mobility index and husbands' migration status. However, both the associations are statistically insignificant. Figure 2 also shows the estimates of the association between women's autonomy index and husbands' migration. The results based on the unadjusted specification indicate a negative association between women's autonomy index and husbands' migration. We observe a positive association between the two after mutual adjustment for controls in the adjusted specification. However, none of the associations are statistically significant.

3.3 Heterogeneity Analysis

Limited evidence exists on the determinants that may influence the relationship between husbands' migration status and women's empowerment. Specifically, it remains unclear whether the finding of a statistically insignificant association between husbands' migration status and women's mobility or autonomy indexes holds across different subgroups. These include younger and older women, women with varying levels of education, women married to husbands with different educational backgrounds, women whose husbands are household heads or not, those in smaller or larger households, and women from different wealth and social groups. To address this, we examine the heterogeneity in the association between husbands' migration status and women's outcomes by analyzing subgroups based on women's age, education, husbands' education, household headship status, household size, wealth category, and social group, using the model specified in Eq. (2). The AMEs of the husbands' migration status for various outcome variables are presented in Figs. 3, 4, 5, and 6.

In line with the overall positive association between husbands' migration and women's current employment (Fig. 1), we observe a statistically significant positive association across a range of subgroups (Fig. 3). These subgroups include both younger and older women, women with lower and higher levels of education, those married to less educated as well as more educated husbands, women whose husbands are household heads or not, those in smaller households, women from both poor and rich wealth category households, and those belonging to ST or OBC backgrounds. The associations among other subgroups, including the oldest age cohort (48 years old), poorest or richest wealth category households, and SC background, are also positive. However, none of these associations is statistically significant.

In Fig. 4, we present the results of the association between husbands' migration and women's employment in the last 12 months across various subgroups. Like current employment, we find a statistically significant positive association for both younger and older women, women with lower and higher levels of education, those

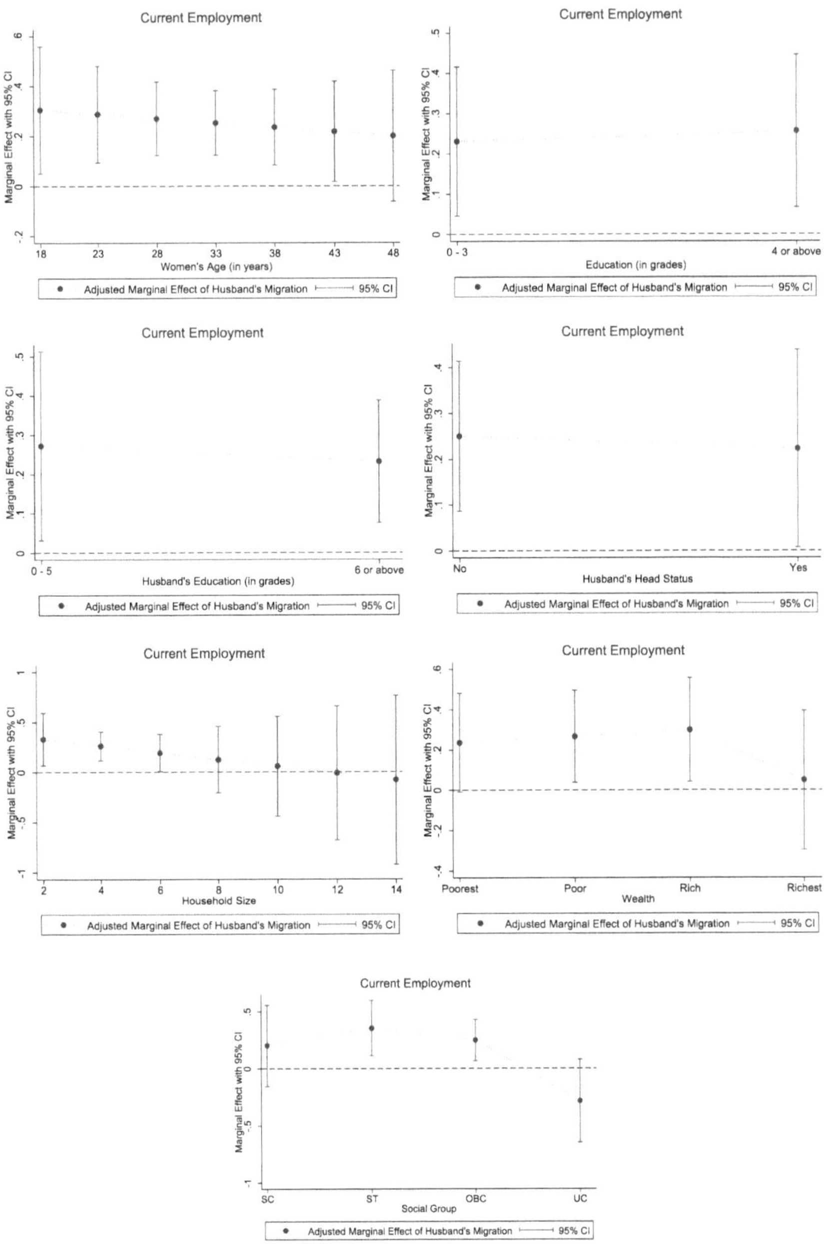

Fig. 3 Heterogeneity analysis: average marginal effects of husbands' migration on wives' current employment

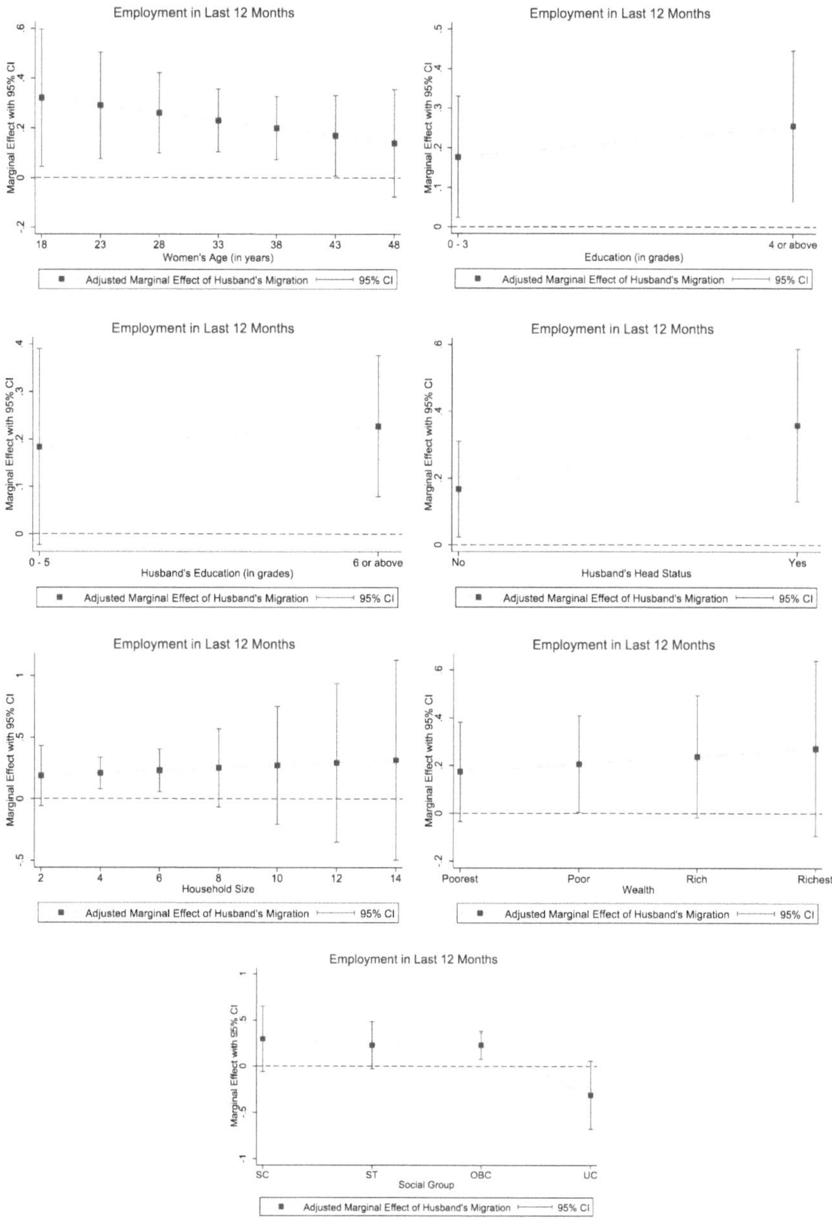

Fig. 4 Heterogeneity analysis: average marginal effects of husbands' migration on wives' employment in the last 12 months

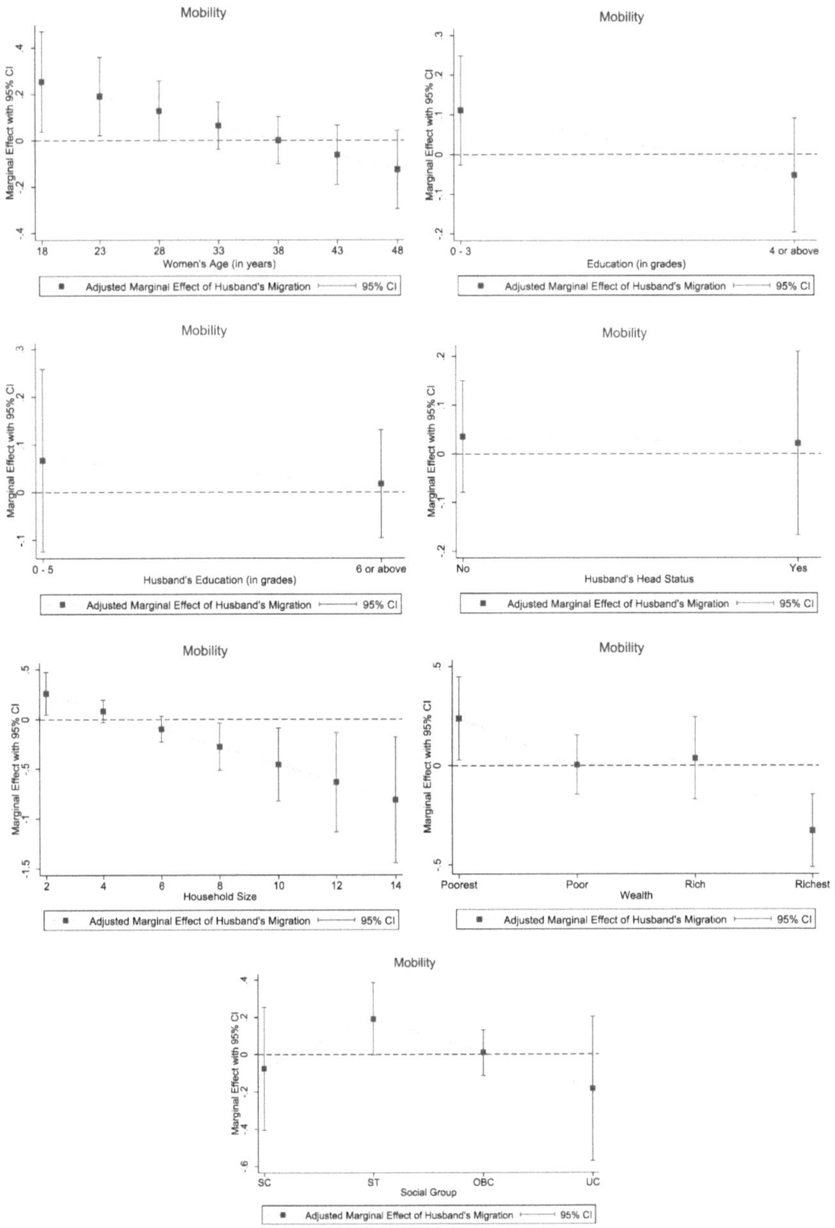

Fig. 5 Heterogeneity analysis: average marginal effects of husbands' migration on wives' physical mobility

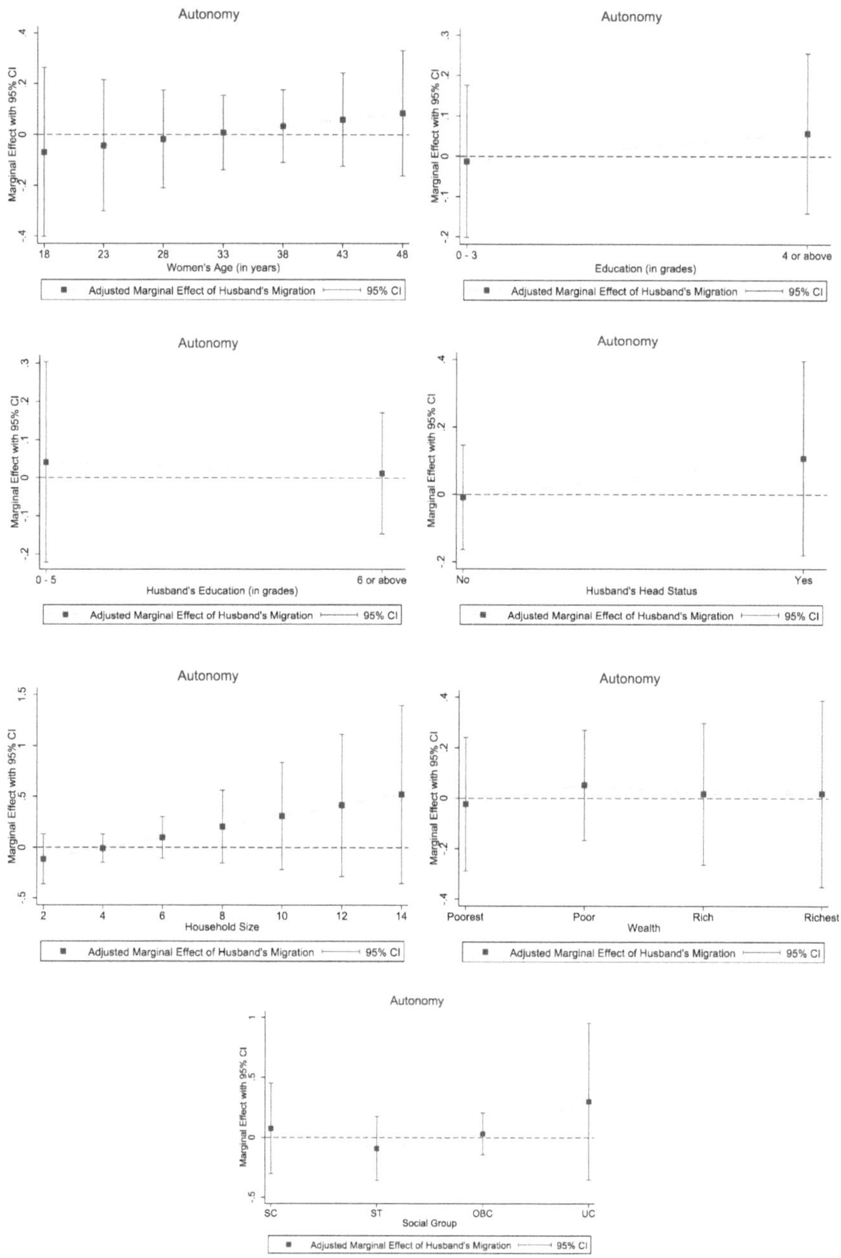

Fig. 6 Heterogeneity analysis: average marginal effects of husbands' migration on wives' decision-making autonomy

married to more educated husbands, women whose husbands are household heads or not, smaller households, women from poorer wealth category households, and those belonging to the OBC background. The associations for other subgroups, however, remain statistically insignificant.

Next, we explore whether the statistically insignificant relationship between husbands' migration and women's mobility index differs by various characteristics (Fig. 5). The association becomes statistically significant and positive among younger women, smaller households, the poorest wealth category households, and women from ST backgrounds. Conversely, we observe a negative relationship among women from larger households and the richest wealth category households. While some women seem to experience enhanced mobility because of their husbands' migration, others do not see significant changes in their ability to move freely. This finding underscores the complexity of women's mobility in the context of the husbands' migration and the conflicting dynamics that come into play.

On the one hand, the out-migration of husbands tends to increase the mobility of left-behind wives as they take on additional responsibilities that their husbands previously managed. This shift in household roles may necessitate increased movement to fulfill economic or social obligations. However, this enhanced mobility might also be closely monitored by extended family members or the community (Kaur, 2022), aiming to limit any unwarranted interactions with other men. Such social surveillance can significantly constrain their freedom and generate a sense of discomfort or unease (McEvoy et al., 2012).

The tension between increased responsibilities and social monitoring suggests that although some women gain greater mobility, they are simultaneously restricted by the norms and expectations of their community. The possibility of facing scrutiny or moral judgment due to their enhanced mobility might pressure these women to limit their movements strictly to essential activities, avoiding social or recreational outings such as visits to parks, cinemas, or friends' homes. This social policing effectively curtails their overall mobility.

Younger women (Bever, 2002), those in smaller households, from the poorest wealth categories, or ST backgrounds (Maharatna, 2000; Mitra, 2008) may experience fewer social barriers or a greater capacity to navigate these challenges. These groups of women might not be as constrained by societal norms or may have developed strategies to cope with the restrictions imposed by their community, thereby displaying a higher likelihood of mobility following their husbands' migration. In contrast, women who do not belong to these subgroups might experience heightened restrictions on their movements due to intensified surveillance and pressure from family or community members. The association between husbands' migration and mobility remains non-existent for these women.

Figure 6 presents the heterogeneity in associations between husbands' migration and wives' autonomy. While positive and negative associations are observed across various subgroups, none are statistically significant. Contrary to earlier findings (Desai & Banerji, 2008; Fakir & Abedin, 2021; Hadi, 2001; Lei & Desai, 2021; Paris et al., 2005; Yabiku et al., 2010), our analysis shows no significant association between husbands' migration and the decision-making autonomy of left-behind wives. This result aligns with the nature of migration observed in the current context, where data indicates that the average migration duration over the last year was under six months. According to Cagliani et al. (2023), husbands often retain decision-making roles despite their physical absence due to short-term migration. This finding suggests that short-term or seasonal migration, driven by limited agricultural and non-agricultural income opportunities (Mitra & Pradhan, 2016; Sharma & Ali, 2014), is unlikely to challenge or alter entrenched gender norms and patriarchal structures that shape household power dynamics. Ram Mohan et al. (2023) points out that these regressive norms continue to dictate household decision-making practices, limiting opportunities for left-behind wives to exercise autonomy.

It is crucial to underscore that this study does not establish causal relationships between husbands' migration and the socioeconomic outcomes of left-behind wives. Instead, our findings provide valuable insights into a complex issue through descriptive analysis. Additionally, caution should be exercised in generalizing these findings beyond the context of this study. The data used here is drawn exclusively from high-migration localities within seven districts in Odisha. As a result, the findings may not reflect the experiences of left-behind wives in other regions or contexts with different migration patterns or socioeconomic characteristics.

4 Conclusion

Our results show that the relationship between husbands' migration and socioeconomic outcomes of left-behind wives is not straightforward. On the one hand, husbands' migration seems to improve the likelihood of employment for women whose husbands are migrants. Moreover, male migration is associated with higher mobility among left-behind wives who are young, belong to smaller households, the poorest wealth category households, and from ST backgrounds. On the other hand, the out-migration of males fails to bring any change in the decision-making autonomy of left-behind wives. In line with Menjívar and Agadjanian (2007), our findings emphasize that the relationship between male migration and outcomes of left-behind wives is complex and cannot be easily characterized in a single direction.

Our findings based on participation in work are plausible given the current context, where husbands' migration due to poverty and distress forces left-behind wives to engage in low-skilled jobs in order to support their families while their husbands are away. This finding suggests that in the absence of opportunities for skill development and access to formal employment, the economic gains from male migration might remain limited and potentially reinforce rather than alleviate gender inequalities in the labor market. The findings related to physical mobility indicate that the association between husbands' migration and left-behind wives' mobility is contingent on many factors, including household composition, socioeconomic status, and social group affiliation. The differential experiences among these subgroups suggest that while some women seem to gain greater independence and mobility, others remain trapped by traditional norms that restrict their freedom of movement, even in the absence of their husbands. Moreover, the anticipated shift in women's autonomy in response to husbands' migration remains elusive due to the short-term nature of husbands' migration. These findings underscore the complex interaction between migration and household power dynamics and illustrate the need to consider the broader social and economic context when estimating the relationship between husbands' migration and left-behind wives' socioeconomic outcomes.

Acknowledgements I am grateful to Amrita Datta for her valuable comments and suggestions to improve this manuscript. I am also thankful to Shreemoyee Saha and Sunny Shankar Ladkat for their research assistance.

Appendix

See Appendix Table 1.

Appendix Table 1 Distribution of individual components of mobility and autonomy indexes of married women aged 18–49 years in 2024, Odisha

Varibles	Proportion				
	Overall	Migrant	Non-migrant	Difference	*p*-value
	(1)	(2)	(3)	(4)	(5)
Physical mobility					
Grocery shop	0.75	0.82	0.70	0.12**	(0.05)
Places of worship	0.73	0.80	0.69	0.11*	(0.09)
Local health centers	0.44	0.53	0.38	0.15**	(0.03)
Places of recreation	0.20	0.27	0.15	0.12**	(0.04)
Friends' or relatives' houses	0.77	0.84	0.71	0.13**	(0.03)
Places located at short distances	0.32	0.41	0.25	0.16**	(0.02)
Index (all the places)	0.18	0.24	0.14	0.10*	(0.06)
Decision-making autonomy					
Cooking	0.91	0.93	0.90	0.03	(0.52)
Purchasing small items (grocery)	0.56	0.58	0.54	0.04	(0.60)
Purchasing expensive items (TV)	0.50	0.43	0.54	−0.11	(0.13)
Purchasing land/property	0.49	0.43	0.52	−0.09	(0.20)
Expenditure on social event	0.61	0.57	0.65	−0.08	(0.24)
Women's healthcare	0.88	0.94	0.84	0.10**	(0.04)
Women's work (outside home)	0.83	0.83	0.83	0.00	(0.95)
Timing of having children	0.93	0.95	0.92	0.03	(0.35)
Number of children	0.93	0.96	0.91	0.05	(0.13)
Index (all the decisions)	0.37	0.31	0.40	−0.09	(0.20)
Observations	205	83	122	205	

*** $p < 0.01$, ** $p < 0.05$, * $p < 0.1$

References

Afridi, F., Dhillon, A., Roy, S., & Sangwan, N. (2025). Social networks, gender norms and women's labor supply: Experimental evidence using a job search platform, QBS Working Paper, No. 2025/02, Queen's University Belfast, Queen's Business School, Belfast. https://www.econstor.eu/bitstream/10419/313325/1/wps2025-02.pdf

Akter, S., Hosen, Md. S., Khan, Md. S., & Pal, B. (2024). Assessing the pattern of key factors on women's empowerment in Bangladesh: Evidence from Bangladesh Demographic and Health Survey, 2007 to 2017–18. *PLOS ONE, 19*(3), Article e0301501. https://doi.org/10.1371/journal.pone.0301501

Azra Batool, S., Ahmed, H. K., & Qureshi, S. N. (2018). Impact of demographic variables on women's economic empowerment: An ordered probit model. *Journal of Women & Aging, 30*(1), 6–26. https://doi.org/10.1080/08952841.2016.1256734

Banerji, M., & Deshpande, A. S. (2021). Does 'love' make a difference? Marriage choice and post-marriage decision-making power in India. *Asian Population Studies, 17*(2), 201–220. https://doi.org/10.1080/17441730.2020.1852713

Bever, S. W. (2002). Migration and the transformation of gender roles and hierarchies in Yucatan. *Urban Anthropology and Studies of Cultural Systems and World Economic Development, 31*(2), 199–230.

Binzel, C., & Assaad, R. (2011). Egyptian men working abroad: Labour supply responses by the women left behind. *Labour Economics, 18*, S98–S114. https://doi.org/10.1016/j.labeco.2011.03.002

Burki, S. J. (1984). International migration: Implications for labor exporting countries. *Middle East Journal, 38*(4), 668–684.

Cagliani, F., Mazzucato, V., & Fourie, E. (2023). Women's social resilience in the context of male out-migration in Dehradun district. *India. Asian and Pacific Migration Journal, 32*(4), 798–820. https://doi.org/10.1177/01171968241228303

Census of India. (2011). *Census of India*. Office of the Registrar General and Census Commissioner, Government of India.

Datta, A., & Mishra, S. K. (2011). Glimpses of women's lives in rural Bihar: Impact of male migration. *The Indian Journal of Labour Economics, 54*(3), 457–477.

De, S. (2019, December 18). Internal migration in India grows, but inter-state movements remain low [WORLDBANK.ORG]. *World Bank Blogs*. Retrieved October 5, 2024, from https://blogs.worldbank.org/en/peoplemove/internal-migration-india-grows-inter-state-movements-remain-low#:~:text=Internal%20Migration%20in%20India%20Grows%2C%20But%20Inter%2DState%20Movements%20Remain%20Low,-Supriyo%20De%20December&text=Internal%20migration%2C%20the%20movement%20of,where%20they%20are%20better%20utilized

De Haas, H., & Van Rooij, A. (2010). Migration as emancipation? The impact of internal and international migration on the position of women left behind in rural Morocco. *Oxford Development Studies, 38*(1), 43–62. https://doi.org/10.1080/13600810903551603

Desai, S., & Banerji, M. (2008). Negotiated identities: Male migration and left-behind wives in India. *Journal of Population Research, 25*(3), 337–355. https://doi.org/10.1007/BF03033894

Duflo, E. (2012). Women empowerment and economic development. *Journal of Economic Literature, 50*(4), 1051–1079.

Eswaran, M., & Malhotra, N. (2011). Domestic violence and women's autonomy in developing countries: Theory and evidence. *Canadian Journal of Economics/Revue Canadienne d'économique, 44*(4), 1222–1263. https://doi.org/10.1111/j.1540-5982.2011.01673.x

Fakir, A. M. S., & Abedin, N. (2021). Empowered by absence: Does male out-migration empower female household heads left behind? *Journal of International Migration and Integration, 22*(2), 503–527. https://doi.org/10.1007/s12134-019-00754-0

Ghimire, D., Zhang, Y., & Williams, N. (2021). Husbands' migration: Increased burden on or more autonomy for wives left behind? *Journal of Ethnic and Migration Studies, 47*(1), 227–248. https://doi.org/10.1080/1369183X.2019.1675502

Goulart, C. M., Purewal, A., Nakhuda, H., Ampadu, A., Giancola, A., Kortenaar, J.-L., & Bassani, D. G. (2021). Tools for measuring gender equality and women's empowerment (GEWE) indicators in humanitarian settings. *Conflict and Health, 15*(1), 39. https://doi.org/10.1186/s13031-021-00373-6

Green, S. H., Wang, C., Ballakrishnen, S. S., Brueckner, H., & Bearman, P. (2019). Patterned remittances enhance women's health-related autonomy. *SSM - Population Health, 9*, Article 100370. https://doi.org/10.1016/j.ssmph.2019.100370

Gulati, L. (1987). Coping with male migration. *Economic and Political Weekly, 22*(44), WS41–WS46.

Gunnarsson, B. (2011). The influence of male migration on female resources, independence, and development in Gambian villages. *Gender & Development, 19*(1), 115–128. https://doi.org/10.1080/13552074.2011.554031

Gupta, K., & Yesudian, P. P. (2006). Evidence of women's empowerment in India: A study of socio-spatial disparities. *GeoJournal, 65*(4), 365–380. https://doi.org/10.1007/s10708-006-7556-z

Hadi, A. (2001). International migration and the change of women's position among left behind in rural Bangladesh. *International Journal of Population Geography, 7*(1), 53–61.

Heller, A., & Kaushik, A. (2020). The consequences of husband's international migration on family left-behind in Tamil Nadu, India. *Journal of International Migration and Integration, 21*(4), 1149–1163. https://doi.org/10.1007/s12134-019-00705-9

Hondagneu-Sotelo, P. (1992). Overcoming patriarchal constraints: the reconstruction of gender relations among Mexican immigrant women and men. *Gender & Society, 6*(3), 393–415.

International Institute for Population Sciences (IIPS), & ICF. (2021). *National family health survey (NFHS-5), 2019–21: India.* Retrieved May 10, 2024, from https://dhsprogram.com/pubs/pdf/FR375/FR375.pdf

Jetley, S. (1987). Impact of male migration on rural females. *Economic and Political Weekly, 22*(44). WS47–WS53.

Kaur, A. P. (2018). International migration and impact of remittances on left behind wives: A case study of the Doaba region of Punjab. In S. I. Rajan & N. Neetha (Eds.), *Migration, gender and care economy* (1st ed.). Routledge. https://doi.org/10.4324/9780429426704-7/international-migration-impact-remittances-left-behind-wives-atinder-pal-kaur

Kaur, A. P. (2022). Migration, a road to empowerment? Agency, resources, and the left behind women in Punjab, India. *Asian Journal of Women's Studies, 28*(2), 167–185. https://doi.org/10.1080/12259276.2022.2052595

Khan, A. G., West, H., Razzaque, A., & Kuhn, R. (2023). The effects of spousal migration on perinatal healthcare utilization. *BMC Pregnancy and Childbirth, 23*(1), 434. https://doi.org/10.1186/s12884-023-05590-w

Khan, M. I., & Valatheeswaran C. (2016). International migration, remittances and labour force participation of left-behind family members: A study of Kerala. *Margin: The Journal of Applied Economic Research, 10*(1), 86–118. https://doi.org/10.1177/0973801015612669

Koirala, S. (2023). Empowering absence? Assessing the impact of transnational male out-migration on left behind wives. *Social Sciences, 12*(2), 80. https://doi.org/10.3390/socsci12020080

Lei, L., & Desai, S. (2021). Male out-migration and the health of left-behind wives in India: The roles of remittances, household responsibilities, and autonomy. *Social Science & Medicine, 280*, Article 113982. https://doi.org/10.1016/j.socscimed.2021.113982

Lokshin, M., & Glinskaya, E. (2009). The effect of male migration on employment patterns of women in Nepal. *The World Bank Economic Review, 23*(3), 481–507. https://doi.org/10.1093/wber/lhp011

Luna, S. S., & Rahman, M. M. (2019). Migrant wives: Dynamics of the empowerment process. *Migration and Development, 8*(3), 320–337. https://doi.org/10.1080/21632324.2018.1520446

Maharatna, A. (2000). Fertility, mortality and gender bias among tribal population: An Indian perspective. *Social Science & Medicine, 50*, 1333–1351.

McAuliffe, M., & Oucho, L. A. (2024). *World Migration Report 2024.* United Nations. Retrieved November 17, 2024, from https://publications.iom.int/books/world-migration-report-2024

McEvoy, J., Petrzelka, P., Radel, C., & Schmook, B. (2012). Gendered mobility and morality in a South-eastern Mexican community: Impacts of male labour migration on the women left behind. *Mobilities, 7*(3), 369–388. https://doi.org/10.1080/17450101.2012.655977

Mendola, M., & Carletto, C. (2012). Migration and gender differences in the home labour market: Evidence from Albania. *Labour Economics, 19*(6), 870–880. https://doi.org/10.1016/j.labeco.2012.08.009

Menjívar, C., & Agadjanian, V. (2007). Men's migration and women's lives: Views from rural Armenia and Guatemala*. *Social Science Quarterly, 88*(5), 1243–1262. https://doi.org/10.1111/j.1540-6237.2007.00501.x

Mitra, A. (2008). The status of women among the scheduled tribes in India. *The Journal of Socio-Economics, 37*(3), 1202–1217. https://doi.org/10.1016/j.socec.2006.12.077

Mitra, A., & Pradhan, B. K. (2016). *Migration, remittances, and changing patterns of livelihood: Evidence from Western Odisha villages* (p. 363). University of Delhi Enclave.

Mohan, R. R., Puskur, R., Chandrasekar, D., & Valera, H. G. A. (2023). Do gender dynamics in intra-household decision making shift with male migration? Evidence from rice-farming households in Eastern India. *Gender, Technology and Development, 27*(2), 157–183. https://doi.org/10.1080/09718524.2022.2140381

Mu, R., & Van De Walle, D. (2011). Left behind to farm? Women's labor re-allocation in rural China. *Labour Economics, 18*, S83–S97. https://doi.org/10.1016/j.labeco.2011.01.009

Paris, T., Singh, A., Luis, J., & Hossain, M. (2005). Labour outmigration, livelihood of rice farming households and women left behind: A case study in Eastern Uttar Pradesh. *Economic and Political Weekly, 40*(25), 2522–2529.

Pattnaik, I., Lahiri-Dutt, K., Lockie, S., & Pritchard, B. (2018). The feminization of agriculture or the feminization of agrarian distress? Tracking the trajectory of women in agriculture in India. *Journal of the Asia Pacific Economy, 23*(1), 138–155. https://doi.org/10.1080/13547860.2017.1394569

Priya, P., Venkatesh, A., & Shukla, A. (2021). Two decades of theorising and measuring women's empowerment: Literature review and future research agenda. *Women's Studies International Forum, 87*, Article 102495. https://doi.org/10.1016/j.wsif.2021.102495

Rodriguez, E. R., & Tiongson, E. R. (2001). Temporary migration overseas and household labor supply: Evidence from urban Philippines. *International Migration Review, 35*(3), 709–725. https://doi.org/10.1111/j.1747-7379.2001.tb00037.x

Samanta, T. (2020). Women's empowerment as self-compassion?: Empirical observations from India. *PLOS ONE, 15*(5), Article e0232526. https://doi.org/10.1371/journal.pone.0232526

Senapati, A. K., & Ojha, K. (2019). Socio-economic empowerment of women through micro-entrepreneurship: Evidence from Odisha. *India. International Journal of Rural Management, 15*(2), 159–184. https://doi.org/10.1177/0973005219866588

Sharma, S., & Ali, Z. (2014). Migration trends from coastal and Western Odisha: A study of migration incidence and issues. In *Studies, stories, and canvas: Seasonal labor migration and migrant workers from Odisha.*

Singh, K. (2024, May 6). How India moves: Understanding patterns of migration within the country. *The Wire*. Retrieved October 5, 2024, from https://thewire.in/urban/how-india-moves-understanding-patterns-of-migration-within-the-country

Singh, R. (2018). Impact of male out-migration on women left behind: A study of two villages in Uttar Pradesh. *Remittances Review, 3*(1), 75–92. https://doi.org/10.33182/rr.v3i1.427

Singh, R. (2022). Origin of world's largest migrant population, India seeks to leverage immigration. *Migration Policy Institute*. Retrieved October 5, 2024, from https://www.migrationpolicy.org/article/india-migration-country-profile

Sinha, B., Jha, S., & Negi, N. S. (2012). Migration and empowerment: The experience of women in households in India where migration of a husband has occurred. *Journal of Gender Studies, 21*(1), 61–76. https://doi.org/10.1080/09589236.2012.639551

Tripathy, S. N. (2021). Distress migration among ultra-poor households in Western Odisha. *Journal of Land and Rural Studies, 9*(2), 241–256. https://doi.org/10.1177/23210249211001975

Yabiku, S. T., Agadjanian, V., & Sevoyan, A. (2010). Husbands' labour migration and wives' autonomy, Mozambique 2000–2006. *Population Studies, 64*(3), 293–306. https://doi.org/10.1080/00324728.2010.510200

Zachariah, K. C., Mathew, E. T., & Rajan, S. I. (2001). Social, economic and demographic consequences of migration on Kerala. *International Migration, 39*(2), 43–71. https://doi.org/10.1111/1468-2435.00149

Chapter 11
Migration, Gender, and Well-Being: Perspectives of "Left-Behind" Women

Shubha Ranganathan, Jayaprakash Mishra, and Muhammed Thwoyyib K. P.

Abstract Drawing on qualitative research comprising semi-structured in-depth interviews and focus group discussions with women from migrant and non-migrant households in Kalahandi and Balangir districts of Odisha, this study explores their multifaceted experiences. The chapter particularly examines their experiences surrounding work, livelihood, health, and family dynamics in the context of migration. The necessity of migration emerges as a coping mechanism in the face of failed public employment schemes and precarious working conditions at destinations. Moreover, the research sheds light on the interconnectedness of migration and increased care responsibilities, especially in the absence of male members in the family, impacting women's access to resources, including healthcare services. It shows the dearth of institutionalized medical facilities, chronic health issues, and the trivialization of health problems among women, accentuated by the absence of state support. Furthermore, our analysis explores the drivers of migration—from economic deprivation to aspirations among young individuals. It also delves into the dynamics of care work within households and the social bonds formed among women due to shared experiences in migrant households. Ultimately, this chapter underscores the intricate intersection of migration, family, health, and livelihood, encapsulating the textured lived realities of women in these migration-prone regions.

Keywords Migration · Gender · Care work · Feminization of agriculture · Left-behind women · Odisha

S. Ranganathan (✉)
Department of Liberal Arts, Indian Institute of Technology Hyderabad, Kandi, Sangareddy, India
e-mail: shubha@la.iith.ac.in

J. Mishra
Thapar School of Liberal Arts and Sciences, Thapar Institute of Engineering and Technology, Patiala, India

Muhammed Thwoyyib K. P.
BML Munjal University, Gurugram, India

A. Datta and S. I. Rajan (eds.), *Migration, Livelihoods and Gender*, International Perspectives on Migration, https://doi.org/10.1007/978-981-95-5465-2_11

1 Introduction and Background

Migration research has heavily focused on male migrants, with a lack of sufficient engagement with women's perspectives and roles in migration. Scholars have drawn attention to the need for adequate engagement with gender through research in two streams: (1) research on women migrants and (2) research on women "left behind". In the case of the former, researchers have pointed out that while the female migration research has largely concentrated on marriage migration—given that it is the single most dominant reason for women's migration—women are also often engaged in intermittent migration beyond marriage migration (Ramamurthy, 2024).

Examples of intermittent female migration patterns include: left-behind women who "follow" their husbands; married women who run away from violent households to the city or their natal villages; single women who run away with a lover and then return to the natal village; and other such kinds of movements that are often not tapped in the conventional research on migration. Priti Ramamurthy (2024) highlights that such intermittent migration patterns are an important reflection of the creativity and agency of women who seek to secure their well-being in relation to the spousal or familial unit.

Research on women "left behind" has typically sought to understand how male out-migration impacts women's empowerment and well-being.[1] Studies have found that the impact of male out-migration on women's economic outcomes is either positive or negative, depending on the circumstances. On the one hand, some research has found that following male out-migration, women are likely to gain in authority and decision-making power (Findley & Williams, 1991). Kumar (2023) found that male out-migration led to an increase in female political engagement with the state, as women became more mobile and involved with the public sphere, accessing information and contributing to discussions in the household. Their access to financial resources also increases. At the same time, Kumar (2023) is careful to point out that these gains in mobility and decision-making are contextual, as male out-migration does not fundamentally change the patriarchal status quo: The moment their husbands return, women's agency and mobility are negatively affected. This is particularly important given the fact that much of this male out-migration is circular, as research on internal labor migration in India has largely documented (see e.g., Das & Sahu, 2019; Datta, 2018; Kumar, 2020). Ultimately, Kumar (2023) argues that there are important shifts in household dynamics with respect to gender, initiated by male out-migration. Other evidence has also found that male out-migration in agricultural contexts can lead to empowerment in some domains, though this is context-specific (World Bank Group & FAO, 2018).

At the same time, research has pointed to the negative effects of male out-migration on the health and well-being of women left behind. With male out-migration, left-behind women are often beset with increased responsibilities in farm labor and

[1] Interestingly, some, like Rajput and Bureau (2024), have critiqued the use of the term 'left-behind'. This term assumes that women should naturally accompany men and ties up their identity with male spouses rather than with their own ties to the village and the land.

household work, resulting in changes in the rural landscape. Studies have found an increase in the workload and stress for women left behind (e.g., Prati et al., 2022; Roy & Nangia, 2005), added responsibilities for women along with limited gains in autonomy and decision-making (Lei & Desai, 2021), and greater involvement of the extended family (Jolly et al., 2003). Sinha et al. (2012) analyzed the survey data from the third round of the National Family Health Survey (NFHS-3) and found that male out-migration has not resulted in improvements in women's empowerment with respect to decision-making. In addition, benefits in terms of women's autonomy and decision-making are related to household dynamics, such as whether they are living in extended or nuclear families (see, e.g., Desai & Banerji, 2008).

Jain (2020) points out that according to the India Human Development Survey (IHDS), over 4.5% of women in rural areas and 1.5% in urban areas have husbands living elsewhere. With their migrant husbands away, women's involvement in and responsibility for both farm labor and household work intensify. But without a concomitant increase in farm holdings, inheritance rights, or land rights, this feminization of agriculture only means that their unpaid care labor is compounded. Some global estimates indicate that women are responsible for 75% of unpaid care and domestic work (da Silva, 2023). Yet, women left behind, as well as single migrant women, are rarely the beneficiaries of welfare programs and migration policies, which tend to focus largely on male migrants (Rajan et al., 2020).

1.1 Understanding Women's Well-Being: Lived Experiences of Women Left Behind

In the migration literature, conventionally, much of the focus has been on male migration streams, including their living and work conditions at the destination sites. Scholars have elaborated on the challenges that migrant workers face in relation to precarious livelihoods, exploitative work conditions, and an uncertain labor market (e.g., Das & Sahu, 2019). The vulnerability and plight of internal migrants also came under the spotlight during the COVID-19 pandemic (Rajan et al., 2020).

Rai (2020) points to the lack of sufficient data on women and children left behind. It is this gap that our study seeks to fill. In looking at the lives of the women who are left behind, research has often focused on the question of whether the absence of male members in the source/destination brings about an increase in the status of women, as they take on more responsibilities at the home front. For instance, Rai (2020) argues that male out-migration does not really bring about empowerment for women left behind and that they still remain in the "clutches of patriarchy" (p. 420). Yet, such perspectives presume that structural changes in the status of women would be brought about by male out-migration, when, in fact, women's empowerment is a far more complex phenomenon. Further, many studies measure empowerment in terms of decision-making and conclude that since men are still largely involved in the decision-making, their absence does not really result in women's empowerment.

At the same time, women participate in decision-making in a variety of ways that are far from obvious.

It is useful here to draw insights from how the empowerment question has similarly been approached in a different context, namely, the role of microfinance initiatives in bringing about women's empowerment. Although not related to migration, the relation between microfinance and women's empowerment has also been approached similarly, where microfinance has often been evaluated in terms of whether it has brought about sustained changes in women's status. Yet, to ask simply whether microfinance—or male out-migration—has empowered women is to miss the intricacies in how power operates in the context of gender. Naila Kabeer (1999) has illustrated that in southern contexts, women's involvement in decision-making is far more complex, consisting of strategies such as bargaining, and negotiating. As she points out,

> Statistical perspectives on decision-making, however, should be remembered for what they are: simple windows on complex realities. They may provide a brief glimpse of processes of decision-making, but they tell us very little about the subtle negotiations that go on between women and men in their private lives. Consequently, they may underestimate the informal decision-making agency which women often exercise. (Kabeer, 1999, p. 447)

Given the fact that women's well-being is firmly located in social and familial relationships, it becomes important to understand how and why women make certain choices within their specific contexts. For instance, research has found that when asked about men's and women's roles in decision-making, women often underplay their roles, asserting that it is men who are in power and have control over decisions, even when in actuality, they control household-level decisions in significant ways (Varghese & Ranganathan, 2022). Consequently, it becomes important to explore the empowerment question not just in an absolute and abstract sense, but in a contextual, processual manner, connected firmly with questions of well-being and agency. It is this relationship between migration, empowerment, and well-being that this chapter focuses on.

1.2 Focus of This Chapter

Against this backdrop, this study unpacks women's empowerment from the perspectives of their work, health, well-being, and agency in relation to male out-migration. When looking at women's well-being, we take a contextualized approach, coming from the assumption that women's well-being is intricately linked to the familial and community structures within which they are situated. Thus, rather than thinking about women's agency in an individualized manner, we seek to locate their well-being and agency in context. This is particularly important given recent reports about the central role of relationships in the lives of migrants and their families (Aggarwal, 2024). In line with scholarship that has argued for the incorporation of the role of emotion into research on migration (see Datta, 2018) and for studying migration in terms of subjectivities and not just income and remittances, we take a qualitative approach in this study, highlighting the experiences of the women left behind.

After outlining our research methods, we elaborate on three distinct yet interconnected themes. First, we examine the impact of migration on work and livelihoods, revealing how the absence of male family members deepens women's economic vulnerabilities. Next, we explore the increased caregiving responsibilities women shoulder in migrant households, highlighting the emotional and physical burdens they endure, including isolation and loneliness. Last, we discuss health and well-being, emphasizing the cyclical relationship between economic instability and health issues in these households. We conclude by discussing the broader implications of our findings and proposing directions for future research. The chapter underscores the urgent need for targeted interventions that address the complex intersections of migration, gender, and health in rural Odisha, aiming to alleviate the compounded challenges faced by women in these contexts.

2 Methodology

2.1 Sampling

Qualitative methods were used to provide an in-depth and nuanced exploration of the relationship between migration, gender, and well-being in Odisha. Fieldwork was carried out in two migration-prone districts, namely Kalahandi and Balangir, situated in Odisha. These districts had been chosen due to their recognition as high migration-prone districts by the Odisha government. Given the fact that married women's well-being is significantly affected by whether they have been married more recently, or for a long time, in selecting the sample, we interviewed younger women from the age group of 18 to 40 years who have been recently married, as well as older women—over the age of 40 years—who have been married for a longer time. Following coding, a thematic analysis was conducted, along the lines of Braun and Clarke (2006), as well as a narrative analysis as outlined by Riessman (2008). Additionally, we drew on ethnographic interpretations from field visits and participant observations.

2.2 Field Sites: Kalahandi and Balangir

Our fieldwork commenced in April 2023 and extended through July 2023. During this period, we conducted interviews with a total of 39 respondents and nine key informants and organized two focus group discussions. In Kalahandi, ten localities were covered, spanning eight out of the district's 13 community development blocks (Bhawanipatna, Golamunda, Kesinga, Lanjigarh Road, Thuamul Rampur, Koksara, Jaipatna, and Kalampur). Through key informant interviews, field sites extended to households, shops, roadside areas, Gram Panchayat offices, and the District Labor Department office.

The Kalahandi district is part of the KBK (Kalahandi-Balangir-Koraput) region, once considered the most backward region of the country. While there has been some progress owing to consistent government intervention (Poverty and Human Development Monitoring Agency [PHDMA], Planning and Convergence Department, Government of Odisha, 2020), the district is still one of India's most backward districts. As per the 2011 Census, 92.26% of the district's population lives in rural areas. There is a high concentration of the Scheduled Caste (SC) and Scheduled Tribe (ST) population, comprising 46.67% of Kalahandi's population (Census of India, 2011). Poverty and widespread malnutrition are prevalent in the district, with a significant proportion of the population living below the poverty line. Though recent official statistics report a steep decline in the poverty headcount ratio and the multidimensional poverty index in Odisha (NITI Aayog, 2023), this was not particularly evident and did not emerge as a significant theme in our research.

This is a district that is heavily dependent on rainfed agriculture. However, the decreased ability of agriculture to generate employment and the resultant poverty and malnutrition have led to the high prevalence of distressed labor migration from the district for decades (Mahanty, 2020). These internal migrants mostly work as unskilled laborers in the brick kiln, construction, aquaculture, and textile industries. The inequities, exploitation, and vulnerability of the migrants at the destination sites have been well-documented (Mahanty, 2020).

Field observations of the topography indicate that the Kalahandi district has extensive ranges of hills covered with forest and rolling highlands. The district is a part of the Eastern Ghats. In a private conversation with the District Labor Commissioner about the migration landscape, he mentioned the four specific blocks in the district that are known for their susceptibility to migration. These are: Golamunda, Dharamgarh, Koksara, and Thuamul Rampur in the Kalahandi district. Furthermore, a striking feature is that 11 out of the 13 community development blocks rely predominantly on *kharif* cultivation due to the absence of adequate irrigation facilities during the *rabi* season. This circumstance leads to a dearth of agricultural employment opportunities throughout the remainder of the year, resulting in a pattern of seasonal migration. The majority of migrants are young male members of households, leaving behind women, children, and the elderly in their places of origin.

In the Balangir district of Odisha, we selected two specific localities, strategically chosen to assess the influence of proximity to the nearest town. The rationale behind this selection lies in the divergent migration profiles, offering a unique opportunity to explore the varying impacts of migration on women in these contrasting contexts. The first locality under study was Umria, situated in the Puintala block of the district, merely 16 km away from the Balangir district headquarters. In contrast, the second locality, Babejuri, was approximately 60 km from the district headquarters, making it a more remote area. A quantitative survey conducted in the initial phase had already indicated that Babejuri had a notably higher migration rate compared to Umria, and the profiles of migrants were distinct. While family migration was common from Babejuri, individuals who migrated from Umria were predominantly unmarried and young. By adopting a focused, in-depth approach in these two villages, we departed from the extensive study strategy employed in Kalahandi, aiming to get specific insights by collecting narratives to understand the lived experiences of people.

These unique characteristics of Umria and Babejuri provided valuable comparative insights for understanding women's experiences related to migration. In Balangir district, our research encompassed a total of 17 interviews, with five conducted in Umria and 12 in Babejuri. Additionally, we organized two focus group discussions and conducted nine key informant interviews, contributing to a rich and diverse dataset that enhanced our understanding of the complexities surrounding migration and its impact on the lives of women in these regions.

In the following sections, we discuss three distinctive yet interconnected themes: health, work and livelihood, and care and family relations. These stories highlight how these are overlapping themes that not only impact one another often, but also generate a kind of vicious cycle for the marginalized communities to make it almost impossible to escape from prolonged deprivation.

2.3 Data Collection Methods

Qualitative data collection was carried out through: in-depth interviews with women, focus group discussions, case studies, participant observation, and key informant interviews. Fieldwork was conducted across 12 localities within these two districts. Among the 39 interviewees, 23 belonged to households with current migrants and 16 were households with returned migrants (Table 1).

2.3.1 Semi-structured Interviews

One-on-one interviews with women have provided a nuanced and intimate exploration of women's experiences, offering valuable insights into the impact of migration on their lives, and the specific challenges that women encountered in employment, health, and personal agency. The main themes that emerged from these in-depth interviews are: work and livelihoods, health and well-being, and care and family relations. Underlying all of these is the extreme economic precarity of the women's lives.

Thirty-nine in-depth interviews were conducted, spanning 12 localities within these two districts. Thirty-two of the participants were under the age of 40 years,

Table 1 Household migration status of women interviewed

Migration status of household	Total
Current migrant household	23
Return migrant household	16

Table 2 Age category of the interview participants

Type of household	Age group 18–40 years	Above 40 years
Current migrant household	18	5
Return migrant household	14	2
Total	32	7

Table 3 Details of focus group discussions (FGDs)

District	Village	Number of participants	Gender of participants
Kalahandi	Balagaon	7	Male
Balangir	Babejuri (at 2 Anganwadi centers)	10	Female

while the remaining seven interviewees belonged to the age group of over 40 years (Table 2).

2.3.2 Focus Group Discussions

We conducted two focus group discussions (FGDs) with men and women, respectively. The first focus group discussion was conducted in the village of Balagaon in Kalahandi with seven men (older and younger). This FGD allowed us to gain insights into how two generations of migrants perceive migration as a strategy for diversifying their livelihoods (Table 3).

A separate FGD with 10 women spanning different age groups was conducted in the village of Babejuri in Balangir district. This discussion was instrumental in gathering insights into the health-related issues and challenges affecting women's overall well-being.

2.3.3 Case Studies

In Balangir, we also used case studies of three families for an in-depth exploration of particular instances. These played a crucial role in providing a well-rounded perspective on how migration impacts households, gender dynamics, and overall well-being (Table 4).

2.3.4 Key Informant Interviews

Key informant interviews (KIIs) allowed us to tap into the local knowledge and expertise of stakeholders such as village- and district-level office-bearers and community members deeply involved in local issues and affairs, providing insights into the

Table 4 Details of case studies

Village	Name	Migration status
Babejuri (Balangir)	Purusothaman Majhi and Jambobati Majhi	Return migrants (returned 20 days ago) who worked in brick kilns in Hyderabad; migrate through *Dalalas* (contractors)
	Dolamani Sahu and Nilamati Sahu	Return migrants (returned one year ago) after six years of migration; worked in brick kilns in Bangalore
	Bursubha Dharua and Sangita Dharua	Return migrants (returned 20 days ago); worked in brick kilns in Vijayawada

Table 5 Details of key informant interviews (KIIs)

Designation	Village/locality/district
An old person from the village who is part of the local politics	Karlaguda
Field staff on the thematic area of health, Mamta NGO	Kadamguda
Sarpanch (village head)	Kaniguma
Gram Rozgar Sevak	Kaniguma
District Labor Officer	Kalahandi
ASHA Worker	Karlaguda

complex web of social and economic relations within the villages and other aspects related to migration and employment. Six KIIs were conducted (Table 5).

3 Emerging Themes and Analysis

3.1 Work and Livelihood

Across both the field sites, work and livelihood issues were significant concerns that plagued women in migrant households. Given that women's well-being was tied to the economic stability of the household, precarious livelihood conditions had a significant impact.

3.1.1 Distress at Home: Economic Precarity and Indebtedness

Non-availability of work and economic distress, in general, emerged as the primary reasons for male out-migration. Basandita Tandi, a mother of two, whom we interviewed in Kalahandi district, said that her husband earned only Rs 150–200 for a day's work in the fields, even after laboring for more than eight hours. This was notwithstanding the fact that the legal minimum wage rate was Rs 352. This meager income was insufficient for managing everyday expenses, and the situation was exacerbated by the burden of a pre-existing debt incurred for their marriage. This issue was reiterated by interviewees from all the sample localities.

For instance, Jyotirmayi Bihari, from Balagaon, whose husband used to migrate away from the district for short-term episodes, reported:

> See, we live in a village and we need money to survive. Whatever work we do is not sufficient to run a family. There are not enough livelihood sources in the village, and the wage rate is also less. We get only 100–150 rupees per day in the village, which is not sufficient to run a family. But one can earn 300 per day outside. My husband earns 300 rupees per day. It is difficult to survive on that amount, but somehow that helps us survive.

Similarly, Rebati Naik from Karlaguda (Kalahandi) spoke about the economic struggles faced by her family, particularly due to the financial burden caused by her son's marriage. The family had to take substantial loans to fund the wedding, resulting in a significant debt burden. In order to repay the loan, they had to rely on another debt in turn, thus placing the family in a cycle of debt.

This situation of Rebati Naik, Basandita Tandi, and Jyotirmayi Bihari reveals a vicious circle of impoverishment and indebtedness within their lives. The only escape from this recurring cumulative debt burden appears to be a higher-paying job, unfortunately, not available in the village or its surrounding areas, as reported by a participant from Mukundapur:

> The only work available here is soil lifting, which is very painful, and no other work is available here. No, it does not provide enough for our survival. In Odisha, if you work for one day, you may have to remain unemployed for eight days.

The only viable solution is migrating to urban centers in other states in search of better employment opportunities. She added:

> What will he do here? He works in agricultural fields during the rainy season. He collects forest produce during the summers. He gathers wood and bamboo from the forest and makes winnowing fans, locally known as Kula. What else can be done?

This excerpt unveils a complex interplay of factors, including reliance on seasonal occupations, limited work availability within the village, and the consequent need for individuals to migrate in pursuit of diversifying livelihood opportunities. This was also pointed out by Laxmi Majhi, a woman in her early 30s, whose husband is a current migrant. The absence of consistent and reliable employment opportunities within the village leaves the household in a state of chronic economic deprivation, as it is difficult to maintain a steady income throughout the year. Consequently, many individuals, including Laxmi's husband, feel compelled to migrate and seek employment in factories and other forms of temporary or irregular labor. As a result, the village faces a continuous cycle of out-migration.

Scholars like Kumar (2020) have written about the practice of livelihood diversification in rural India, where people engage in multiple activities (agricultural and non-agricultural) to make ends meet:

> People often survive on precarious resources, their income is insufficient and unstable, often affected by seasonal cycles, and their labour market is not developed enough so that a household may transfer their entire human resources into a single activity. (p. 221)

Even in Balangir, it was found that men migrated due to the unavailability of work in the village. As one respondent put it, "Why would anyone leave if they were doing well here? People are going out due to distress here."

Villagers often said "*ame gareeb log*" (we are poor people) and attributed migration to their economic distress. When discussing the involvement of youth in agriculture, one young man, who offers private tuition and also does a few other odd jobs, highlighted the lack of profitability and the resultant diminishing aspirations associated with the occupation among youths. Notably, he spoke about how they were often underpaid for their labor and the undervaluation of crops in the market.

Young men preferred to migrate to South India, often using the phrase "Tamil Nadu *jaichon*" to refer to migration from the villages to Bangalore, Tiruppur, or other places. This phrase was often used to signify migration in general. The preference for southern states was largely due to the higher wages earned there.

Women also pushed the men in the family to migrate and earn a livelihood, even though this meant that the burden of housework, livestock, and care work of the children and elderly fell on them. This is brought out in the case of Sadasiba Saltar and Madana Saltar.

Case Illustration: The Saltar Family

Sadasiba Saltar had previously worked in Balangir for two years, around a decade ago. He was a carpenter. He used to live in the town of Balangir for work but used to visit home in the village once a week. After his marriage, he decided to stay back in the village. When his health deteriorated, he stopped working. He has three sons. The eldest one is involved in agriculture, and the middle one is a migrant worker doing odd jobs. The youngest one got a placement after finishing his BCom degree. He works with a cellphone company and lives in Kolkata. He regularly sends money and takes care of the majority of his father's treatment expenses. When we asked why his son decided to go out for work, he smiled and said, "to seek a more joyful life".

He told us that he is from the Gond caste, which is categorized as a Scheduled Tribe. Madana Saltar's son expressed his belief that working outside the village is futile. He argued that even if people acquire skills and receive training elsewhere, it won't be beneficial for their future livelihoods since there are no industries in Odisha or near the village. While many young men migrate for several reasons, men who stay back figure out reasons like these and choose not to leave the village, even though they are often labelled as "lazy" and "good for nothing".

Hearing this, Madana Saltar subtly indicated that her son has not been actively seeking employment and is merely engaged in some superficial work at home. So, while in the field, we come across narratives of women who encourage men in the family to migrate and earn a livelihood instead of wasting time at home, even though this increases their burden at home.

3.1.2 Marginal Landholdings and Dependence on Wage Labor

When thinking about gender and women's well-being, it is important to highlight the broader implications of land distribution, poverty, and the consequent reliance on wage labor within historically deprived communities in Odisha. As Rebati Naik from Kalahandi described:

> I am not an old woman; the face of an old woman that you see now is because of the long years of hard work that I have done. We are very, very poor. My father-in-law has four sons. What share will we have from one acre of land, you tell me? Do you think such a small amount of land will be able to feed us?

The statement about holding and fragmentation of such marginal land reveals the economic strain on the household. The picture gets clearer when we understand that the household belongs to the Scheduled Caste group, and they have been historically landless or had only a marginal amount of land ownership in Odisha.

Another woman, when asked about the reasons for migration, responded:

> There are many reasons, sir. He has migrated because we have no land, no fields, and no jewelry to spend on our future requirements. We have only one option: to go out of the house to work elsewhere. As I told you, he never worked here.

This excerpt emphasizes how disparities in terms of asset/wealth holdings compel poor households to rely on wage labor. Thus, this excerpt delves into the systemic issues of land distribution, economic precarity, and the broader socio-economic factors that drive individuals to seek employment beyond their immediate surroundings.

3.1.3 Experiences with Public Employment Schemes

Migrant families were also affected by the ineffectiveness of government schemes and the inadequacy of wages in the local labor market. When asked about the availability of work through public employment schemes, one woman responded:

> Yes, he [the husband] was getting work here, but he was not receiving a wage equivalent to the labor he put in. Additionally, he is involved in other types of work, such as forest work or MGNREGA and NRGS [govt. employment scheme] projects, but he is not receiving timely payments.

This concern is situated within the broader context of India, where the workforce is often underpaid, and wage rates are kept low. In an article by Jean Drèze, it was noted that the growth rate of real wages for agricultural labor was just 0.8% per year from 2014–2015 to 2022–2023, and for non-agricultural labor, it was only 0.2% (Drèze, 2023b). This lower earning, despite hours of work, negatively impacts the living standards of rural households.

Alongside the issue of untimely payment, the remuneration for these public works is inadequate, as highlighted by one of our respondents, Devanti Chattriya: "The government has declared 352 rupees for one day's work. But here, they are only providing 300 rupees instead of the promised 352 rupees."

As Drèze (2023a) has emphasized, unemployment figures in India for poor people are largely irrelevant because "poor people are rarely unemployed because they can't afford to do nothing" (para. 2). In Devanti Chhatriya's husband's case, he earns a living by selling pigeons, from which he was earning less than Rs 100 per day, which served as the main source of income for their family during the non-agricultural season.

Men who sought employment under the Mahatma Gandhi National Rural Employment Guarantee Act (MGNREGA or NREGA) often expressed frustration with delayed payments and accused the Gram Rozgar Sewak (GRS) of negligence in ensuring timely payments. Apart from NREGA, the only available work is agricultural labor, primarily during the monsoon season. They emphasized that cultivating their lands did not earn them a profit, nor could it be a sustainable and reliable source of income.

3.1.4 Precarious Working Conditions at Destinations

So far, this section on work and livelihood issues has described the challenges in the village that pushed people to migrate. Yet, upon migration, many men also had to experience harsh conditions and exploitation at the destination sites. For instance, Bhoomi Majhi described the challenges that her husband experienced with construction work during the summer. "Yes, it is a very tough job. He works during the hot summer. It's very difficult to work in the summer. We couldn't bear it, and he left the job," said Bhoomi.

This excerpt about the precarious nature of Bhoomi's husband's work provides a glimpse into the harsh conditions that influenced his decision to leave the job. Migrant workers face several challenges at the destination, such as poor and exploitative working conditions without any occupational safety. In serious cases, there have also been deaths at the workplace that impacted entire families as they struggled to get their due compensation. The following two cases illustrate these issues.

Excerpt from Field notes: Deaths at Destination Sites

When we were seated in the District Labor Officer's chamber, a family urgently entered the room. A woman in her early thirties had accompanied an older person. A middle-aged person entered with them and began speaking to the Labor Officer. He was from their village and had come to assist them as they were both illiterate. From their conversation, we gathered that the lady's husband had migrated to Gujarat and died in a workplace accident two years ago. Although the police had registered an FIR, there was a procedural delay in receiving the death certificate from the government since it was in Gujarati. This procedural delay had prevented the deceased person's wife from receiving compensation for accidental death.

In another migrant household, an elderly man in his seventies narrated how his only son, who had gone to Bangalore to work as an electrician in a factory, met with a workplace accident and died. Not even his body was brought to Odisha. Describing these events, the old man broke down in tears. He informed us that they had been trying to contact the employer for compensation. Although the employer initially agreed, he later stopped taking their calls.

These two excerpts from the field notes highlight the gravity of the issues, such as occupational hazards and subsequent deaths of migrant workers in the destination. The dependents did not receive compensation, either from the employer or from the government. This means that issues such as the proper registration, social security, and safe and dignified working conditions of migrants need to be addressed through government policies and regulations.

3.1.5 Women and Work: Gender Gap in Wages

The lack of employment opportunities in rural areas has forced people to take up low-paying jobs, leading to households living in abject poverty. Even in families where both male and female members contributing to the household income, making ends meet is a struggle. Most adult household members were engaged in more than one (and sometimes more than two) activities for a living. Most of the women were engaged in agricultural labor (paid or for the family) or construction work as helpers.

In the excerpt below, Basantida Tandi articulates the challenges of her husband's irregular and volatile income, compelling her to contribute by working in the agricultural fields:

> My husband has been working in different places to make ends meet. I also go to the field whenever there is work, leaving my two children at home. We cannot solely depend on my husband's income since it is very unpredictable. He has not been getting work days for a long time. If there is work for two months, there won't be any work for another month or longer. So, there is no option for me not to do it. Even after returning from the field, I would have to do all the housework. Somehow, I have to manage all this work alone.

The excerpt reveals the dual burden women face in such households, balancing paid work and household responsibilities alone. But this has a detrimental impact on the health and well-being of women. As Rebati Naik aptly put it: "Oh, I have only gotten older and older by engaging in hard work, and hard labor (laughs)." Another respondent in her early 40s, Jaima Komari, from Ampani, described how she continued to seek and take up different kinds of work to run the household.

> Sir, it has been four years. Before the bangles business, I started selling spices in a nearby village. I have worked as a daily wage laborer in the fields and in construction work. During my pregnancy, I went to the jungle to gather firewood and sell it. I never rest. I always engage in some kind of work to run my household.

Similarly, Jyotirmayee Bihari spoke about her long days of work:

I work as a daily wage laborer and agricultural laborer. My mother comes to take care of my children when I go to work. Only depending on money from outside is not sufficient enough to run the family. Other than my husband, there is no one to earn, due to which, sometimes, I also go to work. I work in the fields, uprooting weeds and cutting crops. I also take up construction work for houses. If I go to work at 8 am, I return home at around 4 pm.

Clearly, work and livelihood issues were relevant for women too, as they entered the labor market. At the same time, as expected, there were gender gaps in the pay that women received, as Jaima Komari elucidated:

Jaima Komari: *They pay us around Rs 150 per day. So, if we work in their field for a full day, they pay us Rs 150.*

Field investigator (to a man in the background): *How much are you getting paid?*

Husband: Oh, I get paid Rs 200 because I plough the land with the help of the oxen.

Gender-based wage gaps were common across all sites and localities studied for this analysis.

To conclude, this section on work and livelihood issues has illustrated women's experiences of extreme poverty and deprivation at home. Finances were insufficient, employment opportunities were fewer, and resources were scarce. What makes it even more difficult is the need to support dependent family members, mainly the elderly and children. When there is a crisis in the family because of the death of an earning family member, the situation becomes graver. Most of the stories shared are those of poverty and deprivation. Women often recounted how they had to manage with very little and how extremely difficult it was to navigate family, care, work, and other responsibilities with such few resources. This leads to the next section about care work in the family.

3.2 *Care Work and Family Dynamics*

Across both the field sites of Kalahandi and Balangir, women recounted painful stories of the increased care burdens on them due to the absence of their husbands and other male members in the family. They spoke about the increased care responsibilities on them, as well as the emotional challenges of dealing with loneliness and isolation. The following sections elucidate these concerns.

3.2.1 Migration and Increased Care Responsibilities for Women

The narratives of women, whose male family members migrate for work while they stay home, vividly depict the intricate web of care work, family dynamics, and gendered well-being. Basandita Tandi, whom we have mentioned earlier, remembered the first time when her husband left home for work:

My husband went outside for work for the first time after our marriage in 2015. It was just after two years of our marriage. I was 22 years old at that time. It was quite a bitter experience

> for me. Even though we all expected that he would return soon, he only returned after three months. It was a time of waiting. It was a time of uncertainty. I was always thinking about the future. 'What would I do alone?' and 'How to manage and handle things at home?' I had always been occupied with these thoughts. I had been seeking an answer to these questions in my mind. He would have been helping me with all the work at home when he was here. But I was left behind. He had left me alone and gone to Maharashtra. But, as I had said previously, we had no other option. Even though it was a tough decision, we both had to take that. It was a time of hardship.

Here, the factor of age played an important role. As a younger married woman, Basandita Tandi's standing in the family is far more precarious than an older woman who has been married for longer. Younger and newly married women were far more affected by male out-migration.

We asked Basandita Tandi about her daily responsibilities at home:

> My mother-in-law helps me with cooking and cleaning, but there are particular things for which they need my help and care. My children are young; the elder one is 11 years old, and the younger one is two years old. Their father is not here with us. I am the only person who has to cater to their needs. My elder son is going to school. He is now in the fourth grade. I have to look after things related to his education. Getting him ready for school, sending him to school, and keeping an eye on his academic progress – I am the only person to look after all of these things. My younger one, as you can see, can't do anything on her own. I have to bathe her, give her food, and get her ready. When they get a fever or have any sort of health issue, I have to take care of them. When my husband is here, I must also cater to his needs, such as serving food and keeping his clothes and things ready.

Madana Saltar, mentioned earlier as well, also shared her everyday routine. Like many other women, she appeared to be around 60 years old when she was, in fact, between 50 and 55 years of age. Her day typically starts early at 4 am with household chores such as sweeping, washing utensils, and collecting firewood and dung. She then prepares meals, fetches water, and takes a bath by 7 am. She goes to the field after breakfast if it is the cultivating season. She typically returns home at around 3:30 pm and rests after bathing. Alongside her household responsibilities, she cares for her husband and two sons. Her husband had been experiencing chronic illness that required a lot of expenditure for the treatment. Cooking, household chores, and providing special attention to her husband's ailment are part of her responsibilities. Additionally, Madana Saltar also had to look after the elderly in her household who required assistance.

This narration represents a common scenario where women bear the responsibility of caring for older adults, a dynamic exacerbated in migration contexts where women manage caregiving alongside other household and work responsibilities. All in all, Madana was exhausted from caring for her ailing husband while taking care of the household all by herself. She mentioned that there is no one to assist her except her niece (aged around 12–15 years), who helps with fetching water and other household chores when she is around.

Another woman in Kalahandi, Jyotirmayi, recounted the overwhelming burden of juggling work and childcare:

> I go to work even though I need to take care of my children. I bring water and cook food for them after returning from work. Then I have to wake up early in the morning to get them ready for school, and then I go to work.

Jyotirmayi further elaborated on the financial pressures that necessitated such arduous routines:

> When my elder daughter was about to be born, we needed money, which my husband went out to earn. We are poor and we can't survive without earning our livelihood. During my pregnancy, many problems occurred, and I had to manage them because my husband was away from home. Even today, I go alone to buy rations (groceries), vegetables, and daily needs items. I also go for daily wage work. It is very difficult to survive, and we are poor; without juggling between work and household chores, we can't survive.

Her story illustrates the compounded challenges faced by women during critical life stages, such as pregnancy, in the absence of their husbands. The emotional strain of separation is palpable in Ghanaketi Harijan's words. "I feel sad, but we have many financial crises, so we must stay separate for the money," she said. Another woman, Amrita Tandi, responded, "If your beloved goes away, you feel sad. I cried a lot when he went outside. I feel lonely and helpless." This sentiment resonates with many women, whose well-being has to be constantly negotiated between emotional needs and economic survival.

3.2.2 Migration and marriage in Balangir

When talking about the impact of migration on marital dynamics, there are important differences between Kalahandi and Balangir. In Balangir, there was a tendency for men to migrate *before* marriage. After marriage, they either worked in the village, or nearby areas, or went to Balangir town for employment. For instance, Sushil Putel told us that he used to work outside the district but stopped after getting married five years ago. At the time he was interviewed, he was working locally.

Young men typically went out of the state to work before marriage, saved money, then returned to the village, and used their savings for marriage. This pattern was reiterated by many persons, including Mamta Didi, an Anganwadi worker. Mamta Didi pointed us in the direction of young men and women who went to the nearby towns and outside Odisha for work before marriage. She told us this was because these men were relatively independent of marital responsibilities and child care.

3.2.3 Balancing Care Work and Financial Struggles

As seen earlier, many women struggled with the additional care burdens they shouldered when their husbands were away. At the same time, given the financial hardships, they had few alternatives. Jaima Komari provides a glimpse into the harsh realities of daily life and the constant struggle for financial stability:

> Sir, I save the money sent by my husband, and I take care of all the expenses relating to the house. I cook less rice to save some for the next day's requirement. No one is here to give us any kind of help in our difficult times. We are poor people; we have to save money for the future.

Her narrative not only highlights the financial hardships but also the resilience and resourcefulness required to manage household crises. The logistical challenges of financial management are described by another woman, who notes:

> I opened my bank account in 2016. The bank where I have an account is very far from my home. I used to go there alone, but nowadays I don't go there alone since I have two children to look after. So, I take help from some other person to do my bank work.

Women whose husbands were away struggled with mobility issues in accessing either health or financial services. When asked about how she managed to meet the basic needs, like procuring food, Jyotirmayi's response further illustrated the strenuous physical demands placed on women:

> I go walking. I ask for help from the people I know. If they help, then it is okay; otherwise, I need to carry the rice on my head for 3 km. I divide the rice into two bags and then carry only one at a time because 35 kgs of rice can't be carried on one's head.

These excerpts from interviews with women whose male family members have migrated reveal the extensive care work and responsibilities that fall on them. They highlight how family dynamics shift and the well-being of women is impacted by migration, painting a comprehensive picture of the socio-cultural context of migration in rural Odisha.

3.3 Health and Well-Being

The health and well-being of women were directly related to the financial stability of the family, and good health directly contributed to women's well-being. Unfortunately, serious health concerns were recounted by far too many respondents, both male and female. While our analysis centers on the experiences of women, it is important to note that many men also described severe health problems. In fact, we found that health-related issues were one of the most dominant concerns for migrant families. While health was itself affected by the ability to pay, in turn, poor health was also likely to impact economic precarity and well-being in a cyclical fashion, quite reminiscent of Shaun Grech's analysis of disability and poverty being embroiled in a vicious cycle (Grech, 2015). In the following sections, we describe the three main health-related issues: access to health services, the lack of healthcare facilities, and conditions of chronic illness.

3.3.1 Challenges in Accessing Health Services

One of the most pressing challenges recounted by wives left behind was the difficulty in accessing health services, given the distance, poor public transport, and absence of men. As one woman, Minata Naik, whose husband was a return migrant, said:

> We didn't have access to good facilities and couldn't receive money from the Anganwadi for my delivery. The Anganwadi worker told me that my Aadhar card was incorrect, so I couldn't receive government funds. My two children also did not receive any money from the government.

Public transport facilities to most of the localities were seldom or not available. Poor public transport and limited connectivity made mobility a significant challenge, particularly for women, the aged, and schoolchildren. Sunita Majhi described her challenges with reaching health care facilities in the absence of her husband:

> I was pregnant then, and frequently, I had to go to the hospital or health care center for different needs. There was nobody to take me to the hospital once he left. There were no buses or good roads to reach Bhawanipatna. I had to go alone for all those needs.

Similarly, Jyotirmayi chimed in:

> Medical problems are very difficult to handle. When I was alone during the delivery of my first child, I used to go to the hospital by myself and get all the investigations done alone. I suffered a lot during that time because I had to travel to the hospital by myself.

Because of these issues, women often ended up trivializing and ignoring their symptoms until it was no longer possible, as we describe later.

3.3.2 Lack of Healthcare Facilities

Another dominant concern was the absence of adequate or quality facilities in their proximity. The closest adequate facility was often located at the district or block headquarters. Health centers in the village were chastised for being inadequate. As one group of men put it, their treatments were limited to "prescribing paracetamol." There were incidents narrated about nurses/compounders at the village health center administering the wrong medicines to small babies. Some villages did not have primary health centers, as attested by Anganwadi workers. Apart from this, villagers tended to access unauthorized medical practitioners who sometimes even made home visits in the village.

One informant, Mamata Harijan, highlighted the inadequacy of facilities in the government hospital: "We don't receive many health benefits from the government. We use the Biju Swasthya Kalyan Yojana (BSKY) for treatment in government hospitals." Although she could utilize the BSKY card for cashless treatment, it did not necessarily imply that the hospitals were well-equipped. Also, she, as well as other respondents, often complained about the services they got from the Auxiliary Nurse Midwives (ANMs) and ASHA workers. This suggests issues with last-mile delivery, if not the inadequacy of the schemes the government envisaged.

3.3.3 Chronic Poor Health in the Absence of Services

One of the most disturbing observations from the data collection was the extent to which people were affected by serious, chronic, and debilitating conditions. As researchers, we were struck by the severity of the illnesses that people were affected by, and the extent to which their lives were upturned by chronic illness. Also, the health of women was significantly affected by workload and care responsibilities. Further, women often ignored their own health concerns due to their preoccupation with economic precarity and livelihood issues.

When talking about how women's extensive domestic workload affected their health, Madana Saltar's son recounted his mother's health issues over the past 10–12 years, with her leg frequently swelling for 15–20 days. During these episodes, she would be unable to work and experience significant pain. He shared the story of her recent visit to Raipur, after hospital personnel came to the village in a vehicle and informed everyone about the opportunity to receive low-cost check-ups for any health issues. Five people, including four women and one young man, went together and stayed in Raipur for two to three days. Each person had a different health problem. The man underwent surgery during the visit. Madana Saltar was one of the five villagers who went for the check-up. They conducted various tests on her, and the results showed negative or normal readings for the major tests. They provided an ointment for her swollen leg but did not explain the cause of her condition. They utilized a health insurance card (referred to as the Biju Swasthya Yojana card by the eldest son). Additionally, Madana's husband had been suffering from chronic illness for many years. They had been to several hospitals, including AIIMS Bhubaneswar, and spent a total of around Rs 2 lakh on healthcare but obtained no relief.

When Madana Saltar shared about the ongoing health struggles of her husband, it highlighted the significant financial and emotional burdens faced by families in accessing specialized healthcare. The reliance on their son working in Kolkata underscores a common strategy among rural families to manage healthcare costs through migrant remittances, showcasing the intertwined dynamics of health, migration, and familial support networks in rural India. In their study of migrant workers in Surat—many of whom migrate from Odisha—Das and Sahu (2019) found that remittances were used to deal with emergencies back home by 41.8% of the migrants. These were often for medical emergencies or events like marriages.

What really stood out in our conversation with Madana Saltar was how she spoke about her own health as "not so important." She tends to the goats in the field every day, even when she is unwell or feeling unwell. Once, reeling with dizziness and nausea, she fell down in the fields and was escorted back home by someone else. She was taken to Balangir Hospital, where she was told she had low blood pressure (BP) and prescribed medication, which she took for a few days and stopped after she felt a little better.

This case demonstrates the intersecting challenges faced by rural women like Madana Saltar in Odisha, where migration, gender dynamics, and poverty intersect with healthcare access. Madana's recurrent health issues and reliance on intermittent health camps and distant hospitals show how migration often disrupts consistent healthcare access. The gendered burden of domestic work further exacerbates health inequalities, as women prioritize caregiving over their own health needs. Many women described their bodies as rapidly aging in the face of poverty, deprivation, and migration. And despite government schemes like Biju Swasthya Kalyan Yojana, which aim to provide healthcare support, systemic gaps persist in addressing chronic health conditions among rural populations. Enhancing healthcare infrastructure tailored to the needs of migrant families and improving healthcare literacy are essential steps toward alleviating these disparities and ensuring equitable health outcomes in Odisha's rural migrant communities.

4 Conclusion

The study highlights the significant impact of the non-availability of work and economic distress as primary drivers of male out-migration in rural Odisha. The lack of consistent and reliable employment opportunities within the village leaves households in a state of chronic economic deprivation, making it difficult to maintain a steady income throughout the year. Traditional livelihoods, constrained by insufficient diversified economic activities, fail to support rural households. As a result, many individuals feel compelled to migrate in search of work, often ending up in factories and other forms of temporary or irregular labor. This cycle of out-migration perpetuates economic instability in the village.

Women bear a dual burden in such households, balancing work and household responsibilities alone, which significantly impacts their health and well-being. Their experiences of extreme poverty and deprivation at home and managing large families with limited resources and insufficient finances vividly depict the overwhelming burden of juggling work, childcare, and other responsibilities. Financial pressures necessitate arduous routines, with well-being constantly being negotiated between emotional needs and economic survival. The stark contrast in wages between men and women, prevalent across the district, exacerbates these challenges, making fair remuneration critical in the context of high migration and wage differentials between source and destination areas.

In the context of migration, women's health is particularly compromised. They endure physical strain from balancing domestic workloads and caregiving with external work responsibilities, often neglecting their own health in the process. Women's health remains inadequately addressed due to limited healthcare access and the prioritization of family needs over personal health. Chronic health issues among family members further reveal the intricate relationship between health conditions and the ability to engage in labor for economic sustenance. The lack of proper medical care, compounded by inadequate public transport and limited healthcare infrastructure, exacerbates these issues.

Healthcare inadequacies are evident, with government hospitals often lacking necessary facilities. Despite utilizing health insurance schemes like Biju Swasthya Kalyan Yojana, systemic gaps persist in addressing chronic health conditions among rural populations. Enhancing healthcare infrastructure tailored to the needs of migrant families and improving healthcare literacy are essential steps toward alleviating these disparities. Targeted policies that address the specific health and well-being needs of women in migration contexts are crucial for ensuring equitable health outcomes.

This study demonstrates the intersecting challenges faced by rural women in Odisha, where migration, gender dynamics, and poverty intersect with healthcare access. Despite government schemes, the reliance on intermittent health camps and distant hospitals shows how migration disrupts consistent healthcare access. To ensure equitable health outcomes, policies must focus on improving healthcare infrastructure and addressing the unique needs of rural migrant communities in Odisha.

Acknowledgements The authors would like to thank all the interlocutors for taking out time to participate in the study. We also acknowledge the contribution of Utkal Harpal in field assistance.

References

Aggarwal, I. (2024). For migrant workers in India, healing and well-being are about relationships. *Mad in South Asia*. Retrieved May 12, 2024, from https://madinsouthasia.org/for-migrant-workers-in-india-healing-and-well-being-are-about-relationships/

Braun, V., & Clarke, V. (2006). Using thematic analysis in psychology. *Qualitative Research in Psychology, 3*(2), 77–101. https://doi.org/10.1191/1478088706qp063oa

Census India. (2011). *Kalahandi district population, Odisha*. Retrieved May 12, 2024, from https://www.censusindia2011.com/odisha/kalahandi-population.html

Da Silva, J. M. (2023, June 7). *Why you should care about unpaid care work*. OECD Development Matters. Retrieved May 12, 2024, from https://oecd-development-matters.org/2019/03/18/why-you-should-care-about-unpaid-care-work/

Das, B., & Sahu, G. B. (2019). Coping with cities and connecting with villages: Migrant workers in Surat city. *The Indian Journal of Labour Economics, 62*, 89–112. https://doi.org/10.1007/s41027-019-00158-9

Datta, A. (2018). Pride and shame in the city: Young people's experiences of rural–urban migration in India. *Children's Geographies, 16*(6), 654–665. https://doi.org/10.1080/14733285.2018.1495317

Desai, S., & Banerji, M. (2008). Negotiated identities: Male migration and left-behind wives in India. *Journal of Population Research, 25*(3), 337–355. https://doi.org/10.1007/bf03033894

Drèze, J. (2023a, April 13). Jean Drèze writes: Wages are the worry, not just unemployment. *The Indian Express*. https://indianexpress.com/article/opinion/columns/jean-dreze-writes-wages-are-the-worry-not-just-unemployment-8553226/

Drèze, J. (2023b, May 25). Since 2014, the poorest communities are earning less. *The Indian Express*. https://indianexpress.com/article/opinion/columns/since-2014-the-poorest-communities-are-earning-less-8625367/

Findley, S. E., & Williams, L. (1991). *Women who go and women who stay: Reflections of family migration processes in a changing world*. World Population and Labor Policies Working Paper, 176, ILO. http://www.ilo.org/public/libdoc/ilo/1991/91B09_196_engl.pdf

Government of Odisha. (n.d.). *Demography- Kalahandi.* Retrieved May 12, 2024, from https://kalahandi.odisha.gov.in/about--district/demography

Grech, S. (2015). Disability and poverty in the Global South: Renegotiating development in Guatemala. *Palgrave Macmillan.* https://doi.org/10.1057/9781137307989

Jain, M. (2020, December 4). *"No one knows about me." India's 'left-behind' women.* Article 14. Retrieved May 12, 2024, from https://www.article-14.com/post/no-one-knows-about-me-india-s-left-behind-women

Jolly, S., Bell, E., & Narayanaswamy, L. (2003). *Gender and migration in Asia: Overview and annotated bibliography* (pp. 1–36). Institute of Development Studies. Retrieved May 12, 202, from https://archive.ids.ac.uk/bridge/bridge-publications/bibliographies/A52601.html

Kabeer, N. (1999). Resources, agency, achievements: Reflections on the measurement of women's empowerment. *Development and Change, 30*(3), 435–464. https://doi.org/10.1111/1467-7660.00125

Kumar, N. (2020). Diversification of household labour. In S. I. Rajan & M. Sumeetha (Eds.), *Handbook of internal migration in India* (pp. 220–234). Sage Publications. https://doi.org/10.4135/9789353287788

Kumar, R. (2023, March 23). *Left behind or left ahead? Implications of male migration on female political engagement.* Ideas for India. Retrieved May 11, 2024, from https://www.ideasforindia.in/topics/social-identity/left-behind-or-left-ahead-implications-of-male-migration-on-female-political-engagement.html

Lei, L., & Desai, S. (2021). Male out-migration and the health of left-behind wives in India: The roles of remittances, household responsibilities, and autonomy. *Social Science & Medicine*, 280. https://doi.org/10.1016/j.socscimed.2021.113982

Mahanty, M. (2020). Distress migration. In S. I. Rajan & M. Sumeetha (Eds.), *Handbook of Internal Migration in India* (pp. 235–250). Sage Publications. https://doi.org/10.4135/9789353287788

NITI Aayog (2023). *India National multidimensional poverty index: A progress review.* https://www.niti.gov.in/sites/default/files/2023-08/India-National-Multidimentional-Poverty-Index-2023.pdf

Prati, G., Cazcarro, I., & Hazra, S. (2022). Gender dimensions of the migration, sustainability and care nexus: The case study of the Mahanadi delta, India. *Current Research in Environmental Sustainability, 4*, Article 100104. https://doi.org/10.1016/j.crsust.2021.100104

Rai, N. (2020). Narratives of left-behind women. In S. I. Rajan & M. Sumeetha (Eds.), *Handbook of internal migration in India* (pp. 415–425). Sage Publications. https://doi.org/10.4135/9789353287788

Rajan, S. I., Sivakumar, P., & Srinivasan, A. (2020). The COVID-19 pandemic and internal labour migration in India: A 'crisis of mobility.' *The Indian Society of Labour Economics, 63*(4), 1021–1039. https://doi.org/10.1007/s41027-020-00293-8

Rajan, S. I., & Sumeetha, M. (Eds.) (2020). *Handbook of internal migration in India.* Sage Publications. https://doi.org/10.4135/9789353287788

Rajput, M., & Bureau, A. (2024) Conversation with Manju Rajput. *Gender Talk, NCAER National Data Innovation Center Measurement Brief,* 12–15. Retrieved May 11, 2024, from https://ndic.ncaer.org/wp-content/uploads/2024/01/GenderTalk-2024.pdf

Ramamurthy, P. (2024). Intermittent migration: Female agency within marriage and beyond. *Gender Talk, NCAER National Data Innovation Center Measurement Brief*, 8–10. Retrieved May 11, 2024, from https://ndic.ncaer.org/wp-content/uploads/2024/01/GenderTalk-2024.pdf

Riessman, C. K. (2008). *Narrative methods for the human sciences.* Sage Publications.

Roy, A. K., & Nangia, P. (2005). *Impact of male out-migration on health status of left behind wives—A study of Bihar, India* [Paper Presentation]. International Union for the Scientific Study of Population XXV International Population Conference, Tours, France. https://iussp2005.princeton.edu/papers/51906

Sinha, B., Jha, S., & Negi, N. S. (2012). Migration and empowerment: The experience of women in households in India where migration of a husband has occurred. *Journal of Gender Studies, 21*(1), 61–76. https://doi.org/10.1080/09589236.2012.639551

Varghese, D., & Ranganathan, S. (2022). Informal work from home: Understanding vulnerability and well-being among women in Kudumbashree microenterprises. *Asian Women, 38* (4), 23–50. https://doi.org/10.14431/aw.2022.12.38.4.23

World Bank Group & FAO. (2018). *Male outmigration and women's work and empowerment in agriculture: The case of Nepal and Senegal.* World Bank. https://openknowledge.worldbank.org/handle/10986/30066

Chapter 12
Conclusion

Amrita Datta, S. Irudaya Rajan, and Umi Daniel

Abstract This chapter summarises the key results of the Odisha Migration Study, and discusses the policy implications of this research. First, it underscores the salience of migration statistics and argues that up-to-date migration data, such as that collected by the Odisha Migration Study, provides a wealth of information for policymakers. For instance, in the identified migration corridors and high migration regions, specific policy interventions such as panchayat-level registration of labourers, enhancing the convergence of government schemes and services, provision of legal assistance, and reduction and elimination of the role of contractors in the migration process can be implemented. Third, given the youth domination in migration streams, skill programmes, and safe and informed migration programmes targeting the youth population through migration facilitation centres can be established. Fourth, the social and psychological costs of migration—in both source and destination regions—need to be acknowledged. Fifth, in precarious family migration streams, accompanying migrant children are the worst sufferers in the migration cycle; the government should initiate education, nutrition, health and other services for them both within and outside of the state. Sixth, safeguarding workers' rights is critical in all migration streams, but in particular, vulnerable streams of migration such as Dadan labor and family based migration systems. Seventh, social security for migrant workers must be embedded in the policy architecture at destination states, where migrants contribute significantly to economic growth and development. And last, the chapter argues, that policy attention is also needed in the source regions, where, employment and livelihood opportunities need to be enhanced. A simultaneous push for rural industrialization, the development of the services sector and agricultural diversification can pave the way for stronger rural-urban linkages and balanced development in Odisha.

A. Datta (✉)
Indian Institute of Technology, Hyderabad, India
e-mail: amritadatta@la.iith.ac.in

S. I. Rajan
International Institute of Migration and Development, Thiruvananthapuram, India
e-mail: rajan@iimad.org

U. Daniel
Aide et Action, Bhubaneswar, India
e-mail: umi.daniel@action-education.org

A. Datta and S. I. Rajan (eds.), *Migration, Livelihoods and Gender*, International Perspectives on Migration, https://doi.org/10.1007/978-981-95-5465-2_12

Keywords Migration · Development · Remittances · Livelihoods · Migration Policy · Odisha Migration Study

This book has presented key findings of the Odisha Migration Study, a multidisciplinary empirical research project. This study was undertaken in two phases. In the first phase, the Odisha Migration Survey (OMS) was conducted to determine the overall extent of migration from the state, including detailed breakdowns of intra-state, inter-state, and international migration flows. The OMS also estimated remittances to the state and discussed their impact. Additionally, it delved into several aspects of social and economic development, including education, work and employment, access to government programs, housing and amenities, land ownership and cropping patterns, household food consumption and food security, and women's autonomy and mobility. In the second phase, four standalone studies were conducted: on migration and rural livelihoods, youth aspirations and attitudes towards agriculture, migration, gender, and well-being, and the impact of male migration on "left-behind women". This chapter summarizes the key findings of the book and discusses their implications for migration policy.

1 Summing Up: Odisha Migration Study Findings

Chapter 1 laid out the context of development and migration in Odisha. Situated on the eastern coast of India, Odisha is found to be a state of paradoxes. Blessed with abundant natural resources and a rich cultural heritage, it has also been plagued by pervasive poverty and a history of recurrent natural disasters. The chapter argued that despite high economic growth for more than the past three decades, structural transformation in Odisha has been slow and stunted, with some evidence of structural retrogression. The share of agriculture in the state's gross value added (GVA) declined from 33% in 1993–1994 to 22% in 2019–2020, while the share of industry in the same period increased from 17% to 38%, and that of services, peculiarly, declined from 50% to 40%. However, the corresponding changes in the shares of sectoral employment lagged, and Odisha remained a largely agrarian society. 83.3% of Odisha's population lived in rural areas, where more than half (55%) of the workers were employed in agriculture. The state's development trajectory was characterized by a growing workforce, increasing levels of education of its population, and limited employment opportunities. There is an understanding that migration from Odisha has been increasing, but little is known about its magnitude, patterns, or processes. Chapter 1 then outlined the conceptual framework for this work, anchored in migration, livelihoods, and gender. This was followed by the methodology of the Odisha Migration Study, where, in the first phase, stratified multistage random sampling was used with a sample size of 15,000 households—spread over all 30 districts of the state—in 500 rural and urban localities, with 30 households in each locality.

It highlighted that this was the first large-scale survey conducted in Odisha using computer-assisted personal interviewing (CAPI) across all 30 districts to examine different types of migration and their characteristics, which are covered in Chapters 2–7. It then outlined the methodology of the four studies in Phase II, covered in Chapters 8–11. The chapter ends with a section on the population profile of the state based on the OMS.

Chapter 2 presented characteristics of survey households regarding housing status and amenities, viz., lighting sources, cooking fuel, drinking water, and toilet facilities. It examined access to government programs, with an emphasis on the Public Distribution System (PDS) and the Mahatma Gandhi National Rural Employment Guarantee Act (MGNREGA). This was followed by an analysis of the asset ownership of survey households. The chapter then discussed changes in the income levels of households since the COVID-19 pandemic, focusing on the reasons and magnitude of the decline among households that experienced a fall in income levels. Last, the chapter presented survey results on landownership, irrigation, and cropping patterns.

Chapters 3 and 4 laid out Odisha's migration story. Chapter 3 estimated 2.98 million current migrants and 0.77 million return migrants from Odisha. The chapter reported that approximately 17.1% of households had at least one current migrant, and 4.5% of households included at least one return migrant. It found that out-migration to other states within India was the dominant form of migration from Odisha. Ganjam and Baleshwar were the largest migrant-sending districts to other states, and the predominant migration corridors were: Baleshwar–Tamil Nadu, Bhadrak–Karnataka, and Balangir–Andhra Pradesh. In contrast to the Government of Odisha's data on migration-prone districts from the state, the OMS 2023 found a new set of top districts with the highest migration rates, with only three out of the 11 districts (Ganjam, Khordha, and Nuapada) being common to both lists. Nuapada district had the highest number of return migrants. The chapter emphasized that landlessness was more common among non-migrants, and the proportion of poor households among current migrant households was significantly lower when compared to non-migrant and return migrant households. Current migrants also had better houses compared to the non-migrant and return migrant households, signifying the role of remittances, wealth, and other economic resources in enabling migration. Similarly, economic prosperity among administrative divisions (regions) emerged as a factor facilitating certain migration patterns, wherein rural-urban and urban-urban migration was predominant from the central or coastal region, standing at 80% and 7.4%, respectively. Compare this to the northern region, which had 58.1% of rural-urban migrants and 3.5% of urban-urban migrants. The central/coastal division led in terms of both current migrants (1.57 million) and return migrants (0.29 million). In terms of social groups, current rural-rural migration was higher among SC and ST households compared to OBC and upper caste groups. This suggests that poor and marginalized households with scarce resources used migration as a livelihood strategy for their survival.

Chapter 4 then shed light on the size and impact of remittances and advance payments on the socio-economic conditions of migrant households in Odisha. It found that 68.6% of migrant households in Odisha received remittances, and the average monthly household remittance was Rs 5096. Remittances played a crucial role in supporting families and local economies, underlining the economic diversity and migration patterns within Odisha. The estimated monthly remittances for the entire state of Odisha amounted to Rs 693.47 crores, with Ganjam district emerging as the recipient of the largest share of remittances—estimated to be Rs 112.76 crores per month—closely followed by Bhadrak (Rs 99.23 crores) and Jajpur (Rs 78.3 crores). However, there existed significant disparities in remittance inflows across districts, as the majority of the districts (21) received remittances amounting to less than Rs 20 crores. More than 50% of the migrant households received remittances in most districts, but the quantum of the remittance vastly varied. Remittances significantly impacted the living standards of migrant households in Odisha. Ninety percent of households used remittances for meeting expenses of everyday consumption, and 73% used them for health and medical expenses. Among the various social groups, the OBC community received the highest monthly average remittance of Rs 5527, closely followed by the upper caste households with monthly average remittances of Rs 5397. Among the OBCs, 74.3% of the migrant households received remittances, followed by 71.9% among the SCs. The average monthly remittance for the migrant households in the ST community was Rs 3245, and only 47% of the ST migrant households received remittances. In terms of the rural-urban comparison, 68.8% of the rural migrant households received remittances compared to 52.5% of urban households. The chapter also discussed the practice of advance payments to migrant workers or their families. The data showed variations in the incidence and frequency of advance payments across social groups, wealth quartiles, and regions. The highest proportion of households that reported receiving advances was from the SC community (43%), followed by the OBC community (26%). 11.8% of the poorest migrant households received advance payments, while only 2.1% of the richest households received any advances. Thus, advance-based migration streams were more vulnerable and precarious compared to remittance-based migration streams.

Chapter 5 presented household-level food consumption patterns and dietary practices and identified the prevalence and magnitude of different dimensions of food insecurity. It found that grains were a stable food source for over 90% of households, but food groups like meat, seafood, and fruits were rarely included in the diets of more than two-thirds of households, indicating significant barriers to access. The chapter argued that the limited accessibility to essential food items had profound implications for the nutritional status of these households, potentially leading to deficiencies in vital nutrients. The chapter then discussed survey results related to qualitative dimensions of food access, including perceptions surrounding food consumption and food security. It showed that vulnerable households experienced more severe food insecurity. Socioeconomic characteristics such as social group and wealth status were important factors associated with food insecurity and dietary diversity. Vulnerable groups, including SC and ST households, those residing in lower-quality housing, households in the southern region of Odisha, non-migrant households, those in the lowest wealth quartile, and landless and marginal landholders, were disproportionately affected by food and nutritional insecurity. The chapter concluded that the prevalence of food and nutritional insecurity among the vulnerable population underscored the pressing need for government intervention to address accessibility and affordability.

Chapter 6 presented an overview of educational attainments of the general and youth population in Odisha. It found that the highest percentage (13.4%) have completed secondary education (Class 10), 12.6% of the population was illiterate, and illiteracy was higher among women (16.5%) compared to men (8.9%). Overall, males had higher educational attainments than females, and furthermore, this gender disparity was more pronounced at higher levels of education, such as graduate and professional education. There was a stark rural-urban as well as a regional divide in educational attainments. The coastal region had better educational attainments in Odisha compared to the northern and southern regions, and educational outcomes varied for different caste groups, as overall educational attainments were better for upper castes, followed by OBCs, SCs, and STs. The chapter thus showed the different ways in which inequality in educational attainments existed in Odisha, highlighting the disparities in educational attainments by different categories like gender, region, and caste.

Chapter 7 covered the work and employment scenario in Odisha. It estimated the Workforce Participation Rate (WPR) in the state to be 45.5% and found that the WPR varies considerably by sex (the male WPR was 73.3% and the female WPR was 15.9%). It found that migrants had a higher WPR than residents, and that the WPRs were higher for individuals in the younger age cohort, marginalized communities such as the SC and ST, and those in the poorest and poor wealth quartiles. For both men and women, WPR by age took an inverted U curve, where it was lower among younger age cohorts, peaked between the ages of 25–44, and then declined again for older age cohorts. The chapter found that agriculture was the predominant occupation in Odisha, employing 40.1% of all workers. This was followed by service occupations (36.7%), construction (19%), and manufacturing and mining (3.7%). The data suggested a feminization of employment in agriculture, as 57.7% of female workers were engaged in the agricultural sector, as compared to 39.9% male workers. The occupational profile of workers varied significantly by residential status, and migration was associated with a *gendered* movement away from agriculture to non-agricultural occupations, predominantly in the services sector.

Chapter 8, in the context of a changing rural economy and society, studied the role of agriculture, non-agriculture, and remittances on the livelihoods of rural households. Based on data from a primary survey and qualitative case studies, it examined the distribution of household income and explored how individuals and households combined multiple sources of livelihoods and income. At the aggregate level, the study found that local non-agriculture was the most important source of income, followed by agriculture, migrant remittances, and government transfers. Nearly one-third of the households had migrants, but remittances contributed only 14.3% to average incomes among all households. Households with migrants had lower incomes than households without migrants, pointing to the distress-oriented nature of migration from rural Odisha. The chapter developed livelihood- and income-based household typologies to find that the *type of livelihood* mattered: income levels and distribution of income vary significantly among agriculture-based households, non-agriculture-based households, remittance-based households, and government transfer-based households.

Chapter 9 explored *youth aspirations and attitudes towards agriculture* in the context of smallholder rainfed cultivation in a high-migration region of Odisha. It found that despite harsh structural realities of farming being adversely impacted by climate variability, water scarcity, increasing input costs, and declining agricultural profits, young people valued agriculture for the food security it provided. Farming was not just an activity but was considered an occupational, social, and cultural identity, despite monetary income from farming being meagre in comparison to income from remittances or local non-farm incomes. Young people valued land, and those with land—no matter how small their land tract may have been—considered themselves fortunate and committed to cultivation. Even if they migrated, young people remained involved in agriculture, and migration did not supplement agriculture; instead, it complemented agriculture. Youth migration led to an increase in women's work on family farms, and as sharecroppers; women have a heavier workload and take on more farm tasks, including farm management. Among youth migrants across social classes, the desire to remain in the village, or eventually return to the village, was very strong. For young migrants, including highly educated migrants and those earning comfortable incomes in destination regions, the imagination of their future remained tied to the village, closely linked with agriculture. At the same time, youth cultures of temporary migration were widespread—a rite of passage, particularly for those who were less educated—due to an aversion to agriculture at a young age and the lack of employment options in source regions.

Chapters 10 and 11 studied the impact of male migration on *left-behind women*. Chapter 10 undertook a quantitative analysis; it found a positive association between male migration and left-behind women's employment outcomes, though no association was observed with their physical mobility and decision-making autonomy. The chapter found significant individual- and household-level variations in the relationship between male migration and women's mobility. In the context of resource-constrained regions with prevalent migration, the chapter argued that the relationship between husbands' migration and left-behind wives' socioeconomic outcomes cannot be generalized in a singular direction. It suggested that while distress-driven migration of husbands compels left-behind women to take up employment to sustain household livelihoods, this shift fails to translate into enhanced autonomy for left-behind women due to the short-term nature of the migration.

Chapter 11, based on a qualitative study, focused on the lived realities and women's experiences surrounding work, livelihood, health, and family dynamics in the context of migration. It argued that the necessity of migration emerged as a coping mechanism in the face of economic deprivation, failed public employment schemes, and aspirations among young individuals. The chapter emphasized the interconnectedness of migration and increased care responsibilities, particularly in the absence of male members of the family. It also highlighted the social bonds formed among women due to shared experiences in migrant households. In the context of health, the chapter found a dearth of institutionalized medical facilities, chronic health issues, and the trivialization of health problems among women, exacerbated by the absence of state support.

2 Policy Implications

This research has several implications for policy. The first is related to migration statistics. There exist no credible statistics on internal migration in India. Both the Census and National Sample Survey (NSS) data vastly underestimate migration, and these data are now dated. The last Census was undertaken in 2011; the 2021 Census never took place, and the next Census is quite delayed. For the state of Odisha, the OMS is the first-of-its-kind migration survey that has estimated intra-state, inter-state, and international migration. For evidence-based policymaking, it is crucial that migration data is collected methodically and that such databases are updated regularly.

Up-to-date migration data provides a wealth of information for policy-makers. For instance, once migration corridors are identified, policy interventions can be undertaken in *both* source and destination regions. In this study, Ganjam–Gujarat, Baleshwar–Tamil Nadu, Bhadrak–Karnataka, and Balangir–Andhra Pradesh/Telangana emerge as the most important migration corridors. In the past, the governments of Odisha and Andhra Pradesh have signed a Memorandum of Understanding (MoU) specifically targeted toward the vulnerable brick kiln migrant workers. Apart from devising methods to improve migrant registration, such collaborations have also aimed to enhance the convergence of government schemes and services, provide legal assistance, and reduce and eliminate the role of contractors in the migration process. Such MOUs need to be revived and multiplied. In addition, in source regions, Panchayat-level registration of laborers under the Inter-state Migrant Workmen Act of 1979 can be undertaken, and the district labor office may keep the database of all inter- and intra-state migrant laborers.

Third, data from the OMS shows that, like other source states in Eastern India, such as Bihar and Jharkhand, migration from Odisha is youth-dominated. The OMS data also suggests that over time, the average age of migrants has declined. This, in turn, has implications for the education and skilling of young persons and prospective migrants. In high migration pockets, skill programs, and safe and informed migration programs targeting the youth population through migration facilitation centres can be established. The government can set up migration information centres in the key high labor-sending cities and states through NGOs. Simultaneously, these centres should sensitize young workers to their labor rights, and spread awareness and advocacy related to child migration and trafficking.

Fourth, male-dominated migration *means* that family members live and work in different locations for long periods of time. This has profound implications for family members—children, women, the elderly, and migrants. Policies need to acknowledge and address the social and psychological impacts of male migration in both source and destination regions. Fifth, in precarious family migration streams, accompanying migrant children are the worst sufferers in the migration cycle. The government should initiate education, nutrition, health, and other services for accompanying migrant children both within and outside the state.

Sixth, accurate and reliable data helps us identify and locate vulnerable migration streams. In such streams, it is all the more necessary for the state to be proactive so as to safeguard migrant workers' rights, prevent them from being exploited, and be able to rescue migrants in distress. In Odisha, this is particularly relevant in the case of *Dadan* labor and family-based migration systems. The OMS data shows that some streams of migration from the southern and northern regions, such as rural-rural migration and advance-based migration, are quite precarious. In contrast, migration from the advanced coastal region is to urban areas and is remittance-based.

At the same time, in the coastal and some of the southern regions, large-scale migration is induced due to extreme climate and frequent natural disasters. The government should identify the climate hotspots (like Ganjam, Bhadrak, Baleshwar, and Kendrapara) and initiate climate resilience and vulnerability reduction measures for people affected by climate change. Special government projects aiming at livelihood enhancement, agriculture promotion, social protection, and climate resilience intervention can help reduce distress migration in the migration-prone districts identified by the government and in the high migration districts as per the OMS.

Seventh, for all types of migration and migrant workers, social security needs to be firmly incorporated in the legal and policy framework. After all, migrant workers contribute not only to the development of destination regions but also to the source regions, by way of remittances. India's social security architecture, particularly in destination regions, must reach and benefit the rapidly growing population of migrant workers who have largely been outside the ambit of social security due to their double disadvantage of being *migrant* and *informal* workers. Correcting this anomaly in our development process will contribute toward reducing inequalities and promoting migrant well-being and economic justice.

Last, while migrant rights and dignity must be protected, and workers should be able to exercise their choice to migrate to their preferred destination, policy attention is also needed in the source regions. In the context of a predominantly agrarian society characterized by distress-oriented migration, state intervention in the agricultural sector is critical. It needs to address structural issues—such as the provision of irrigation—which will help this region transition from single to multiple cropping and allow for crop diversification. In turn, this would enhance not only food and nutritional security but also the commercialization of agriculture and increase farming incomes. Given the widespread prevalence of sharecropping, access to land needs to be institutionalized. This, in turn, will help young farmers directly access formal credit and agricultural markets (*mandis*). The recognition of young women as farmers is critical for them to be able to access agricultural credit and inputs and become successful farmers. Agricultural extension and training for women need to be prioritized, particularly in the context of high male migration and feminization of agriculture. Ultimately, the agricultural sector and the rural non-farm economy should provide work and employment to rural youth in a context where young people prefer to stay in rural areas if decent livelihood options are available. Thus, employment and livelihood opportunities in source regions need to be enhanced. A *simultaneous* push for rural industrialization, the development of the services sector, and agricultural diversification can pave the way for stronger rural-urban linkages and balanced development in Odisha.

MIX
Papier aus verantwortungsvollen Quellen
Paper from responsible sources
FSC® C105338

If you have any concerns about our products,
you can contact us on
ProductSafety@springernature.com

In case Publisher is established outside the EU,
the EU authorized representative is:
Springer Nature Customer Service Center GmbH
Europaplatz 3, 69115 Heidelberg, Germany

Printed by Libri Plureos GmbH
in Hamburg, Germany